The Unofficial Guide to Radiology: 100 Practice Abdominal X-Rays with Full Colour Annotations and Full X-Ray Reports

FIRST EDITION

Authored by
DANIEL WEINBERG MBCHB (Hons) MPHIL
Radiology Registrar
Central Manchester NHS Foundation Trust

REBECCA BEST BSc (Hons) MBBCh
Academic Foundation Doctor
Queen Elizabeth University Hospital, Glasgow, UK

LYDIA SHACKSHAFT
Medical Student
Kings College London, UK

Edited by
MARK RODRIGUES BSc (Hons) MBCHB (Hons) FRCR
Radiology Registrar,
Edinburgh Royal Infirmary, Edinburgh, UK

ZESHAN QURESHI BM BSc (Hons) MSc BM MRCPCH FAcadMEd MRCPS (Glasg)
Paediatric Registrar,
King's College Hospital, London UK.

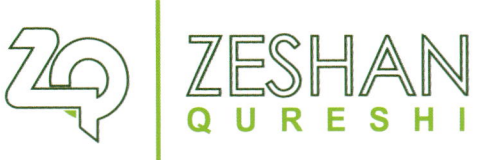

ISBN 978-1910399033

Edited by Mark Rodrigues and Zeshan Qureshi
Authored by Daniel Weinberg, Rebecca Best, Lydia Shackshaft

Published by Zeshan Qureshi. First published 2020.

Original design by Zeshan Qureshi and SWATT Design Ltd. Page make-up by Amnet.

Cover Design by Anne Bonson-Johnson.

A catalogue record for this book is available from the British Library.

Editor's Acknowledgements:

We would like to thank all the authors for their hard work, and our panel of student reviewers for their
unique input. We are extremely grateful for the support given by medical schools across the UK, Europe
and Australia. We would also like to thank the medical students that have inspired this project, believed
in this project, and have helped contribute to, promote, and distribute the book across the UK.

Printed in India
Production managed by Jellyfish Print Solutions Ltd

DEDICATION

Daniel would like to dedicate this book to his lovely partner Sarah, for her tremendous support over the years he has known her. Daniel would also like to thank his parents Ray and Karen for spurring him on to apply for a career in medicine and their endless support and guidance throughout his career to date. He would not have ever been in a position to write this book without them.

Rebecca would like to dedicate this book to her sisters Lana and Louise, who inspire her every day with their enthusiasm, kindness and resilience.

Lydia would like to dedicate this book to her beautiful Mum, for every single thing her mum did to get Lydia where she is today; for always putting Lydia's education before her own desires, for her never-ending encouragement and her belief that Lydia could achieve anything, and for sharing with Lydia her absolute wonder at the world.

INTRODUCTION

Whilst it could be argued that the abdominal X-ray is becoming an outdated radiological investigation in modern day medicine with the advent and ever-increasing use of CT and MRI, it remains a readily available and relatively low dose test to investigate and assist in clinical decision-making for patients of all ages. Furthermore, given a particular clinical concern, the abdominal X-ray is a useful adjunct in conjunction with the clinical assessment in determining which patients may require further cross-sectional imaging. In a low pre-test probability patient, this may preclude the need for further evaluation with CT, thereby reducing the patient's radiation dose.

The Royal College of Radiologists has published iRefer guidelines to assist clinicians in requesting the most appropriate imaging test for patients. These guidelines provide invaluable information, including the clinical indications that abdominal X-rays should be requested for. These include, however are not limited to: preliminary evaluation for bowel obstruction, radiopaque foreign body evaluation, evaluation of radiopaque lines and tubes and assessment for renal calculi.

Despite its universal importance, X-ray interpretation is often an overlooked subject in the medical school curriculum, making it difficult and daunting for many medical students and junior doctors. *The Unofficial Guide to Radiology: 100 Practice Abdominal X-Rays, with Full Colour Annotations and Full X-Ray Reports* aims to help address this.

The key to interpreting X-rays is having a systematic method for assessment, and then getting lots of practice looking at and presenting X-rays. The best-selling core radiology text *The Unofficial Guide to Radiology* was specifically designed for medical students, radiographers, physician's associates, and junior doctors. It outlines a comprehensive system for assessing X-rays, in addition to clinical and radiology based MCQs to contextualise the radiographs to real clinical scenarios. Its approach led to recognition from the British Medical Association, the British Institute of Radiology and the Royal College of Radiologists. This follow-up textbook builds upon these foundations, providing readers with the opportunity to practise and consolidate their abdominal X-ray assessment and presenting skills.

There are lots of radiology textbooks available, but many have important limitations. Most have small, often poor quality images which are not ideal for displaying the radiological findings. The findings are usually only described in a figure below the image, and it may be difficult to know exactly what part of the image corresponds to which finding! Many textbooks deal with X-rays in isolation rather than in a useful clinical context.

We have designed this book to allow readers to practice interpreting X-rays in as useful and clinically relevant a way as possible. There are:

- 100 large, high quality abdominal X-rays to assess.
- Cases presented in the context of a clinical scenario and covering a wide range of common and important findings (in line with the Royal College of Radiologists' Undergraduate Radiology Curriculum).
- Detailed on-image colour annotations to highlight key findings.
- Comprehensive systematic X-ray reports.
- Relevant further investigations and management.

The cases in the book are divided by difficulty into standard, intermediate and advanced. Each begins with a clinical scenario and an abdominal X-ray for you to interpret. You can then turn over the page, and find a fully annotated version of the same X-ray with a comprehensive report. Each systematically structured report is colour coded to match the corresponding labelled image.

Each report is based on a systematic approach to assessing the abdominal X-ray, and is as follows:

- Technical features
- Bowel gas pattern
- Bowel wall
- Pneumoperitoneum
- Solid organs
- Vascular
- Bones
- Soft tissues
- Other
- Review areas
- Summary
- Investigations and management

Realistic clinical history

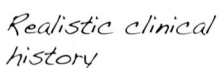

SCENARIO 1

A 36 year old female presents to ED with a 2 day history of generalised abdominal pain. She has not opened her bowels in that time and feels nauseated but has not vomited. Her past medical history is significant for a recent toothache, for which she has been taking cocodamol and she is a non-smoker. On examination, she has saturations of 99% in room air and a temperature of 36.9°C. Her HR is 82 bpm, RR is 15 and blood pressure is 115/66 mmHg. The abdomen is distended with tenderness over the right side and voluntary guarding. Bowel sounds are normal. Urine dipstick is unremarkable and a pregnancy test is negative.

An abdominal X-ray is requested to assess for possible bowel obstruction.

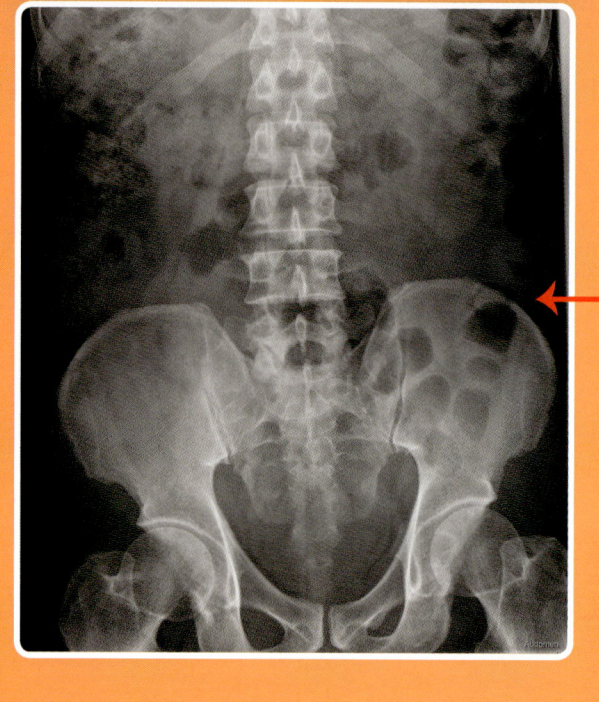

Large, high quality image to assess

15

REPORT – FAECAL RESIDUE

Detailed report following a standard format

REPORT
Patient ID: Anonymous.
Projection: AP supine.
Rotation: Adequate.
Penetration: Adequate – the spinous processes are visible.
Coverage: Adequate – the anterior ribs are visible superiorly and the inferior pubic rami are visible.

BOWEL GAS PATTERN
The bowel gas pattern is normal.
There is moderate volume of faecal residue present predominantly from the caecum to proximal transverse colon.

BOWEL WALL
There is no evidence of mural thickening or intramural gas within the large or small bowel.

PNEUMOPERITONEUM
There is no evidence of free intra-abdominal gas.

SOLID ORGANS
The solid organ contours are within normal limits with no solid organ calcification.

VASCULAR
No abnormal vascular calcification.

BONES
There is degenerative change visible in the distal lumbar spine with osteophyte formation.

There is degenerative change in the weight-baring region of the sacroiliac joints bilaterally.

No fractures or destructive bone lesions are visible in the imaged skeleton.

SOFT TISSUES
The psoas muscle outline is visible bilaterally.

The extra-abdominal soft tissues are unremarkable.

OTHER
There are no radiopaque foreign bodies.

There are no vascular lines, drains or surgical clips.

REVIEW AREAS
Gallstones / Renal calculi: No radio-opaque calculi.
Lung bases: Not fully included.
Spine: Degenerative change in the distal lumbar spine and weight-baring sacroiliac joints.
Femoral heads: Normal.

x-ray review areas specifically highlighted

Clear annotations highlighting the major x-ray findings

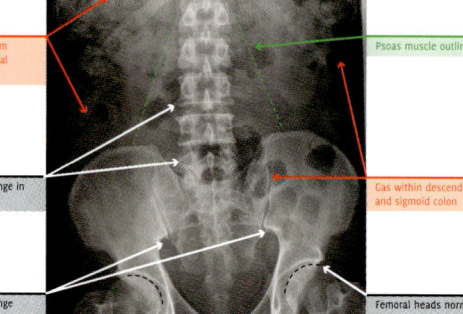

Faecal residue from caecum to proximal transverse colon

Psoas muscle outlines

Degenerative change in spine

Gas within descending and sigmoid colon

Degenerative change sacroiliac joints

Femoral heads normal

SUMMARY
This X-ray demonstrates a moderate volume of faecal residue predominantly in the ascending and proximal transverse colon. There are mild degenerative changes in the distal lumbar spine and weight-baring sacroiliac joints bilaterally. There is no evidence of bowel obstruction or pneumoperitoneum.

be given regarding lifestyle adjustments, including adequate fluid intake, sufficient dietary fibre and exercise if clinically appropriate.

If the patient is otherwise well, no further investigation or imaging is required.

INVESTIGATIONS AND MANAGEMENT
If the patient is clinically constipated, current medications should be reviewed and laxatives considered. Advice should

Investigations & management plan put the x-ray in the context of the overall clinical management

16

With this textbook, we hope you will become more confident and competent interpreting abdominal X-rays, both in exam situations and in clinical practice.

We also hope that this is just the beginning; we want you to get involved! This textbook has been a collaboration with junior doctors and students just like you. You have the power to contribute something valuable to medicine; we welcome your suggestions and would love for you to get in touch. A good starting point is our Facebook page, which is growing into a forum for medical education.

Please get in touch and be part of the medical education project.

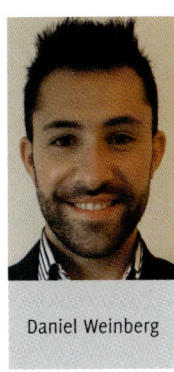

Daniel Weinberg

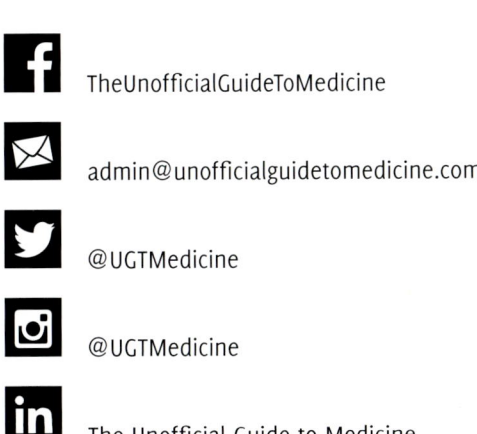

TheUnofficialGuideToMedicine

admin@unofficialguidetomedicine.com

@UGTMedicine

@UGTMedicine

The Unofficial Guide to Medicine

FOREWORD

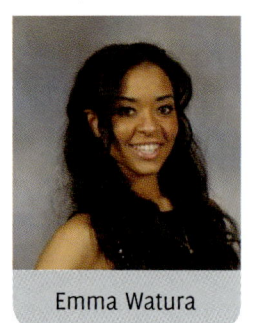

Emma Watura

To support good quality patient care, it is important to develop a structured approach to interpreting radiological images and presenting the findings. *The Unofficial Guide to Radiology: 100 Practice Abdominal X-rays with Full Colour Annotations and Full X-Ray Reports* offers plenty of opportunity to practise image interpretation and test yourself using large, high quality images.

Each X-ray is accompanied by a realistic scenario, making it more relevant to clinical practice. A variety of cases are covered, ranging from standard to advanced level. Therefore, students can begin at a level suitable for them and progress accordingly. The summaries provided for each case are great examples of how to present X-ray findings to colleagues or examiners. In addition, useful advice is given for further investigations and management.

A systematic method for assessing and reporting abdominal X-rays is demonstrated throughout. Each report is laid out with anatomical subtitles. This is a good method to learn as it ensures all review areas are inspected. The X-rays are clearly annotated with concise notes and a colour code, making *The Unofficial Guide to Radiology* easy to read and appealing to medical students, junior doctors and other healthcare professionals.

I would recommend this textbook to anyone hoping to enhance their knowledge and competence in interpreting abdominal X-rays. I look forward to referring to *The Unofficial Guide to Radiology* more often in the future to improve my confidence in radiological image interpretation.

EMMA WATURA
Medical Student, The University of Birmingham, UK
Medical Student Representative, The Society of Radiologists in Training

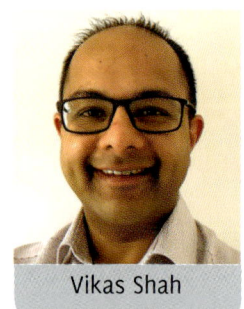

Vikas Shah

The investigation of abdominal disease is evolving rapidly, and with imaging modalities such as CT and MRI being more easily accessible, the role of the plain film radiography has declined in recent years. However, the abdominal x-ray (AXR) is still a widely utilised test. The interpretation of AXRs, like most other plain films in the acute setting, falls primarily to junior doctors. The AXR is one of the toughest imaging tests to interpret accurately due to the multiple overlapping structures of varying density within a complex 3-dimensional compartment, displayed as a 2-dimensional image. However, despite the decline of the AXR, it remains an important and valuable tool and a working knowledge of correct interpretation can only have positive benefits for patient outcomes.

There are several aspects of this textbook that will make it essential reading for multiple different professional groups. Rather than focussing purely on the x-ray findings, the authors have provided valuable clinical context by offering some history and examination findings, and ending each case with a summary and suggestions on the next investigative and management steps. This approach will be particularly useful for medical students and junior doctors. An important facet of any radiology book is high-resolution images, found in abundance here. The accompanying annotated images with the key findings listed in a systematic manner ensures a consistent format running throughout the book. There is ample coverage of the common abnormalities encountered, as well as those that are less common but important not to miss.

The authors are to be commended for producing an easily digestible, visually pleasing and methodically structured book, providing plentiful material to enable more confident interpretation of the AXR. Undergraduates, qualified doctors, physician associates and radiographers will all have something to take away from this book, and I am delighted to give it my full endorsement.

VIKAS SHAH
Consultant Radiologist
University Hospitals of Leicester

ABBREVIATIONS

AAA	abdominal aortic aneurysm	**IV**	intravenous
ACE	Antegrade colonic enema	**IVC**	inferior vena cava
AP supine	anteriorposterior supine	**LFT**	liver function tests
AXR	abdominal x ray	**MDT**	multidisciplinary team
BPM	beats per minute	**MRI**	magnetic resonance imaging
CMV	cytomegalovirus	**NBM**	nil by mouth
COPD	chronic obstructive pulmonary disease	**NG**	Nasogastric
CRP	c-reactive protein	**NICU**	neonatal intensive care unit
CT scan	computerised tomography scan	**PCR**	polymerase chain reaction
CXR	chest x ray	**PEG**	percutaneous endoscopic gastrostomy
EBV	ebstein-barr virus	**PEG-J**	percutaneous endoscopic transgastric jejunostomy
ECG	electrocardiogram	**PR**	rectal exam
ED	emergency department	**RIG**	radiologically inserted gastrostomy tube
ESR	erythrocyte sedimentation rate	**RR**	respiratory rate
ET tube	endotracheal tube	**SCBU**	special care baby unit
FBC	full blood count	**SSRI**	selective serotonin reuptake inhibitor
FISH	florescence in situ hybridisation	**TFT**	thyroid function tests
GCS	Glasgow coma scale	**U and E**	urea and electrolytes
GP	general practitioner	**USS**	ultrasound scan
HR	heart rate	**VP**	ventriculoperitoneal
IUCD	intrauterine contraceptive device		

CONTRIBUTORS

AUTHORS

Daniel Weinberg
MBChB (Hons) MPhil

Radiology Registrar
Central Manchester NHS Foundation Trust

Rebecca Best
BSc (Hons) MBBCh

Academic Foundation Doctor
Queen Elizabeth University Hospital, Glasgow, UK

Lydia Shackshaft

Medical Student
Kings College Hospital, UK

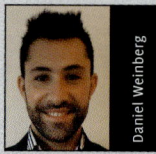  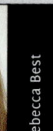 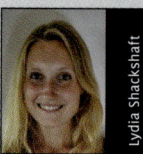

EDITORS

Mark Rodrigues
BSc (Hons) MBChB (Hons) FRCR

Radiology Registrar, Edinburgh Royal
Infirmary, Edinburgh, UK

Zeshan Qureshi
BM BSc (Hons) MSc BM MRCPCH
FAcadMEd MRCPS(Glasg)

Paediatric Registrar,
King's College Hospital, London UK.

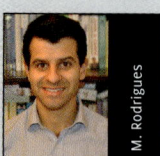 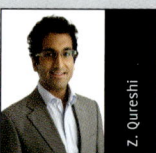

STUDENT REVIEWERS

Lydia Wilson   University of Birmingham, UK

Triya Chakravorty   University of Oxford, UK

SENIOR REVIEWERS

Professor Sathi Sukumar   Consultant Radiologist, Central Manchester NHS Foundation Trust, UK

Dr Haider Alwan-Walker   Consultant Radiologist, Central Manchester NHS Foundation Trust, UK

Dr Velauthan Rudralingam   Consultant Radiologist, Central Manchester NHS Foundation Trust, UK

Dr Sue Liong   Consultant Radiologist, Central Manchester NHS Foundation Trust, UK

Dr Matt Wood   Obstetrics and Gynaecology Registrar, West Midlands Deanery, UK

Dr Patrice Eastwood   Paediatric Surgical Registrar, Royal Belfast Hospital for Sick Children, Belfast, UK

Dr Greta McLachlan   Surgical Registrar, Frimley Park Hospital, UK

Dr Christopher Gee   Consultant Orthopaedic and Trauma Surgeon, NHS Lanarkshire, UK

Dr Patrick Byrne   Consultant Physician & GP, Belford Hospital, Fort William, UK

CONTENTS

STANDARD

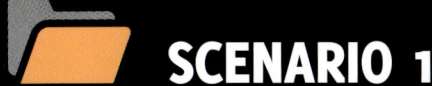

SCENARIO 1

A 36 year old female presents to ED with a 2 day history of generalised abdominal pain. She has not opened her bowels in that time and feels nauseated but has not vomited. Her past medical history is significant for a recent toothache, for which she has been taking cocodamol and she is a non-smoker. On examination, she has saturations of 99% in room air and a temperature of 36.9°C. Her HR is 82 bpm, RR is 15 and blood pressure is 115/66 mmHg. The abdomen is distended with tenderness over the right side. Bowel sounds are normal. Urine dipstick is unremarkable and a pregnancy test is negative.

An abdominal X-ray is requested to assess for possible bowel obstruction.

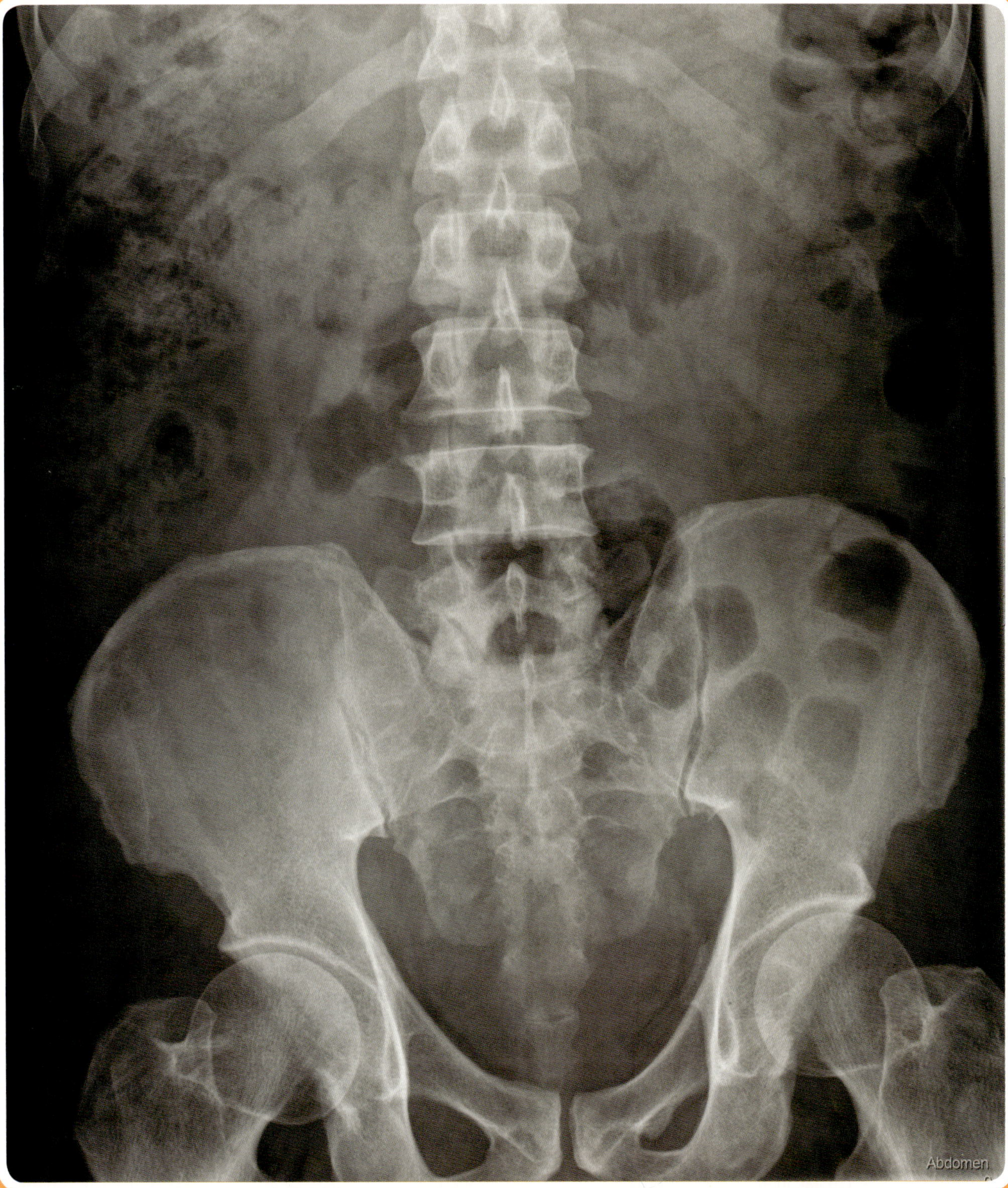

Abdomen

REPORT
Patient ID: Anonymous.
Projection: AP supine.
Rotation: Adequate.
Penetration: Adequate – the spinous processes are visible.
Coverage: Inadequate - the upper abdomen is not fully included.

BOWEL GAS PATTERN
The bowel gas pattern is normal.

There is moderate volume of faecal residue present predominantly from the caecum to the proximal transverse colon.

BOWEL WALL
There is no evidence of mural thickening or intramural gas within the large or small bowel.

PNEUMOPERITONEUM
There is no evidence of free intra-abdominal gas.

SOLID ORGANS
The solid organ contours are within normal limits with no solid organ calcification.

VASCULAR
No abnormal vascular calcification.

BONES
There is degenerative change visible in the distal lumbar spine with osteophyte formation.

There is degenerative change in the weight-bearing region of the sacroiliac joints bilaterally.

No fractures or destructive bone lesions are visible in the imaged skeleton.

SOFT TISSUES
The psoas muscle outline is visible bilaterally.

The extra-abdominal soft tissues are unremarkable.

OTHER
There are no radiopaque foreign bodies.

There are no vascular lines, drains or surgical clips.

REVIEW AREAS
Gallstones / Renal calculi: No radiopaque calculi.
Lung bases: Not fully included.
Spine: Degenerative change in the distal lumbar spine and weight-bearing sacroiliac joints.
Femoral heads: Normal.

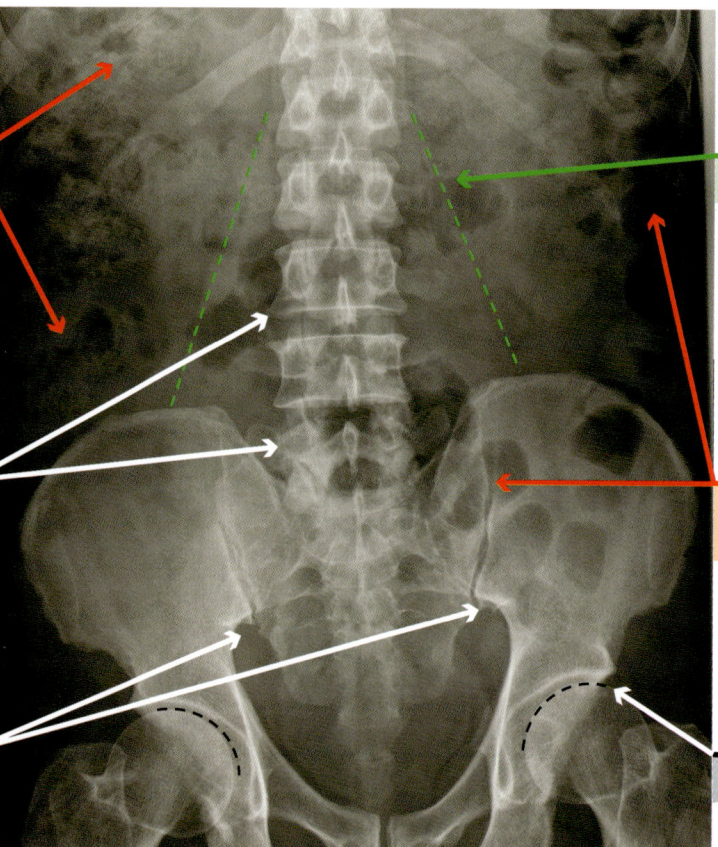

Faecal residue from caecum to proximal transverse colon

Degenerative change in spine

Degenerative change sacroiliac joints

Psoas muscle outlines

Gas within descending and sigmoid colon

Femoral heads normal

SUMMARY
This X-ray demonstrates a moderate volume of faecal residue predominantly in the ascending and proximal transverse colon. There are mild degenerative changes in the distal lumbar spine and weight-bearing sacroiliac joints bilaterally. There is no evidence of bowel obstruction or pneumoperitoneum.

INVESTIGATIONS AND MANAGEMENT
If the patient is clinically constipated, current medications should be reviewed and laxatives considered. Advice should be given regarding lifestyle adjustments, including adequate fluid intake, sufficient dietary fibre and exercise if clinically appropriate.

If the patient is otherwise well, no further investigation or imaging is required.

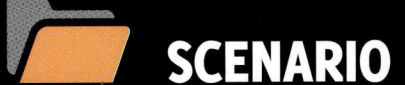

SCENARIO 2

A 60 year old male presents to ED with generalised abdominal pain. He has no significant past medical history and is a non-smoker. On examination, he has saturations of 97% in room air and a temperature of 36.7°C. His HR is 83 bpm, RR is 17 and blood pressure is 118/80 mmHg. The abdomen is soft and there is tenderness in both flanks with normal bowel sounds. Urine dipstick shows blood +++.

An abdominal X-ray is requested to assess for possible renal calculi.

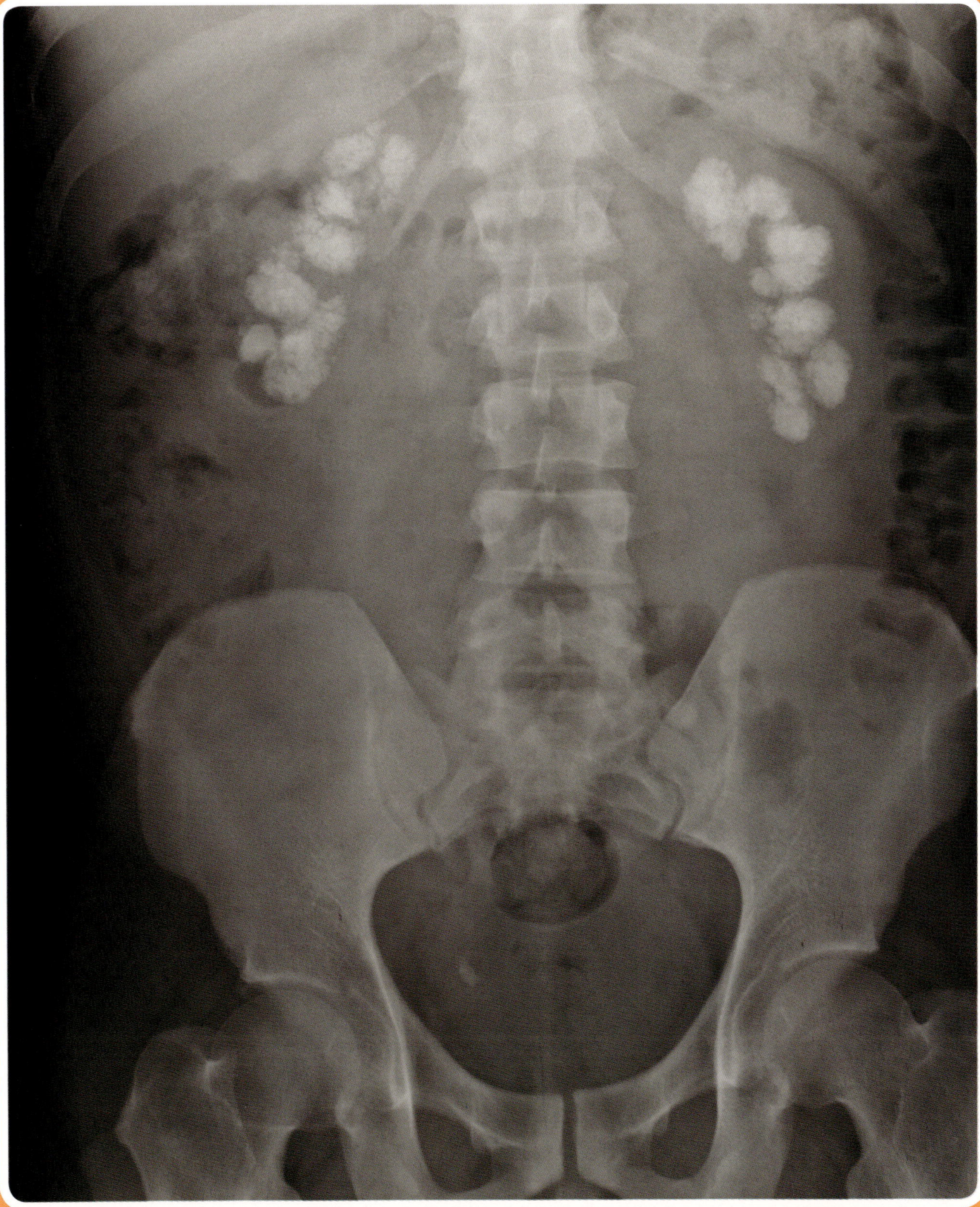

REPORT
Patient ID: Anonymous.
Projection: AP supine.
Penetration: Adequate – the spinous processes are visible.
Coverage: Adequate – the anterior ribs are visible superiorly and the inferior pubic rami are visible.

BOWEL GAS PATTERN
The bowel gas pattern is normal.

There is a moderate volume of faecal residue present in the ascending colon and distal transverse colon.

BOWEL WALL
There is no evidence of mural thickening or intramural gas within the large or small bowel.

PNEUMOPERITONEUM
There is no evidence of free intra-abdominal gas.

SOLID ORGANS
There are multiple large well-defined radiopaque densities projected over the renal medullae of both kidneys.

VASCULAR
No abnormal vascular calcification.

BONES
There are no abnormalities of the imaged thoracic and lumbar spine, or within the pelvis.

SOFT TISSUES
The psoas muscle outline is visible bilaterally.

The extra-abdominal soft tissues are unremarkable.

OTHER
There is a radiopaque density projected over the region of the right urinary bladder, which most likely represents a bladder calculus.

There are no radiopaque foreign bodies.

There are no vascular lines, drains or surgical clips.

REVIEW AREAS
Gallstones / Renal calculi: There are multiple calcific densities projected over the renal medullae.
Lung bases: Not fully included.
Spine: Normal.
Femoral heads: Normal.

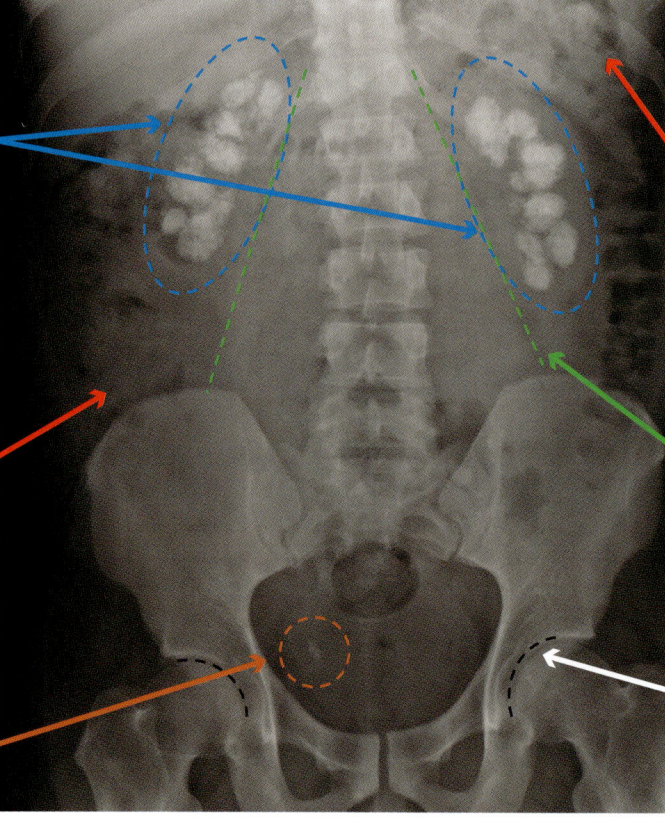

Calcific densities over regions of both kidneys

Faecal residue throughout ascending colon

Bladder calculus

Faecal residue in distal transverse colon

Psoas muscle outlines

Femoral heads normal

SUMMARY
This X-ray demonstrates multiple radiopaque densities projected over the renal medullae of both kidneys in keeping with medullary nephrocalcinosis. There is a further radiopaque density projected over the urinary bladder, which most likely represents a urinary bladder calculus. There is a moderate volume of faecal loading in the ascending colon and distal transverse colon.

INVESTIGATIONS AND MANAGEMENT
The patient should be resuscitated using an ABCDE approach.

Adequate analgesia and hydration should be provided.

Urgent bloods should be taken, including FBC, U&Es, CRP, LFTs, blood gas, and bone profile.

The patient should be assessed for acute kidney injury, and if present, an ultrasound of the urinary tract in the first instance would be beneficial in assessing for hydronephrosis.

A CT scan of the kidneys, ureters and bladder may be useful for better visualisation of the anatomy.

The patient should be referred to urology for further assessment of the medullary nephrocalcinosis and presumed urinary bladder calculus.

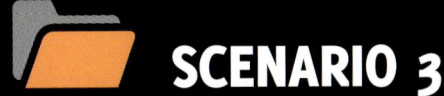

SCENARIO 3

A 45 year old female presents to ED with acute abdominal pain. She has a history of recurrent pulmonary embolisms and is a non-smoker. On examination, she has saturations of 97% in room air and a temperature of 39°C. Her HR is 92 bpm, RR is 22 and blood pressure is 125/80 mmHg. The abdomen is rigid with voluntary guarding and there is generalised tenderness with normal bowel sounds. Urine dipstick is unremarkable and a pregnancy test is negative. The patient is noted to be obese.

An abdominal X-ray is requested to assess for possible bowel obstruction.

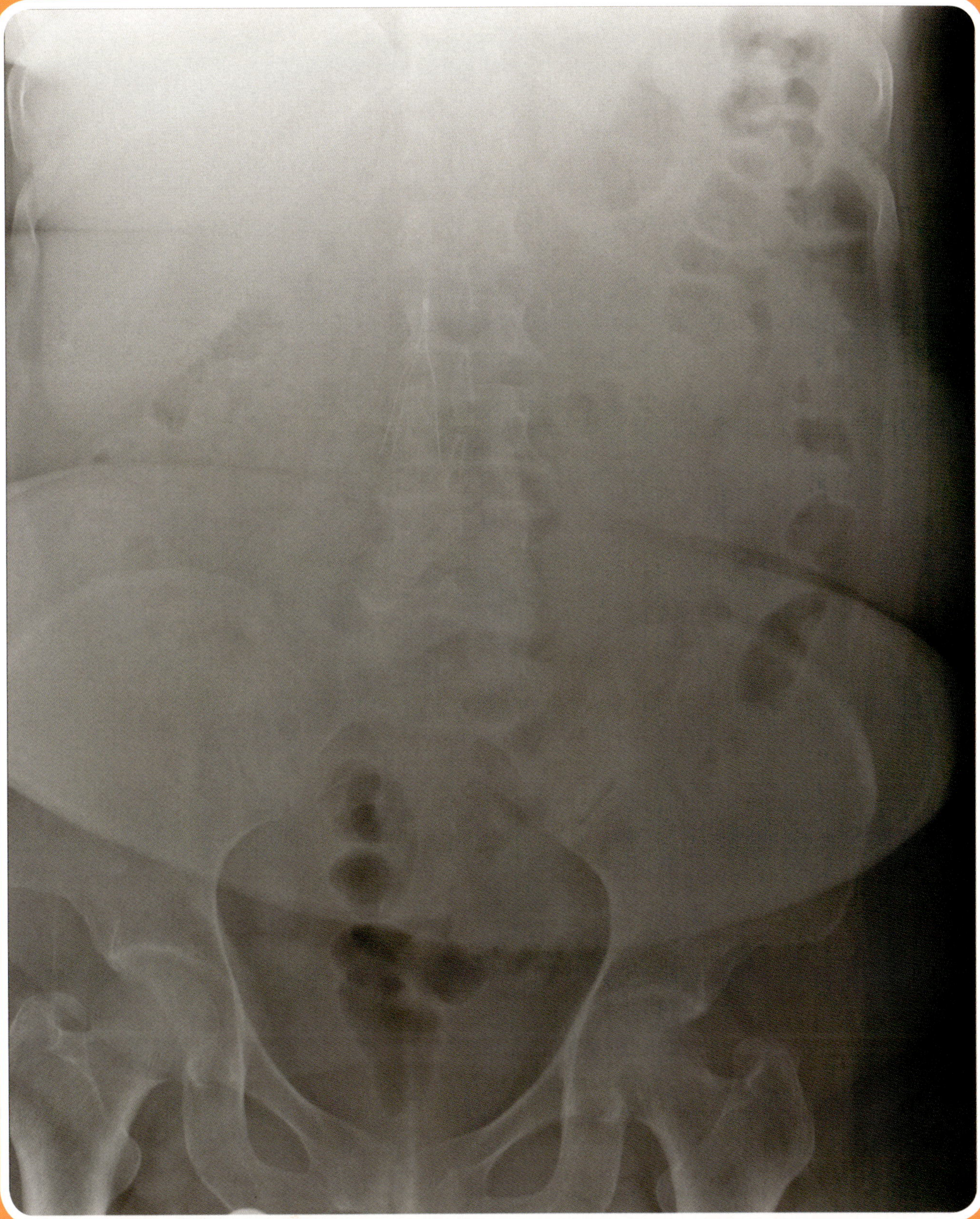

REPORT

Patient ID: Anonymous.
Projection: AP supine.
Rotation: Adequate.
Penetration: Adequate – the spinous processes are visible.
Coverage: Adequate – the anterior ribs are visible superiorly and the inferior pubic rami are visible.

BOWEL GAS PATTERN

The bowel gas pattern is normal.

BOWEL WALL

There is no evidence of mural thickening or intramural gas within the large or small bowel.

PNEUMOPERITONEUM

There is no evidence of free intra-abdominal gas.

SOLID ORGANS

The solid organ contours are within normal limits with no solid organ calcification.

VASCULAR

No abnormal vascular calcification.

BONES

There is mild degenerative change seen in the spine.

SOFT TISSUES

The psoas muscle outline is visible bilaterally.

There are cutaneous fat folds projecting over the region of the abdomen.

OTHER

There is a radiopaque foreign object projected over the region of the right pedicles of lumbar vertebrae L2 and L3, within the region of the abdominal inferior vena cava, in keeping with an inferior vena cava filter.

There are no drains or surgical clips.

REVIEW AREAS

Gallstones / Renal calculi: No radiopaque calculi.
Lung bases: Not fully included.
Spine: Normal.
Femoral heads: Normal.

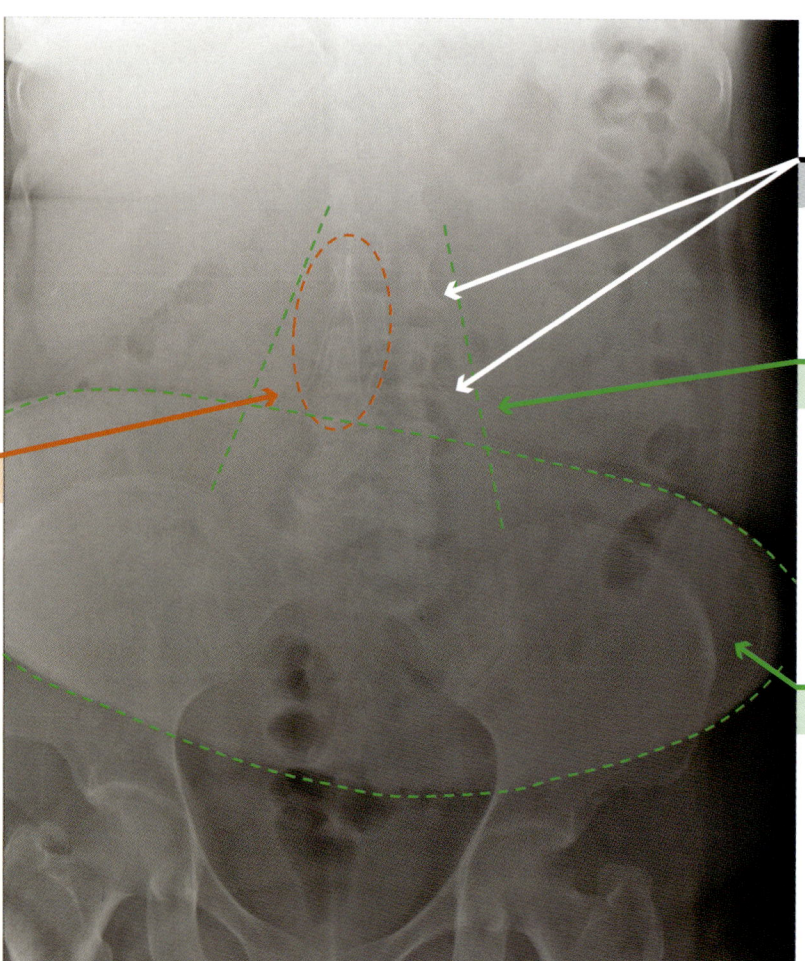

Degenerative changes

Psoas muscle outlines

IVC filter

Cutaneous fat folds

SUMMARY

This X-ray demonstrates no evidence of bowel obstruction. The IVC filter and mild degenerative changes in the spine are incidental findings.

INVESTIGATIONS AND MANAGEMENT

The patient should be resuscitated using an ABCDE approach.

Adequate analgesia and hydration should be provided.

Urgent bloods should be taken including FBC, U&Es, LFTs, amylase, bone profile, coagulation, blood cultures, blood gas and CRP.

Broad spectrum antibiotics should be prescribed, the patient should be made NBM and started on IV fluids.

There are no clear findings on the abdominal X-ray to explain the patient's clinical presentation. A CT scan of the abdomen/pelvis with IV contrast may be considered for further evaluation of the abdomen and the general surgical team should be involved.

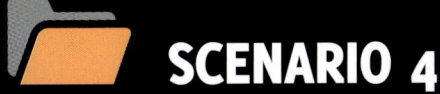

SCENARIO 4

A 69 year old male presents to ED with longstanding abdominal and pelvic pain that has worsened over the last 72 hours. He has been taking co-codamol. He feels nauseated but has not vomited, and his bowels have not opened for 3 days. His past medical history is significant for severe COPD, which has been treated with steroids in the past, and ischaemic heart disease. He is an ex-smoker. On examination, he has saturations of 94% in room air and a temperature of 37.0°C. His HR is 74 bpm, RR is 16 and blood pressure is 130/75 mmHg. His abdomen is soft and there is no tenderness. Rectal examination reveals hard stools and a urine dipstick is unremarkable.

An abdominal X-ray is requested to assess for possible bowel obstruction.

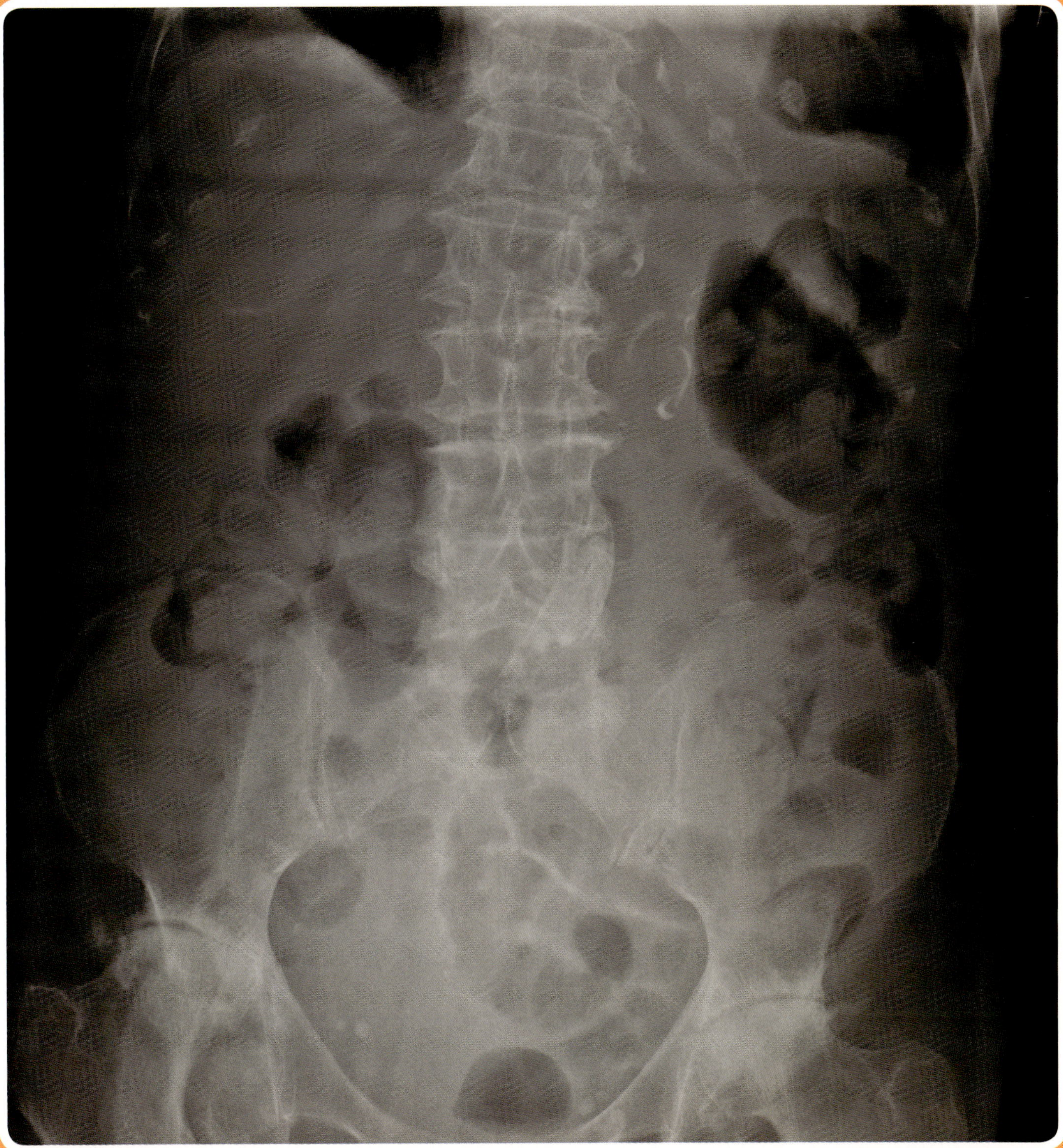

REPORT
Patient ID: Anonymous.
Projection: AP supine.
Rotation: Adequate.
Penetration: Adequate – the spinous processes are visible.
Coverage: Inadequate – the pubic symphysis and inferior pubic rami have not been fully included.

BOWEL GAS PATTERN
Bowel gas pattern is normal.

There is a moderate volume of faecal residue throughout the colon. The rectum contains gas.

BOWEL WALL
There is no evidence of mural thickening or intramural gas within the large or small bowel.

PNEUMOPERITONEUM
There is no evidence of free intra-abdominal gas.

SOLID ORGANS
The solid organ contours are within normal limits with no solid organ calcification.

VASCULAR
There is atherosclerotic calcification of the abdominal aorta and iliac arteries.

BONES
There is moderate to severe degenerative change in the imaged lumbar spine, with lateral osteophytes visible.

There is severe bilateral degenerative change in the hip joints, including complete loss of joint space, subchondral sclerosis and subchondral lucencies in keeping with subchondral cyst formation.

Both femoral heads are deformed, with flattened, abnormal contours.

There is widespread age-related costochondral calcification.

SOFT TISSUES
The psoas muscle outline is not visible on the left side, which is non-specific.

The extra-abdominal soft tissues are unremarkable.

OTHER
There are several rounded calcific radiopaque densities projected over the region of the pelvis, which most likely represent phleboliths.

There are no vascular lines, drains or surgical clips.

REVIEW AREAS
Gallstones / Renal calculi: No radiopaque calculi.
Lung bases: Normal left lung base. Right lung base is not visible.
Spine: Degenerative change in lumbar spine.
Femoral heads: Bilateral degenerative and dysplastic changes.

Costochondral calcification

Degenerative change in lumbar spine and osteophytes

Joint space narrowing

Subchondral cysts and sclerosis

Faecal residue throughout colon

Calcified aorta and iliac vessels

Subchondral sclerosis

Flattening of femoral heads

Phleboliths

SUMMARY
This X-ray demonstrates a normal bowel gas pattern with a moderate volume of faecal residue throughout the colon, however no evidence of obstruction. There are severe bilateral degenerative changes in the hip joints involving the femoral heads and acetabula in keeping with stage IV avascular necrosis. The degenerative changes in the lumbar spine, costochondral calcification and phleboliths are also incidental findings.

INVESTIGATIONS AND MANAGEMENT
The patient should be resuscitated using an ABCDE approach.

Adequate analgesia and hydration should be provided. Co-codamol may be contributing to the constipation.

Urgent bloods should be taken, including FBC, U&Es, CRP, LFTs, coagulation, amylase, blood gas, and group and save.

If the patient is clinically constipated, current medications should be reviewed and laxatives considered. Advice should be given regarding lifestyle adjustments, including adequate fluid intake, sufficient dietary fibre and exercise if clinically appropriate.

Additionally, the patient should be referred to the orthopaedic outpatient clinic for assessment of the avascular necrosis and degenerative changes, and for consideration of treatment, such as total hip replacement. An AP pelvis should be performed to assess the hip properly.

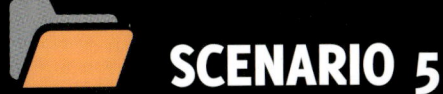

A 32 year old female presents to ED with a 2 day history of lower abdominal pain. She has not opened her bowels in that time, feels nauseated, and reports vomiting numerous times. Her past medical history is significant for generalised anxiety disorder, for which she takes fluoxetine (an SSRI). She is a non-smoker. On examination, she has saturations of 99% in room air and a temperature of 36.8°C. Her HR is 74 bpm, RR is 19 and blood pressure is 120/72 mmHg. The abdomen is distended and there is tenderness in the lower abdomen with voluntary guarding. Bowel sounds are sluggish. Urine dipstick is unremarkable and a pregnancy test is negative.

An abdominal X-ray is requested to assess for possible bowel obstruction.

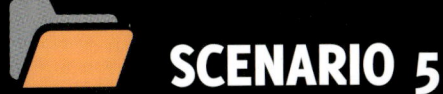

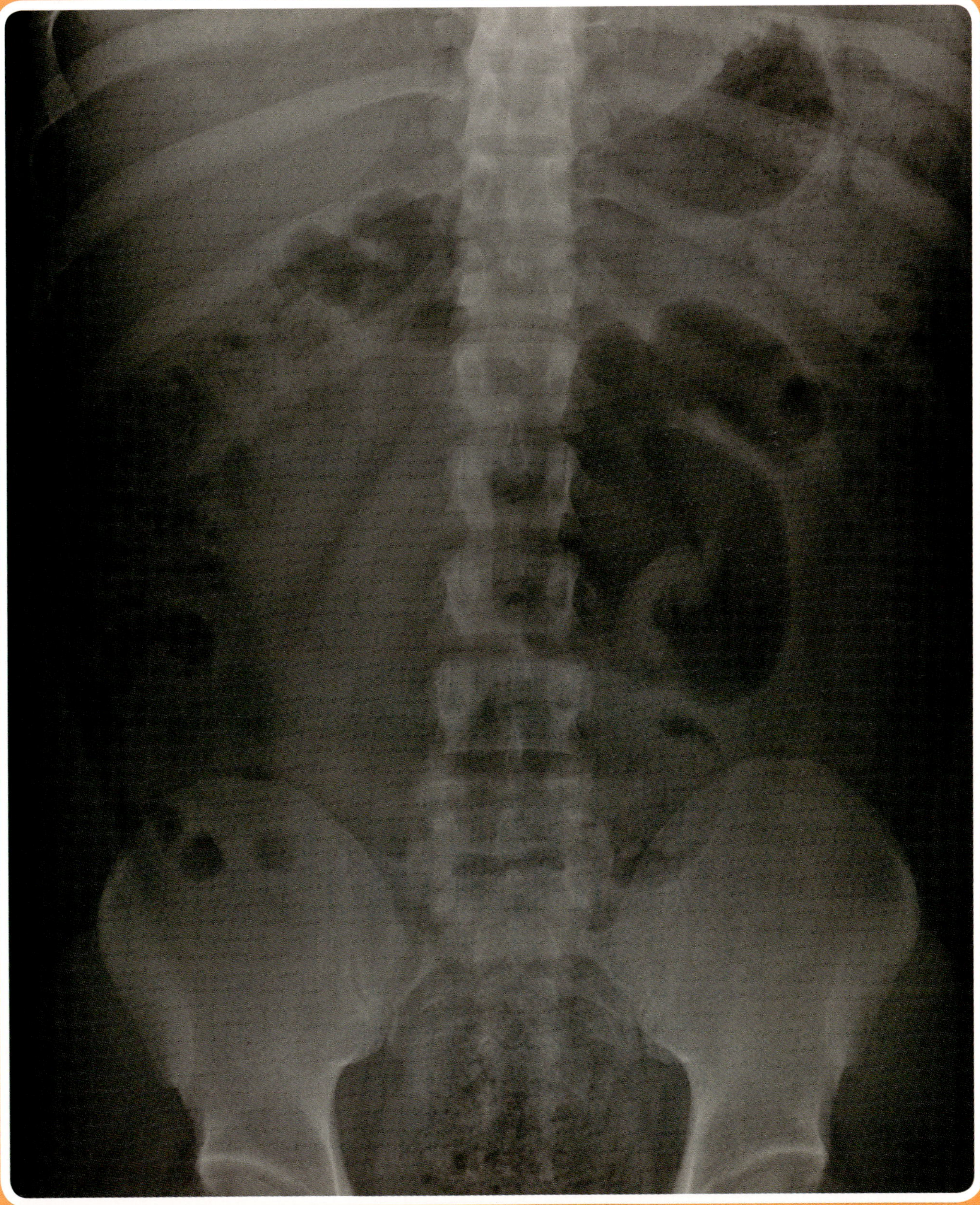

REPORT – FAECAL RESIDUE RECTUM

REPORT
Patient ID: Anonymous.
Projection: AP supine.
Rotation: Adequate.
Penetration: Adequate – the spinous processes are visible.
Coverage: Inadequate – the pubic symphysis and inferior pubic rami have not been fully included.

BOWEL GAS PATTERN
The sigmoid colon is mildly distended with gas but no bowel obstruction is evident.

There is a significant volume of faecal residue present throughout the large bowel. The rectum is prominent and contains faeces.

BOWEL WALL
There is no evidence of mural thickening or intramural gas within the large or small bowel.

PNEUMOPERITONEUM
There is no evidence of free intra-abdominal gas.

SOLID ORGANS
The solid organ contours are within normal limits with no solid organ calcification.

VASCULAR
No abnormal vascular calcification.

BONES
There are no abnormalities of the imaged thoracic and lumbar spine, or within the pelvis.

SOFT TISSUES
The psoas muscle outline is preserved.

The extra-abdominal soft tissues are unremarkable.

OTHER
There are no radiopaque foreign bodies.

There are no vascular lines, drains or surgical clips.

REVIEW AREAS
Gallstones / Renal calculi: No radiopaque calculi.
Lung bases: Not fully included.
Spine: Normal.
Femoral heads: Normal.

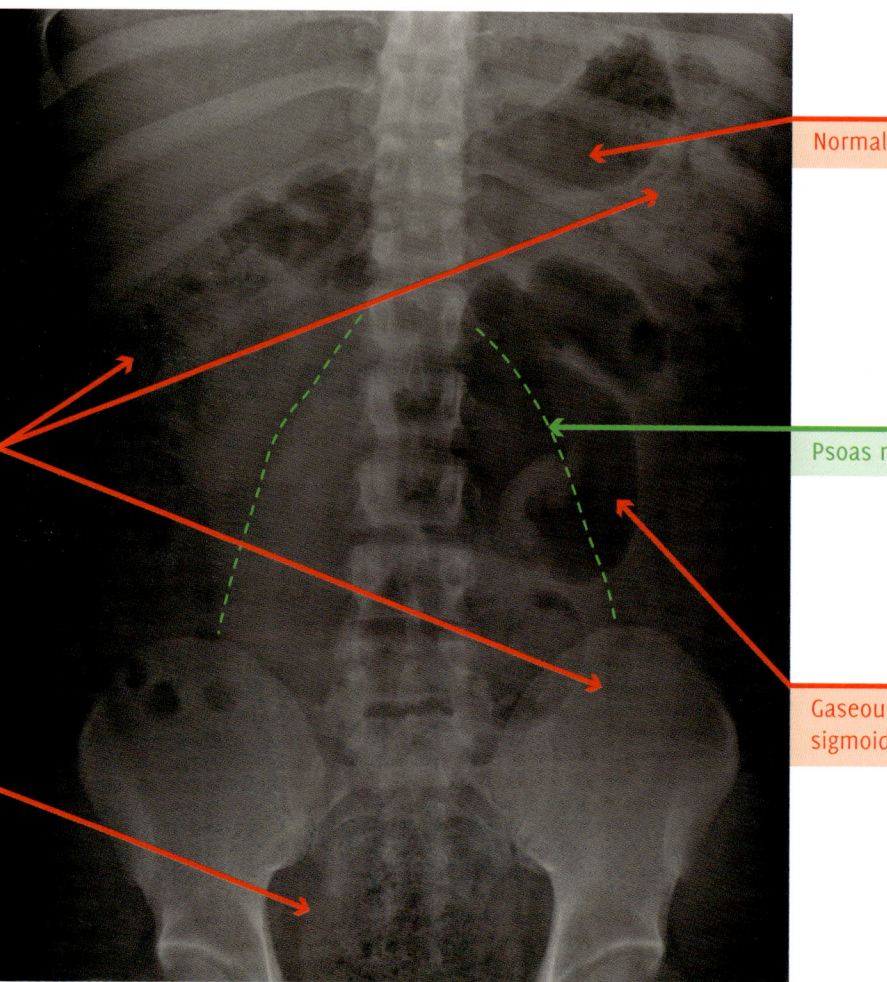

Normal stomach bubble

Faecal residue throughout large bowel

Psoas muscle outlines

Dilated rectum containing faeces

Gaseous prominent sigmoid loop

SUMMARY
This X-ray demonstrates a significant volume of faecal residue throughout the large bowel, with prominence of the rectum containing faeces. There is a mildly prominent gaseous sigmoid loop; however no evidence of bowel obstruction or pneumoperitoneum.

INVESTIGATIONS AND MANAGEMENT
If the patient is clinically constipated, current medications should be reviewed and laxatives considered. An enema may be required acutely. Advice should be given regarding lifestyle adjustments, including adequate fluid intake, sufficient dietary fibre and exercise if clinically appropriate.

If the patient is otherwise well, no further investigation or imaging is required.

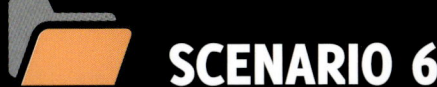
A 69 year old female presents to ED with worsening abdominal distension. She has not opened her bowels for the past 48 hours. Her past medical history is significant for a previous hysterectomy 10 years ago for endometrial cancer and she is a non-smoker. On examination, she has saturations of 96% in room air and a temperature of 37.6°C. Her HR is 102 bpm, RR is 30 and blood pressure is 110/65 mmHg. The abdomen is rigid and there is generalised tenderness with tinkling bowel sounds. Urine dipstick is unremarkable.

An abdominal X-ray is requested to assess for possible bowel obstruction.

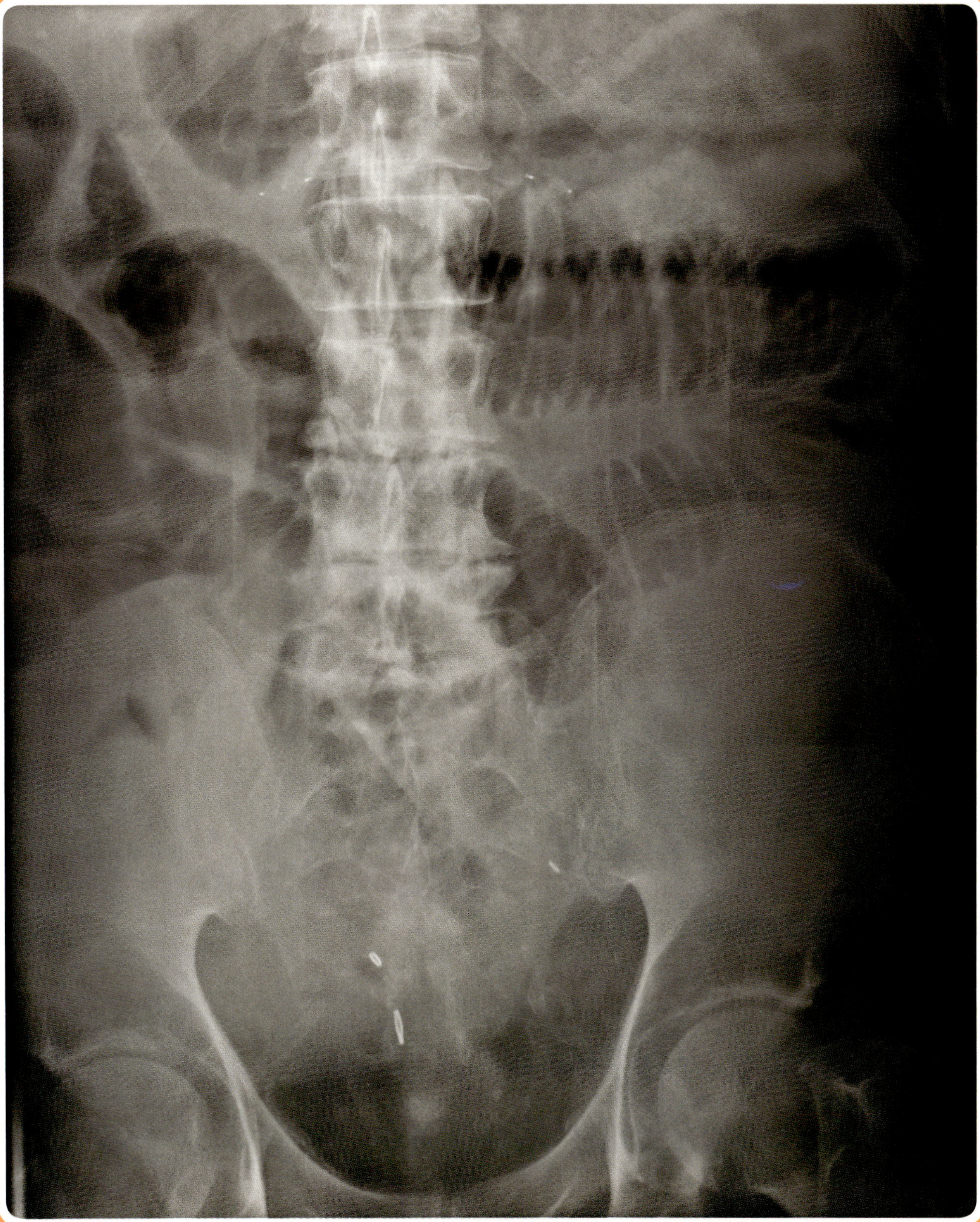

REPORT
Patient ID: Anonymous.
Projection: AP supine.
Rotation: Adequate.
Penetration: Adequate – the spinous processes are visible.
Coverage: Inadequate – the pubic symphysis, right flank and upper abdomen have not been fully included.

BOWEL GAS PATTERN
There are multiple loops of dilated bowel seen centrally in the abdomen, which demonstrate valvulae conniventes in keeping with small bowel obstruction.

BOWEL WALL
There is no evidence of mural thickening or intramural gas within the large or small bowel.

PNEUMOPERITONEUM
There is no evidence of free intra-abdominal gas.

SOLID ORGANS
The solid organ contours are within normal limits with no solid organ calcification.

VASCULAR
There is calcification of the iliac arteries bilaterally.

BONES
There is moderate degenerative change in the lower lumbar spine with osteophyte formation and intervertebral disc space narrowing.

SOFT TISSUES
The psoas muscle outline is not visible bilaterally, which is non-specific.

The extra-abdominal soft tissues are unremarkable.

OTHER
There are three radiopaque densities projected over the pelvis that appear to be surgical clips, in keeping with previous gynaecological surgery.

There are no vascular lines or drains.

REVIEW AREAS
Gallstones / Renal calculi: No radiopaque calculi.
Lung bases: Not fully included.
Spine: Moderate degenerative change in lower lumbar spine.
Femoral heads: Normal.

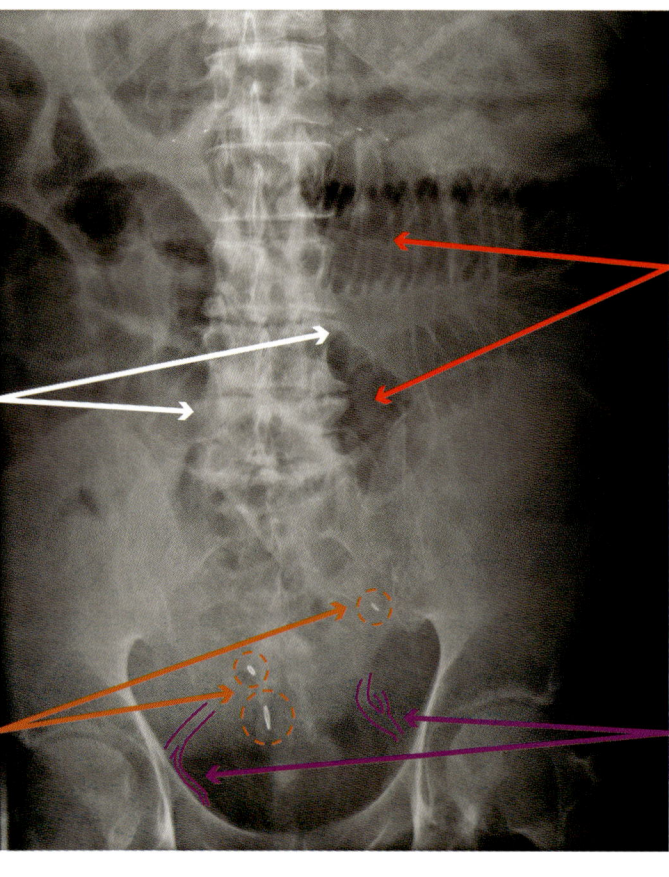

Small bowel dilatation with valvulae conniventes

Degenerative change in the spine

Surgical clips

Calcified iliac arteries

SUMMARY
This X-ray demonstrates multiple loops of dilated bowel seen centrally within the abdomen demonstrating valvulae conniventes, in keeping with small bowel obstruction. No cause for this is visible, however, given the clinical history, this is likely secondary to adhesions from previous surgery. The bilateral iliac artery calcifications, moderate degenerative changes in the lower lumbar spine and pelvic surgical clips are incidental findings.

INVESTIGATIONS AND MANAGEMENT
The patient should be resuscitated using an ABCDE approach.

Adequate analgesia and hydration should be provided.

The patient should be kept NBM and an NG tube inserted on free drainage to relieve the pressure in the small bowel. IV fluids should be commenced.

Urgent bloods should be taken, including FBC, U&Es, CRP, LFTs, coagulation, blood gas, and group and save.

The general surgical team should be contacted urgently and a CT scan of the abdomen/pelvis with IV contrast should be considered for better visualisation of the anatomy and further assessment.

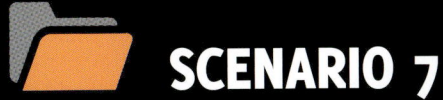

SCENARIO 7

A 25 year old female presents to ED with worsening abdominal pain. Her past medical history is significant for severe constipation (on multiple laxatives) and she is a non-smoker. A spinal cord stimulator has been inserted previously for severe neuropathic pain. On examination, she has saturations of 97% in room air and a temperature of 37.2°C. Her HR is 97 bpm, RR is 24 and blood pressure is 132/74 mmHg. The abdomen is soft with generalised tenderness and normal bowel sounds. Urine dipstick is unremarkable and a pregnancy test is negative.

An abdominal X-ray is requested to assess for possible bowel obstruction.

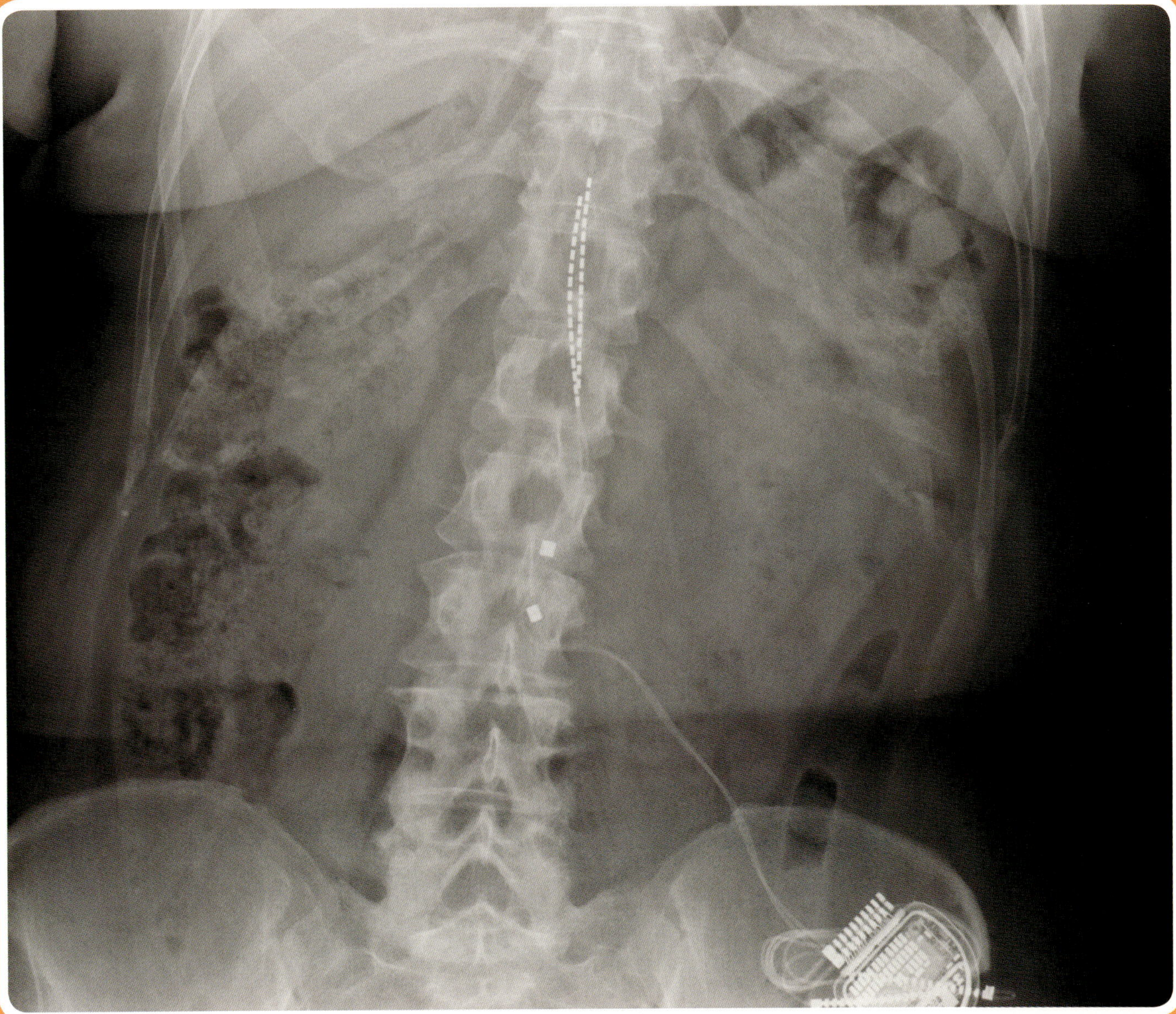

REPORT
Patient ID: Anonymous.
Projection: AP supine.
Rotation: Adequate.
Penetration: Adequate – the spinous processes are visible.
Coverage: Inadequate – the pubic symphysis, inferior pubic rami and hip joints have not been included.

BOWEL GAS PATTERN
The bowel gas pattern is normal.

There is extensive faecal residue present throughout the ascending colon.

BOWEL WALL
The descending colon is featureless.

There is no evidence of mural thickening or intramural gas within the large or small bowel.

PNEUMOPERITONEUM
There is no evidence of free intra-abdominal gas.

SOLID ORGANS
The solid organ contours are within normal limits with no solid organ calcification.

VASCULAR
No abnormal vascular calcification.

BONES
There is very mild lumbar scoliosis seen convex to the right, centred at the L2/L3 level. No fractures or destructive bone lesions are visible in the imaged skeleton.

SOFT TISSUES
The psoas muscle outline is visible bilaterally.

The extra-abdominal soft tissues are unremarkable.

OTHER
There is a radiopaque foreign object projected over the region of the left iliac fossa, with wires extending up towards the midline of the spine, in keeping with a spinal cord stimulator.

The preperitoneal fat is clearly visible, which should not be mistaken for free gas.

There are no vascular lines, drains or surgical clips.

REVIEW AREAS
Gallstones / Renal calculi: No radiopaque calculi.
Lung bases: The right lung base is not fully included.
Spine: Very mild lumbar scoliosis seen convex to the right, centred at L2/L3.
Femoral heads: Not visible.

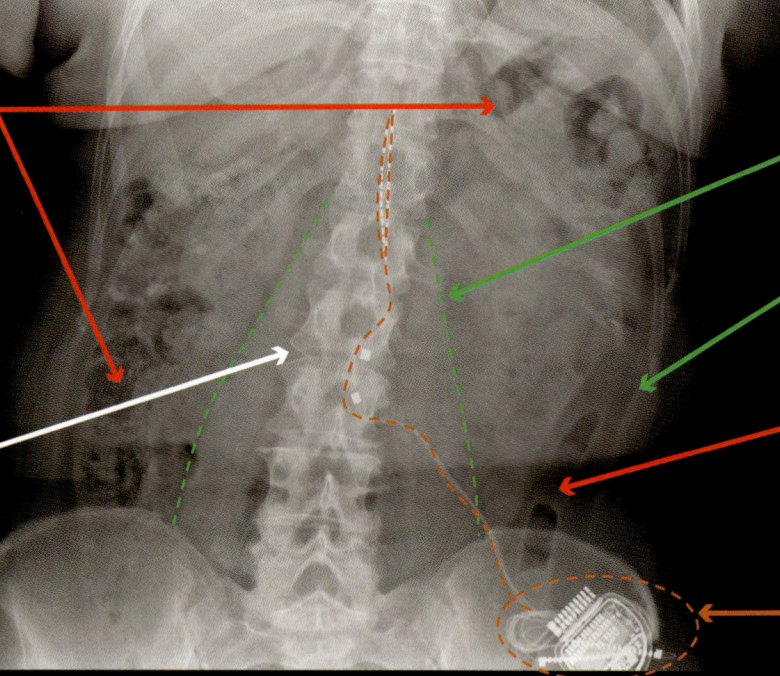

Faecal residue throughout ascending and transverse colon

Scoliosis

Psoas muscle outlines

Preperitoneal fat

Collapsed colon with reduced haustra markings

Spinal cord stimulator

SUMMARY
This X-ray demonstrates extensive faecal residue within the ascending and transverse colon, which given the clinical history is suggestive of constipation. It also demonstrates a spinal cord stimulator in situ. The very mild lumbar scoliosis seen convex to the right, centred at the L2/L3 level is an incidental finding.

INVESTIGATIONS AND MANAGEMENT
Adequate analgesia and hydration should be provided.

If the patient is otherwise well, no further investigations or imaging is required.

If the patient is clinically constipated, current medications should be reviewed and additional laxatives considered. Advice should be given regarding lifestyle adjustments, including adequate fluid intake, sufficient dietary fibre and exercise if clinically appropriate.

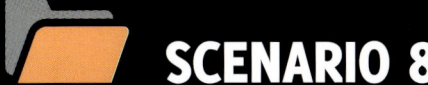
A 50 year old female is currently admitted on the urology ward with ureteric colic. Her past medical history is significant for renal calculi and she previously had a right-sided ureteric stent inserted. She is a non-smoker. On examination, she has saturations of 96% in room air and a temperature of 36.5°C. Her HR is 82 bpm, RR is 13 and blood pressure is 118/80 mmHg. The abdomen is soft and there is mild tenderness in the right iliac fossa with normal bowel sounds. Urine dipstick is unremarkable.

An abdominal X-ray is requested to assess the position of the ureteric stent and to assess for possible renal calculi.

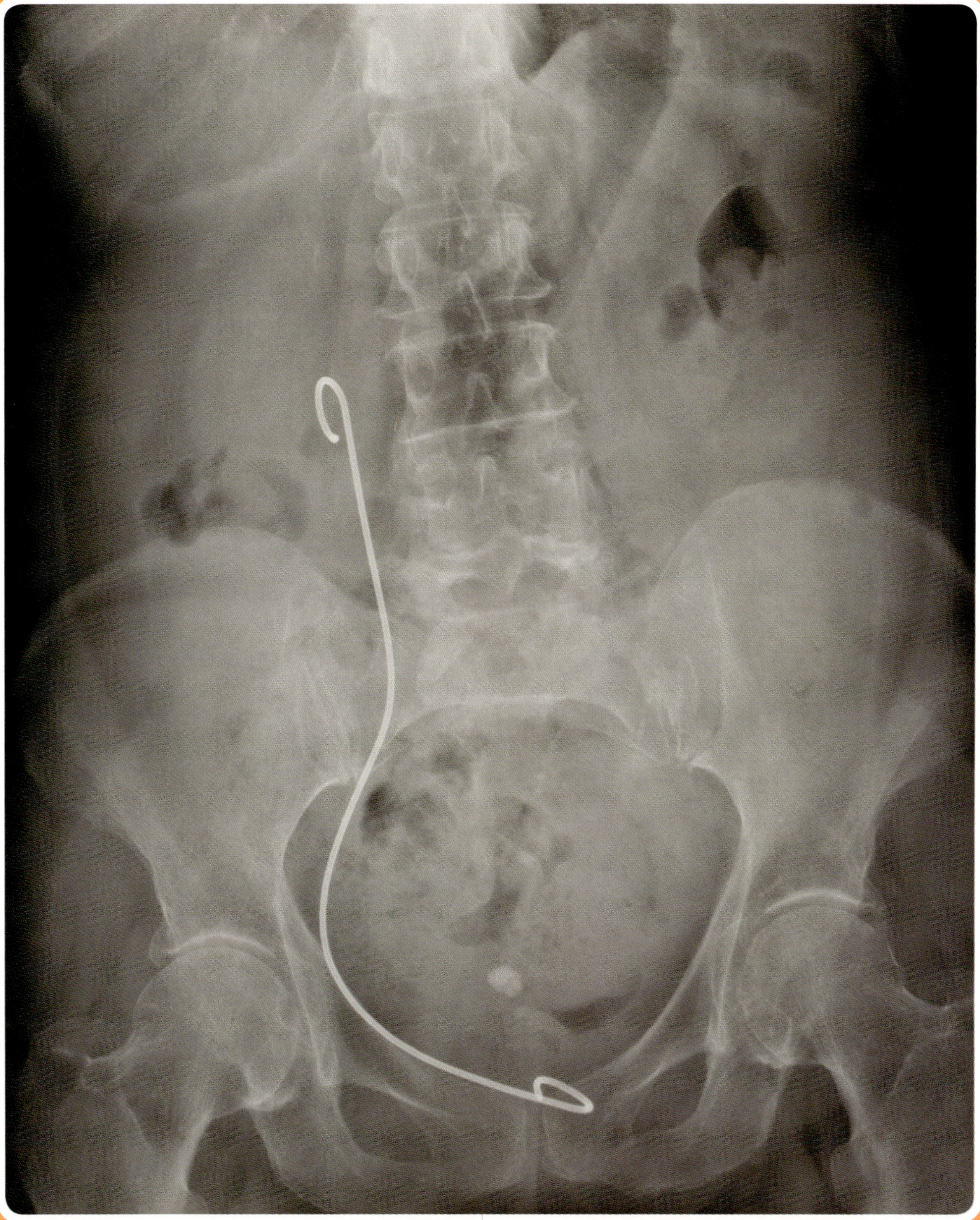

REPORT
Patient ID: Anonymous.
Projection: AP supine.
Rotation: Adequate.
Penetration: Adequate – the spinous processes are visible.
Coverage: Adequate – the anterior ribs are visible superiorly and the inferior pubic rami are visible.

BOWEL GAS PATTERN
The bowel gas pattern is normal.

BOWEL WALL
There is no evidence of mural thickening or intramural gas within the large or small bowel.

PNEUMOPERITONEUM
There is no evidence of free intra-abdominal gas.

SOLID ORGANS
The solid organ contours are within normal limits with no solid organ calcification.

VASCULAR
No abnormal vascular calcification.

BONES
There is mild degenerative change seen in the spine.

SOFT TISSUES
The psoas muscle outline is visible bilaterally.

The extra-abdominal soft tissues are unremarkable.

OTHER
There is a radiopaque line projected over the region of the right ureter in keeping with a correctly sited JJ ureteric stent. The proximal end is projected over the right renal pelvis and the distal end over the bladder.

There is a well-defined radiopaque density projected over the region of the bladder, which most likely represents a bladder calculus. Other differentials include calcified pelvic lymph node, ovarian teratoma calcification or fibroid calcification.

There are no other radiopaque foreign bodies.

There are no vascular lines or surgical clips.

REVIEW AREAS
Gallstones / Renal calculi: Likely bladder calculus.
Lung bases: Normal.
Spine: Mild degenerative changes.
Femoral heads: Normal.

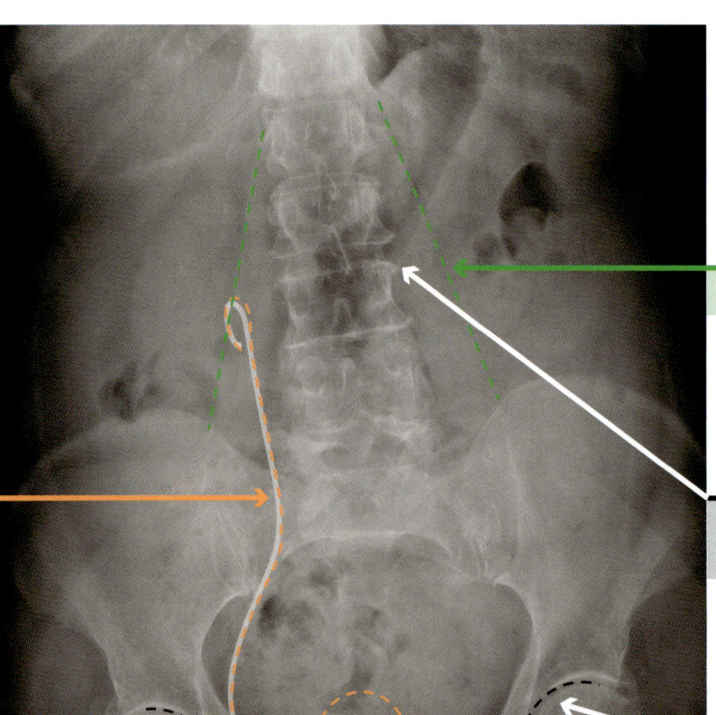

JJ ureteric stent

Bladder calculus

Psoas muscle outlines

Degenerative change in the spine

Femoral heads normal

SUMMARY
This X-ray demonstrates a right-sided appropriately sited JJ ureteric stent and a well-defined radiopaque density projected over the region of the bladder most likely in keeping with a calculus.

INVESTIGATIONS AND MANAGEMENT
Adequate analgesia and hydration should be provided.

Urgent bloods should be taken, including FBC, U&Es, CRP, LFTs, blood gas, and bone profile.

The patient should be assessed for acute kidney injury, and if present, an ultrasound of the urinary tract in the first instance would be beneficial in assessing for hydronephrosis.

Smaller stones may pass spontaneously, but referral to urology may be required for further assessment.

A CT scan of the kidneys, ureters and bladder may be useful for better visualisation of the anatomy. The appearances should be compared with previous imaging to assess for interval change.

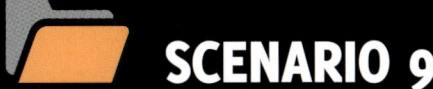

SCENARIO 9

An 84 year old male presents to ED with generalised abdominal pain on a background of a 2 month history of hip pain and reduced mobility. His past medical history is significant for prostate cancer and he is a non-smoker. A nephrostomy tube has previously been inserted on the left for hydronephrosis. On examination, he has saturations of 99% in room air and a temperature of 36.7°C. His HR is 92 bpm, RR is 20 and blood pressure is 115/65 mmHg. The abdomen is soft and there is mild generalised tenderness with normal bowel sounds. Urine dipstick is unremarkable. There is tenderness over the right hip and pain on hip flexion.

An abdominal X-ray is requested to assess for possible bowel obstruction.

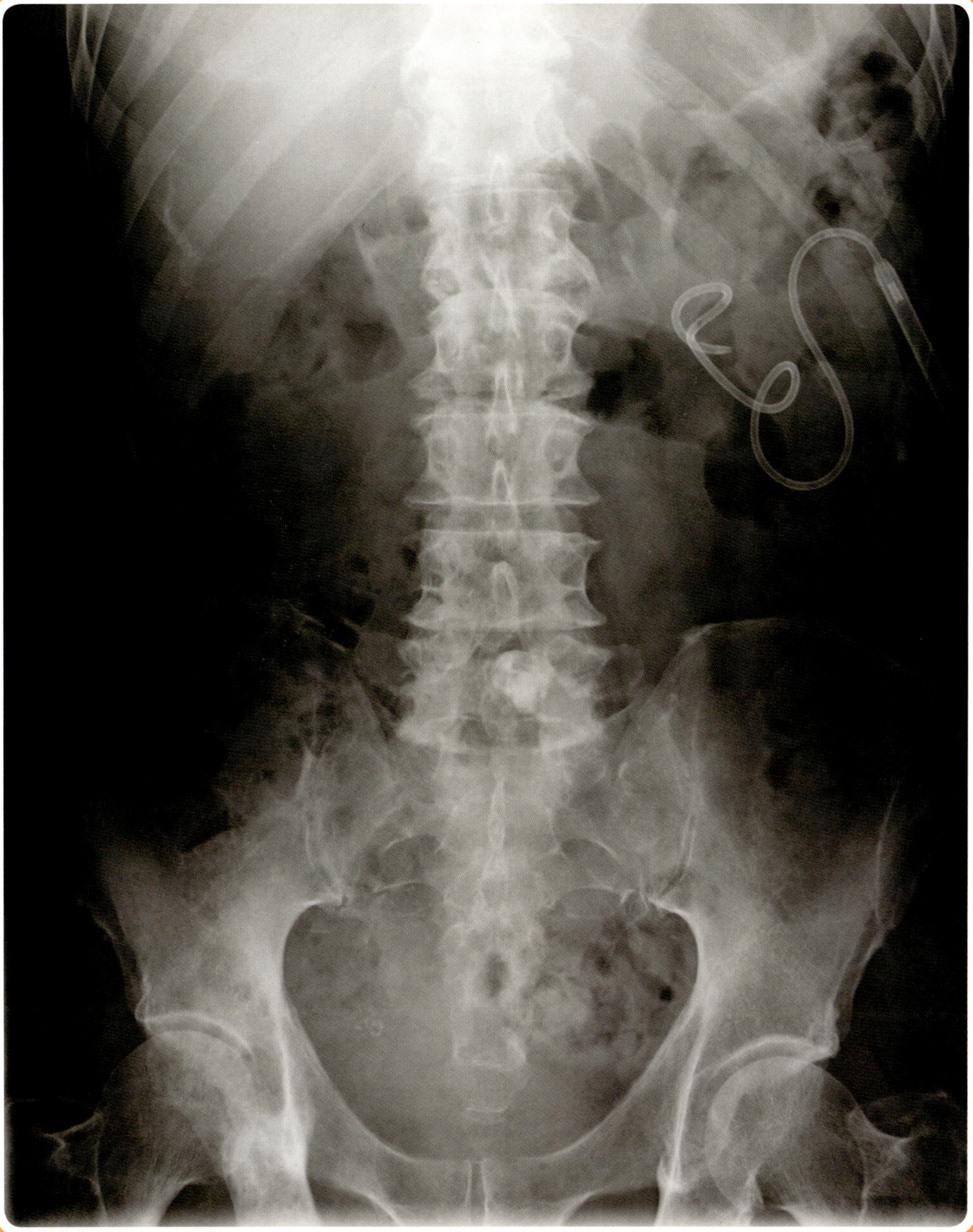

REPORT

Patient ID: Anonymous.
Projection: AP supine.
Rotation: Adequate.
Penetration: Adequate – the spinous processes are visible.
Coverage: Inadequate – the pubic symphysis and inferior pubic rami have not been fully included.

BOWEL GAS PATTERN

The bowel gas pattern is normal.

BOWEL WALL

There is no evidence of mural thickening or intramural gas within the large or small bowel.

PNEUMOPERITONEUM

There is no evidence of free intra-abdominal gas.

SOLID ORGANS

There is a left-sided catheter projected over the region of the left kidney, in keeping with a nephrostomy tube.

VASCULAR

There is calcification of the right-sided iliac arteries.

BONES

There is a well-circumscribed sclerotic lesion projected over the L5 vertebral body with loss of the L5 spinous process, which most likely represents a vertebral metastasis given the clinical history.

There is a sclerotic ill-defined lesion projected over the region of the inferior aspect of the right acetabulum with sclerosis of the ilioischial line. The location is not typical for degenerative change and most likely represents a further metastasis given the clinical history.

No fractures are visible in the imaged skeleton.

SOFT TISSUES

The psoas muscle outline is visible bilaterally.

The extra-abdominal soft tissues are unremarkable.

OTHER

There is a left-sided catheter projected over the region of the left kidney, in keeping with a nephrostomy tube.

There are no other vascular lines, drains or surgical clips.

REVIEW AREAS

Gallstones / Renal calculi: No radiopaque calculi.
Lung bases: Not fully included.
Spine: Lesion at L5 vertebral body as previously described.
Femoral heads: Sclerotic lesion at inferior aspect of right acetabulum as previously described.

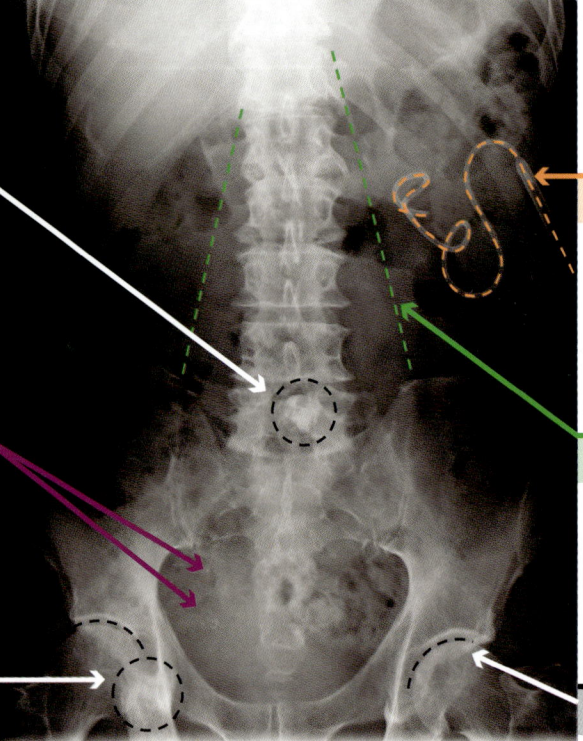

Lesion at L5

Calcified iliac arteries

Sclerotic bone lesion

Nephrostomy tube

Psoas muscle outlines

Femoral head normal

SUMMARY

This X-ray demonstrates two sclerotic bone lesions: one in the L5 vertebra and one at the right-sided acetabulum. These are suspicious for metastases given the clinical history of prostate cancer. There is a left-sided nephrostomy catheter in situ. There is no evidence of bowel obstruction.

INVESTIGATIONS AND MANAGEMENT

The patient should be resuscitated using an ABCDE approach.

Adequate analgesia and hydration should be provided.

Bloods should be taken, including FBC, U&Es, CRP, LFTs, bone profile, blood gas, and tumour markers.

If no recent scan has been performed, an up to date staging CT scan of the chest, abdomen and pelvis with IV contrast should be considered to evaluate for disease progression.

The patient should be referred to urology and oncology services for further management, which may include biopsy and MDT discussion.

Treatment, which may include surgery, radiotherapy, chemotherapy, or palliative treatment, will depend on the outcome of the MDT investigations and the patient's wishes.

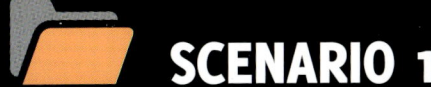

A 30 year old male presents to ED with left sided loin pain radiating to the left groin. His past medical history is significant for previous renal calculi and he is a non-smoker. He has previously had a left-sided ureteric stent inserted. On examination, he has saturations of 96% in room air and a temperature of 36.8°C. His HR is 102 bpm, RR is 24 and blood pressure is 130/80 mmHg. The abdomen is soft with tenderness in the left loin radiating to the left groin. Bowel sounds are normal. Urine dipstick shows blood +++.

An abdominal X-ray is requested to assess for possible renal calculi.

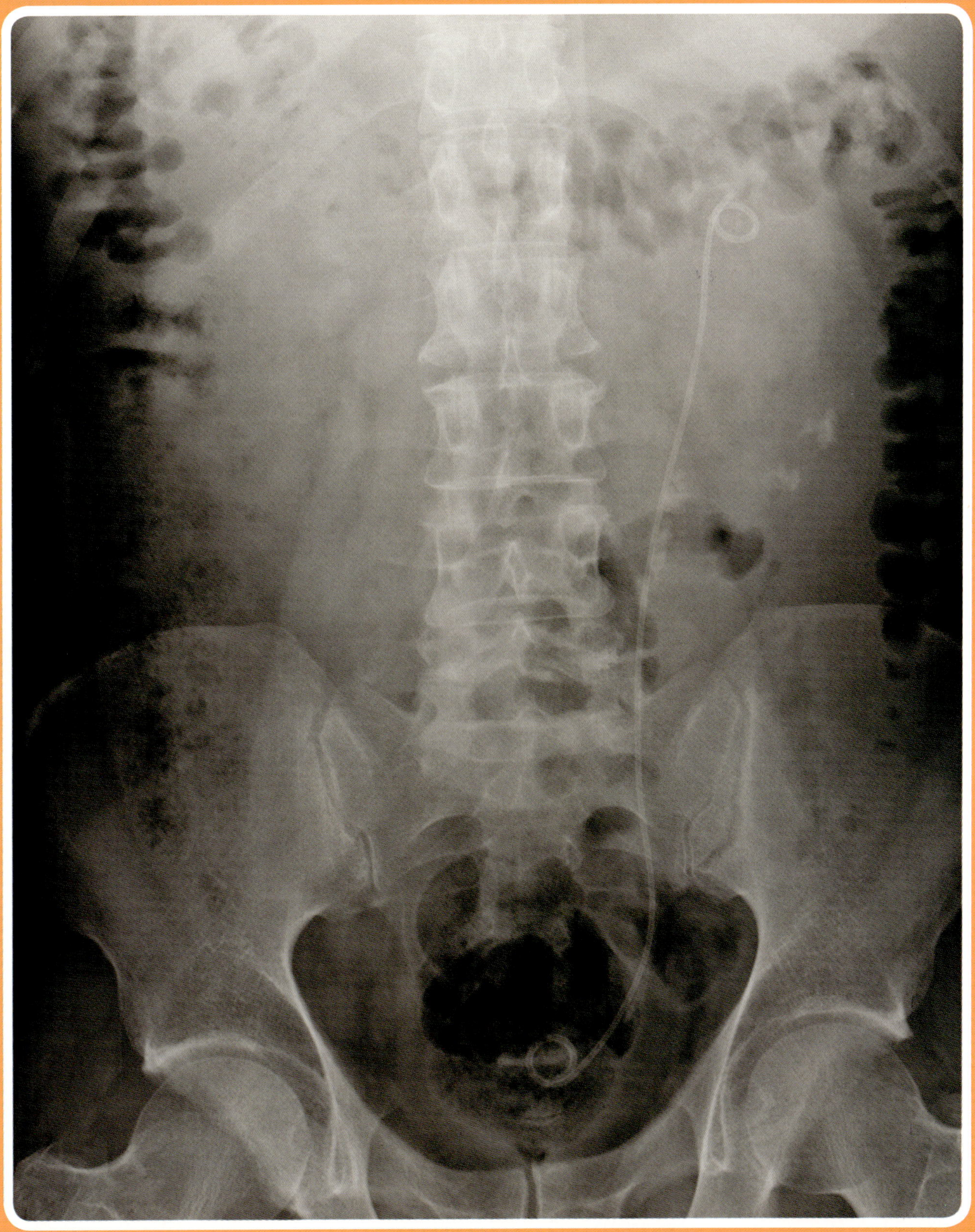

REPORT – LEFT JJ STENT AND RENAL CALCULI

REPORT
Patient ID: Anonymous.
Projection: AP supine.
Rotation: Adequate.
Penetration: Adequate – the spinous processes are visible.
Coverage: Inadequate – the inferior pubic rami have not been fully included.

BOWEL GAS PATTERN
The bowel gas pattern is normal.

There is a mild volume of faecal residue present throughout the ascending colon.

BOWEL WALL
There is no evidence of mural thickening or intramural gas within the large or small bowel.

PNEUMOPERITONEUM
There is no evidence of free intra-abdominal gas.

SOLID ORGANS
There are 2 small radiopaque densities projected over the region of the inferior pole of the left kidney, in keeping with renal calculi.

VASCULAR
No abnormal vascular calcification.

BONES
There are no abnormalities of the imaged thoracic and lumbar spine, or within the pelvis.

SOFT TISSUES
The psoas muscle outline is visible bilaterally.

The extra-abdominal soft tissues are unremarkable.

OTHER
There is a radiopaque line projected over the region of the left ureter, which represents a correctly sited JJ ureteric stent.

There are several radiopaque densities projected to the left side of the ureteric stent at the level of L3/4, in keeping with ureteri calculi.

There are no vascular lines, drains or surgical clips.

REVIEW AREAS
Gallstones / Renal calculi: Renal calculi in inferior pole of left kidney and left ureter.
Lung bases: Not fully included.
Spine: Normal.
Femoral heads: Normal.

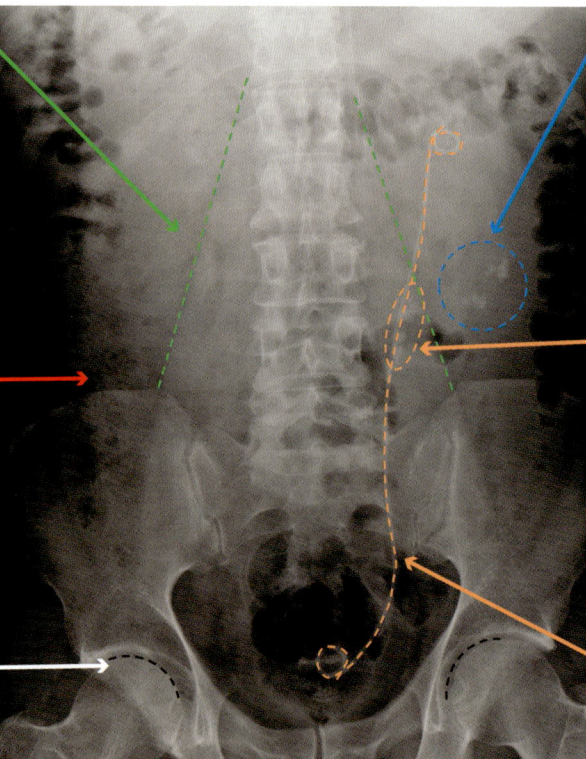

Psoas muscle outlines

Faecal residue in ascending colon

Femoral heads normal

Renal calculi

Calcification within left ureter

JJ ureteric stent

SUMMARY
This X-ray demonstrates 2 small radiopaque densities projected over the region of the inferior pole of the left kidney, in keeping with renal calculi. It also demonstrates a left-sided JJ ureteric stent in situ with associated ureteric calculi. There is a mild volume of faecal residue within the ascending colon.

INVESTIGATIONS AND MANAGEMENT
The patient should be resuscitated using an ABCDE approach.

Adequate analgesia and hydration should be provided.

Urgent bloods should be taken, including FBC, U&Es, CRP, LFTs, blood gas, and bone profile.

The patient should be assessed for acute kidney injury, and if present, an ultrasound of the urinary tract in the first instance would be beneficial in assessing for hydronephrosis.

Smaller stones may pass spontaneously, but referral to urology is required for possible further intervention. A CT scan of the kidneys, ureters and bladder might be useful for better visualisation of the anatomy.

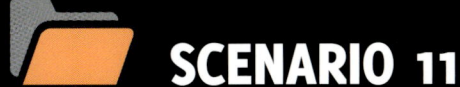

SCENARIO 11

A 45 year old female presents to ED with pain on urination. Her past medical history is significant for previous bowel surgery and she is a non-smoker. On examination, she has saturations of 98% in room air and a temperature of 36.8°C. Her HR is 85 bpm, RR is 16 and blood pressure is 120/80 mmHg. The abdomen is soft and there is tenderness in the right flank with normal bowel sounds. Urine dipstick shows blood ++ and a pregnancy test is negative.

An abdominal X-ray is requested to assess for possible renal calculi.

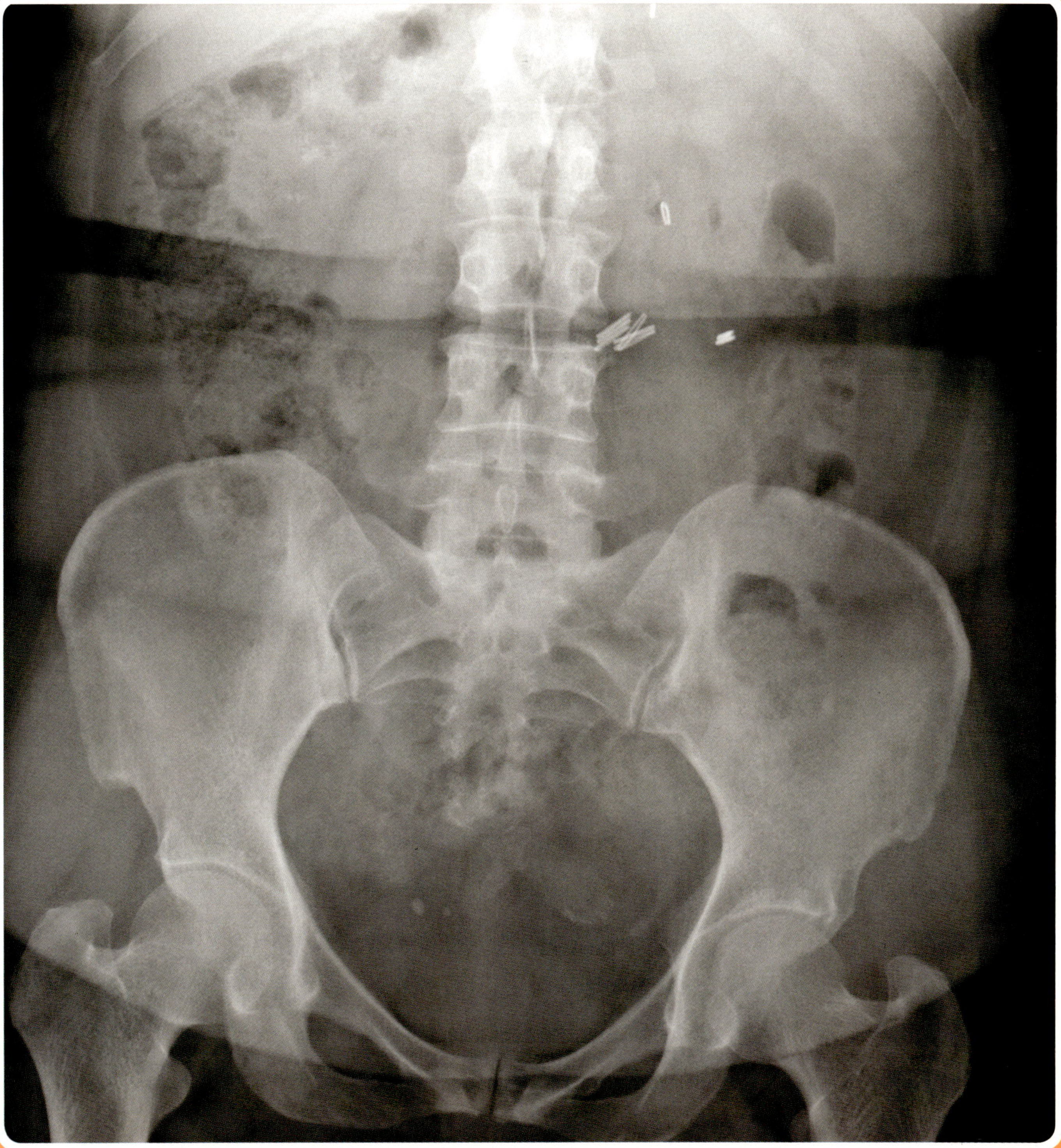

REPORT
Patient ID: Anonymous.
Projection: AP supine.
Rotation: Adequate.
Penetration: Adequate – the spinous processes are visible.
Coverage: Adequate – the anterior ribs are visible superiorly and the inferior pubic rami are visible.

BOWEL GAS PATTERN
There is a paucity of bowel gas but no bowel dilatation is visible.

There is a moderate volume of faecal residue present throughout the large bowel, extending from caecum to rectum.

BOWEL WALL
There is no evidence of mural thickening or intramural gas within the large or small bowel.

PNEUMOPERITONEUM
There is no evidence of free intra-abdominal gas.

SOLID ORGANS
There are several small radiopaque densities projected over the region of the right kidney, in keeping with renal calculi.

VASCULAR
No abnormal vascular calcification.

BONES
There are no abnormalities of the imaged thoracic and lumbar spine, or within the pelvis.

SOFT TISSUES
The psoas muscle outline is visible bilaterally.

The extra-abdominal soft tissues are unremarkable.

OTHER
There are no vascular lines or drains. There are several rounded radiopaque densities projected over the region of the pelvis, which most likely represent phleboliths.

There are several surgical clips, including in the epigastric region and to the left of L2/3 to L3/4.

REVIEW AREAS
Gallstones / Renal calculi: Several likely renal calculi in the region of the right kidney.
Lung bases: Not fully included.
Spine: Normal.
Femoral heads: Normal.

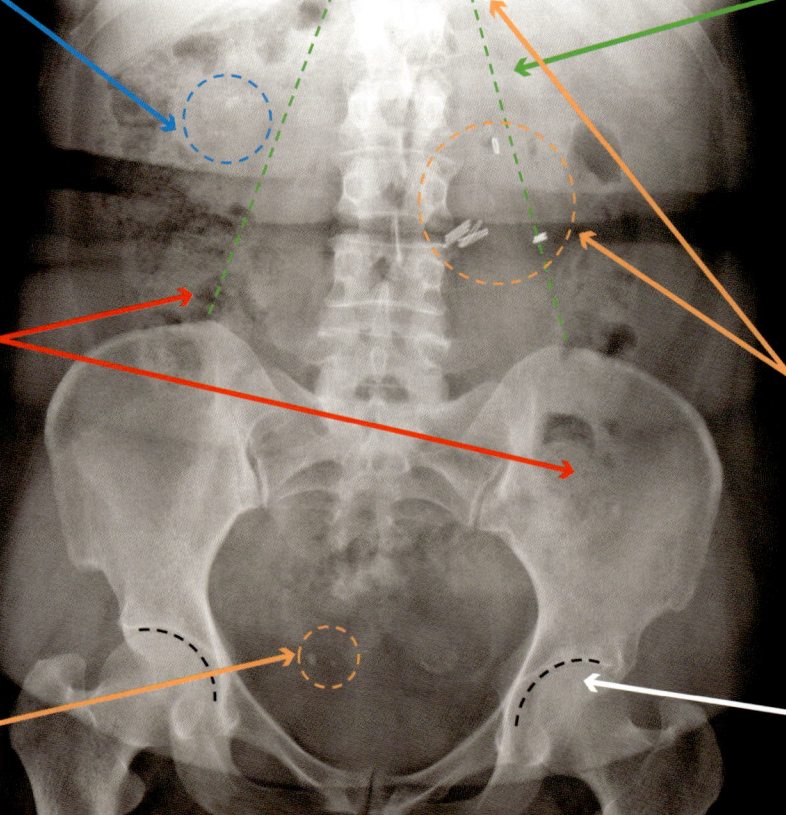

Renal calculi — Psoas muscle outlines — Faecal residue throughout large bowel — Surgical clips — Phleboliths — Femoral heads normal

SUMMARY
This X-ray demonstrates several small radiopaque densities projected over the region of the right kidney, in keeping with renal calculi. The moderate volume of faecal residue throughout the large bowel, pelvic phleboliths, and surgical clips projecting over the epigastrium and to the left of L2/3 and L3/4 are incidental findings.

INVESTIGATIONS AND MANAGEMENT
The patient should be resuscitated using an ABCDE approach.

Adequate analgesia and hydration should be provided.

Urgent bloods should be taken, including FBC, U&Es, CRP, LFTs, blood gas, and bone profile.

The patient should be assessed for acute kidney injury, and if present, an ultrasound of the urinary tract in the first instance would be beneficial in assessing for hydronephrosis.

Smaller stones may pass spontaneously, but referral to urology may be required for possible further intervention. A CT scan of the kidneys, ureters and bladder would be useful for better visualisation of the anatomy, depending on the clinical picture and blood test results.

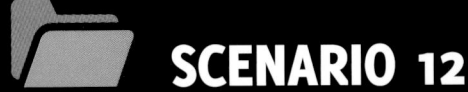

SCENARIO 12

A 15 year old female presents to ED with severe constipation, having not opened her bowels for 6 days or passed flatus for 24 hours. She feels nauseated and reports vomiting that morning. She has no significant past medical history and is a non-smoker. On examination, she has saturations of 99% in room air and a temperature of 37.1°C. Her HR is 82 bpm, RR is 16 and blood pressure is 110/65 mmHg. The abdomen is mildly distended and there is tenderness and voluntary guarding in the lower abdomen with normal bowel sounds. Urine dipstick is unremarkable and a pregnancy test is negative.

An abdominal X-ray is requested to assess for possible bowel obstruction.

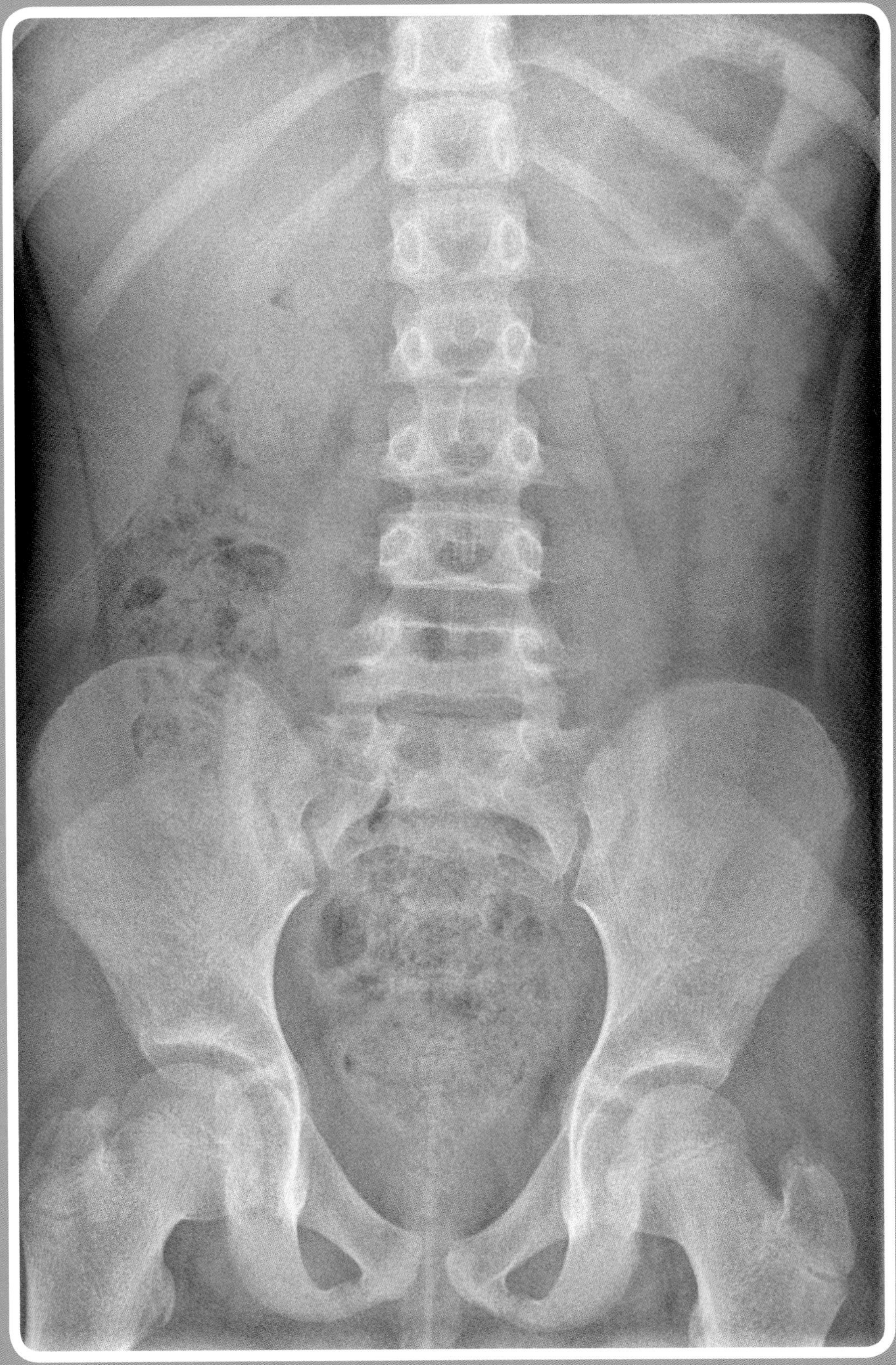

REPORT
Patient ID: Anonymous.
Projection: AP supine.
Rotation: Adequate.
Penetration: Adequate – the spinous processes are visible.
Coverage: Adequate – the anterior ribs are visible superiorly and the inferior pubic rami are visible.

BOWEL GAS PATTERN
There is a paucity of bowel gas but no bowel dilatation is visible.

There is a moderate volume of faecal residue present predominantly in the ascending and distal sigmoid colon and rectum.

BOWEL WALL
There is no evidence of mural thickening or intramural gas within the large or small bowel.

PNEUMOPERITONEUM
There is no evidence of free intra-abdominal gas.

SOLID ORGANS
The right lobe of the liver extends inferiorly beyond the lower margin of the right kidney, with a tongue-like appearance, in keeping with a Riedel's lobe.

VASCULAR
No abnormal vascular calcification.

BONES
There are no abnormalities of the imaged thoracic and lumbar spine, or within the pelvis. There are growth plates at the femoral head, trochanters and acetabulum as the ossification centres have not yet fused, which is a normal finding in a child of this age.

SOFT TISSUES
The psoas muscle outline is visible bilaterally.

The extra-abdominal soft tissues are unremarkable.

OTHER
There is a urethral urinary catheter in situ.

There are no radiopaque foreign bodies.

There are no vascular lines, drains or surgical clips.

REVIEW AREAS
Gallstones / Renal calculi: No radiopaque calculi.
Lung bases: Not fully included.
Spine: Normal.
Femoral heads: Normal.

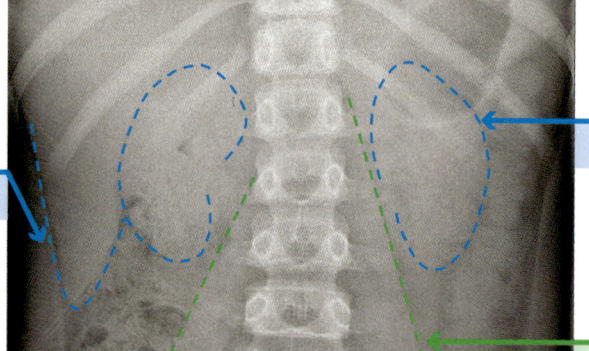

Reidel's lobe of the liver

Normal renal contours

Psoas muscle outlines

Faecal residue in ascending and sigmoid colon/rectum

Femoral heads normal

Urinary catheter

Unfused growth centres

SUMMARY
This X-ray demonstrates a moderate volume of faecal residue predominantly in the ascending and distal sigmoid colon and rectum. There is a normal variant Riedel's lobe of the liver. There is no evidence of bowel obstruction or pneumoperitoneum.

INVESTIGATIONS AND MANAGEMENT
If the patient is clinically constipated, current medications should be reviewed and laxatives considered. Advice should be given regarding lifestyle adjustments, including adequate fluid intake, sufficient dietary fibre and exercise if clinically appropriate.

If the patient is otherwise well, no further investigation or imaging is required.

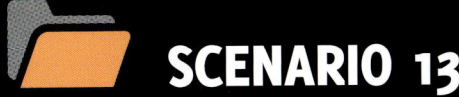

An 11 year old female attends the gastroenterology outpatient clinic for a routine follow up appointment. Her past medical history is significant for chronic constipation, for which she takes laxatives. On examination, she has saturations of 98% in room air and a temperature of 36.7°C. Her HR is 80 bpm, RR is 20 and blood pressure is 110/70 mmHg. The abdomen is soft, but slightly distended, with mild tenderness with normal bowel sounds.

An abdominal X-ray is requested to assess for possible bowel obstruction.

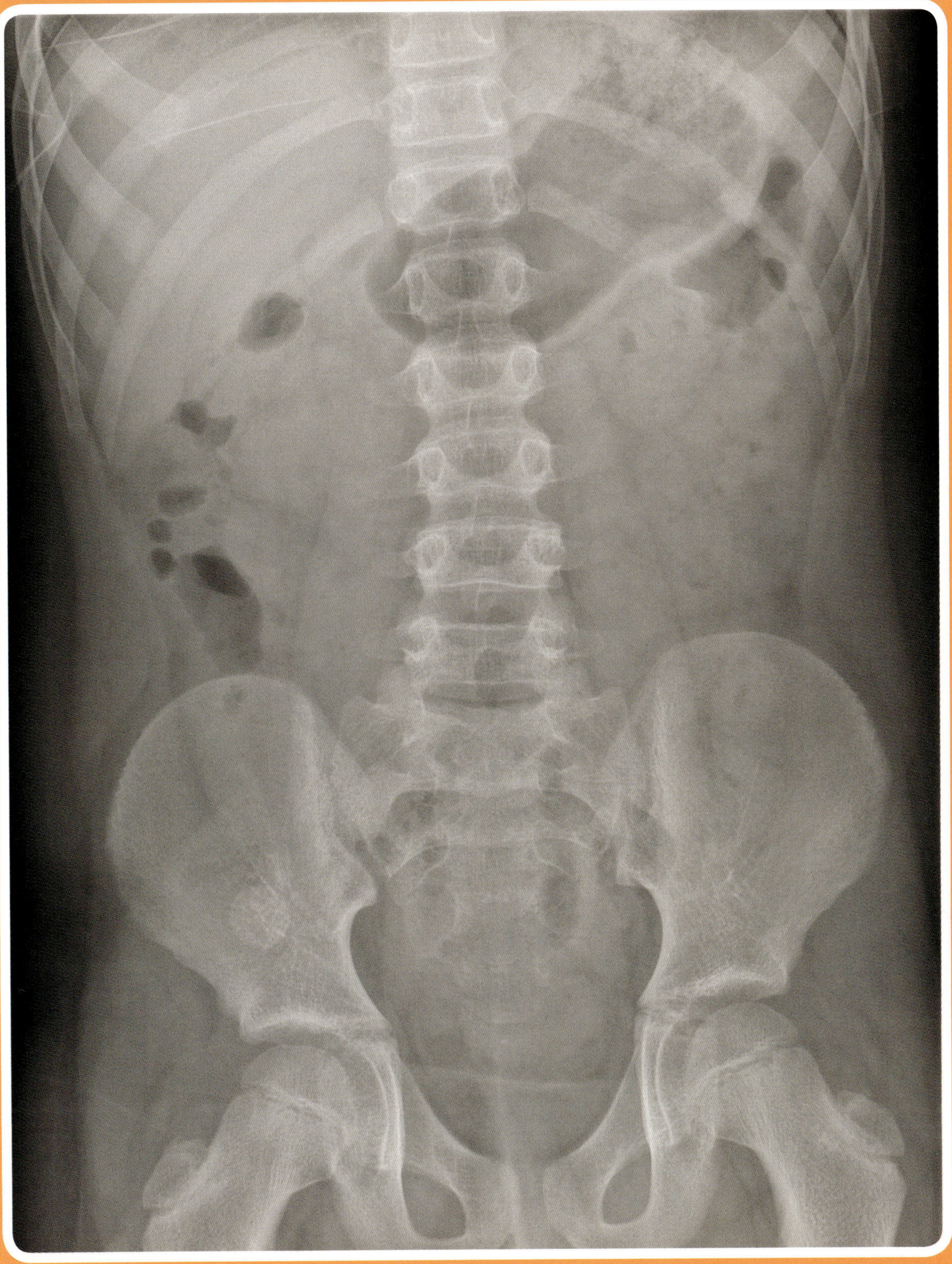

REPORT
Patient ID: Anonymous.
Projection: AP supine.
Rotation: Adequate.
Penetration: Adequate – the spinous processes are visible.
Coverage: Adequate – the anterior ribs are visible superiorly and the pubic rami are visible inferiorly.

BOWEL GAS PATTERN
The bowel gas pattern is normal.

BOWEL WALL
There is no evidence of mural thickening or intramural gas within the large or small bowel.

PNEUMOPERITONEUM
There is no evidence of free intra-abdominal gas.

SOLID ORGANS
The solid organ contours are within normal limits with no solid organ calcification.

VASCULAR
No abnormal vascular calcification.

BONES
There are no abnormalities of the imaged thoracic and lumbar spine, or within the pelvis.

There are growth plates at the femoral head, greater trochanter and acetabulum as the ossification centres have not yet fused, which is a normal finding in a child of this age.

SOFT TISSUES
The psoas muscle outline is visible bilaterally.

The extra-abdominal soft tissues are unremarkable.

OTHER
There is a rounded radiopaque density projected over the right iliac fossa, which most likely represents the stopper of an Antegrade Colonic Enema (ACE) stoma given the history of chronic constipation.

There are no vascular lines, drains or surgical clips.

REVIEW AREAS
Gallstones / Renal calculi: No radiopaque calculi.
Lung bases: Not fully included.
Spine: Normal.
Femoral heads: Normal – growth plates present.

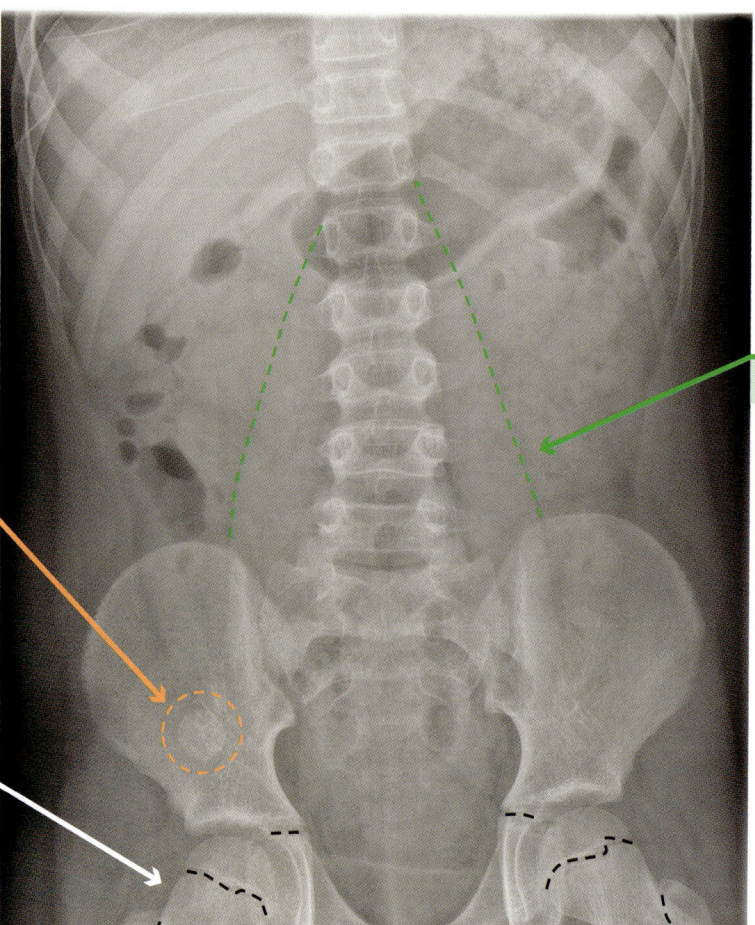

Psoas muscle outlines

Antegrade Colonic Enema stoma stopper

Growth plates

SUMMARY
This X-ray demonstrates no evidence of bowel obstruction. There is a a rounded radiopaque density projected over the right iliac fossa, most likely to represent the stopper of an Antegrade Colonic Enema stoma.

INVESTIGATIONS AND MANAGEMENT
Adequate analgesia and hydration should be provided.

If the patient is otherwise well, no further investigation or imaging is required. Referral to the paediatric continence team would be helpful to review her laxative regime.

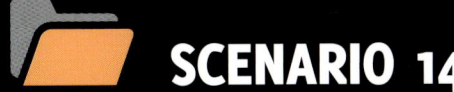

SCENARIO 14

A 12 year old female presents to ED with abdominal distension and vomiting. She has a PEG-J tube in situ to manage severe gastro-oesophageal reflux. On examination, she has saturations of 99% in room air and a temperature of 37.1°C. Her HR is 90 bpm, RR is 18 and blood pressure is 120/80 mmHg. The abdomen is soft, bowel sounds are normal, the jejunostomy site is clean, and there is some mild diffuse tenderness with no evidence of peritonism. Urine dipstick and pregnancy test are both negative.

An abdominal X-ray is requested to assess for the position of the jejunostomy tube, and for possible bowel obstruction.

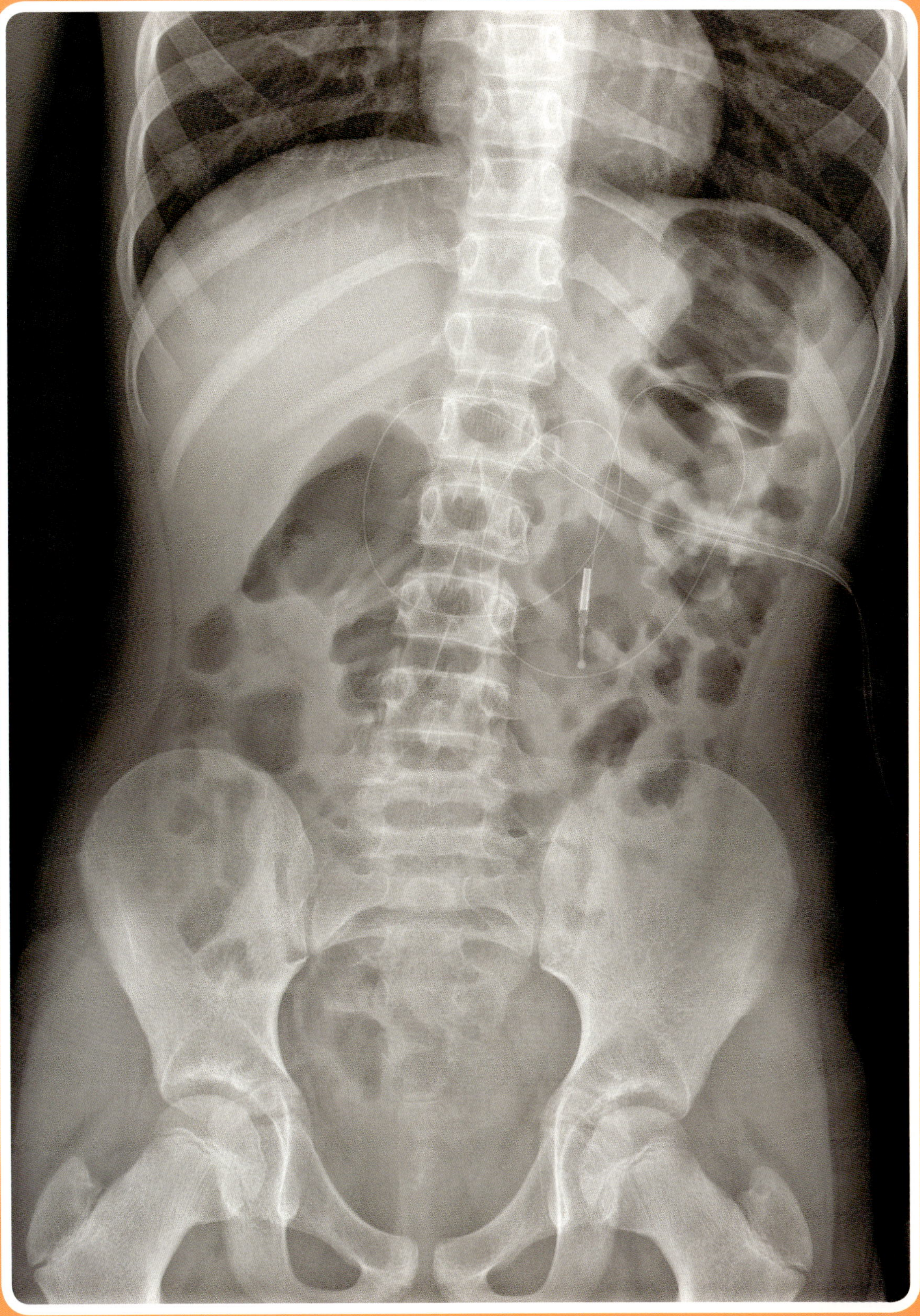

REPORT

Patient ID: Anonymous.
Projection: AP supine.
Rotation: Adequate.
Penetration: Adequate – the spine is visible.
Coverage: Adequate – the anterior ribs are visible superiorly and the inferior pubic rami are visible.

BOWEL GAS PATTERN

Bowel gas pattern is normal.

BOWEL WALL

There is no evidence of mural thickening or intramural gas within the large or small bowel.

PNEUMOPERITONEUM

There is no evidence of free intra-abdominal gas.

SOLID ORGANS

The solid organ contours are within normal limits with no solid organ calcification.

VASCULAR

No abnormal vascular calcification.

BONES

There are no abnormalities of the imaged thoracic and lumbar spine, or within the pelvis.

There are growth plates at the femoral head, greater trochanter and acetabulum (triradiate cartilage) as the ossification centres have not yet fused which is a normal finding in a child of this age.

SOFT TISSUES

The psoas muscle outline is visible bilaterally.

Extra-abdominal soft tissues are unremarkable.

OTHER

There is a radiopaque port and two internal-external lines projecting in the left upper quadrant. The tip of the shorter line is projected over the stomach in keeping with a percutaneous endoscopic gastrostomy (PEG) and the longer line follows the same course through the expected course of the duodenum with its tip projecting over the proximal jejunum in keeping with a percutaneous endoscopic transgastric jejunostomy (PEG-J).

There are no vascular lines, drains or surgical clips.

REVIEW AREAS

Gallstones / Renal calculi: No radiopaque calculi.
Lung bases: Normal.
Spine: Normal. The sacrum is not yet fused which is a normal finding in a child of this age.
Femoral heads: Normal – growth plates present.

- PEG tube tip
- PEG-J port
- Psoas muscle outlines
- PEG-J (two tubes - one to the stomach and one to the jejunum)
- Triradiate cartilage
- PEG-J tube tip
- Growth plates

SUMMARY

This abdominal X-ray demonstrates appropriately sited PEG and PEG-J lines, although you cannot be certain from a single view. The bowel gas pattern is normal and there is no evidence of bowel obstruction.

INVESTIGATIONS AND MANAGEMENT

The patient should be resuscitated using an ABCDE approach.

Adequate analgesia and anti-emetics should be provided.

The patient should be made NBM, the gastrostomy limb of the PEG-J put on free drainage, and the patient should be started on IV fluids.

Urgent bloods should be taken for FBC, U&Es, CRP, bone profile, LFTs, coagulation, blood gas, blood cultures, and cross match.

The paediatric general surgical team should be involved, and if there is no improvement, a contrast study could be considered.

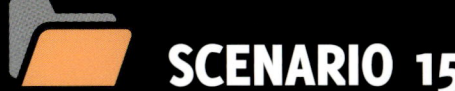

SCENARIO 15

A 45 year old male presents to ED with worsening abdominal distension. He has not passed flatus or opened his bowels for over 48 hours. He has no significant past medical history. On examination, he has saturations of 97% in room air and a temperature of 37.6°C. His HR is 94 bpm, RR is 20 and blood pressure is 134/92 mmHg. The abdomen is rigid and there is generalised tenderness with tinkling bowel sounds. Urine dipstick is unremarkable.

An abdominal X-ray is requested to assess for possible bowel obstruction.

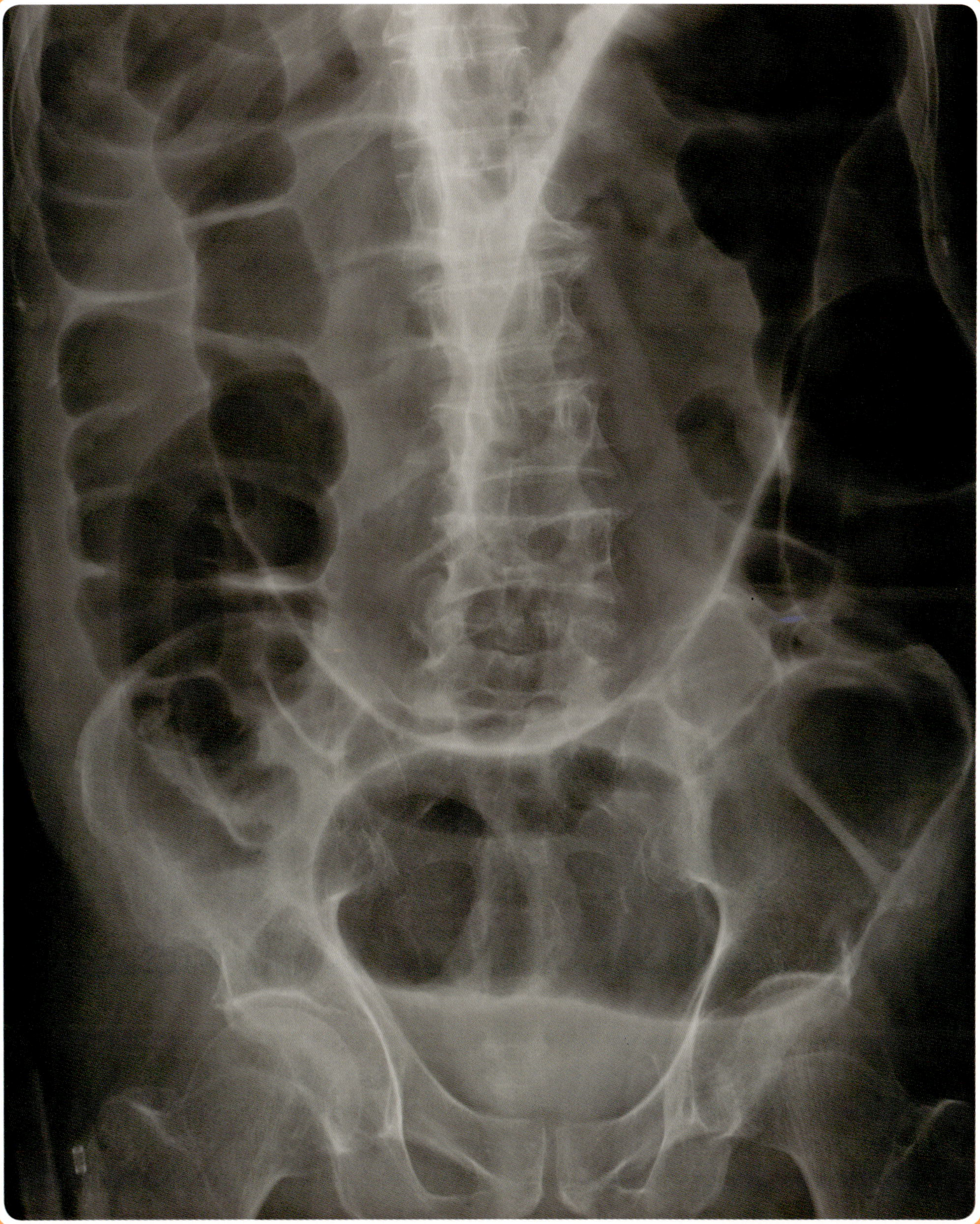

REPORT – LARGE BOWEL OBSTRUCTION

REPORT
Patient ID: Anonymous.
Projection: AP supine.
Rotation: Adequate.
Penetration: Adequate – the spinous processes are visible.
Coverage: Inadequate – the anterior ribs have not been included.

BOWEL GAS PATTERN
There are multiple loops of dilated bowel seen in the abdomen demonstrating haustra, in keeping with large bowel obstruction. A dilated small bowel loop is visible in the right lower quadrant.

Bowel gas is not seen in the rectum.

BOWEL WALL
There is no evidence of mural thickening or intramural gas within the large or small bowel.

PNEUMOPERITONEUM
There is no evidence of free intra-abdominal gas.

SOLID ORGANS
The solid organ contours are within normal limits with no solid organ calcification.

VASCULAR
No abnormal vascular calcification.

BONES
There are degenerative changes in the lumbar spine with lateral osteophytes at L1/2 and a mild scoliosis convex to the left at L4/L5. The L3 and L4 vertebral bodies have reduced height with concave endplates, in keeping with endplate fractures of indeterminate age.

SOFT TISSUES
The psoas muscle outline is visible bilaterally.

The extra-abdominal soft tissues are unremarkable.

OTHER
There are no radiopaque foreign bodies.

There are no vascular lines, drains or surgical clips.

REVIEW AREAS
Gallstones / Renal calculi: No radiopaque calculi.
Lung bases: Not fully included.
Spine: Degenerative changes and endplate fractures as described.
Femoral heads: Normal.

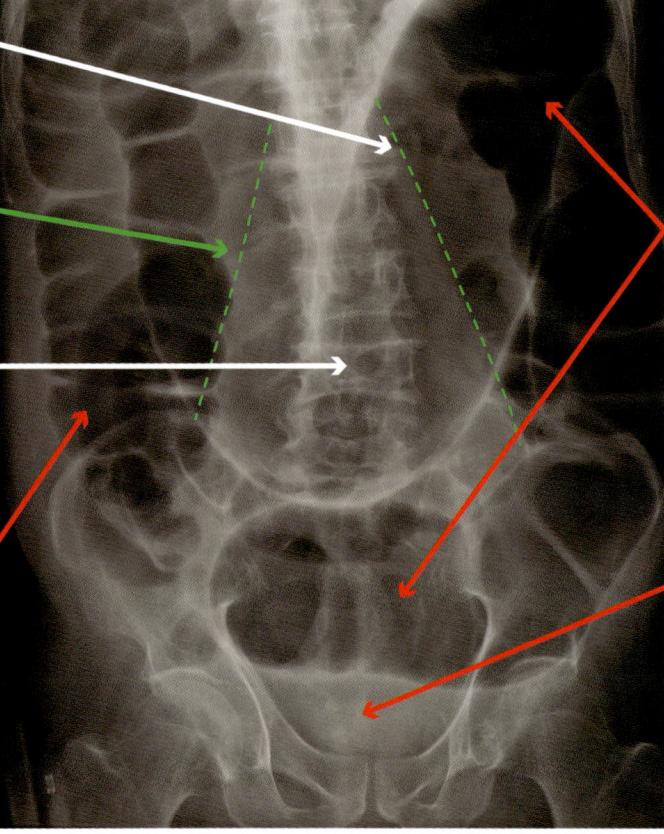

Osteophyte

Psoas muscle outlines

Reduced height

Dilated small bowel loop

Large bowel dilatation of ascending, transverse and descending colon

Empty rectum

SUMMARY
This X-ray demonstrates multiple loops of dilated bowel seen within the abdomen demonstrating haustra, in keeping with large bowel obstruction, as well as a loop of dilated small bowel. The absence of gas in the small intestine indicates a competent ileo-caecal valve creating a closed-loop obstruction. The absence of bowel gas in the rectum suggests a distal obstructing point. Given the absence of previous abdominal or pelvic surgery, findings may be secondary to a benign or malignant stricture. Vertebral endplate fractures of indeterminate age are also noted, which may be related to malignancy.

INVESTIGATIONS AND MANAGEMENT
The patient should be resuscitated using an ABCDE approach.

Adequate analgesia and hydration should be provided.

The patient should be kept NBM and an NG tube inserted on free drainage. IV fluids should be commenced.

Urgent bloods should be taken, including FBC, U&Es, CRP, LFTs, coagulation, blood gas, and group and save.

The general surgical team should be contacted urgently and a CT scan of the abdomen/pelvis with IV contrast should be considered for better visualisation of the anatomy and further assessment. With regard to the bony changes, further history should be taken, and previous images reviewed.

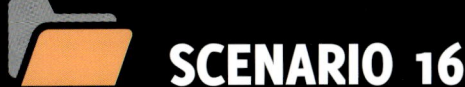

SCENARIO 16

A 36 year old female presents to her doctor with a 6 week history of mild generalised abdominal pain. Her past medical history is significant for Type I diabetes mellitus and a previous cholecystectomy. She is a non-smoker. On examination, she has saturations of 98% in room air and a temperature of 36.6°C. Her HR is 65 bpm, RR is 15 and blood pressure is 120/68 mmHg. The abdomen is soft with mild generalised tenderness with normal bowel sounds. Urine dipstick is unremarkable and a pregnancy test is negative.

An abdominal X-ray is requested to assess for possible bowel obstruction.

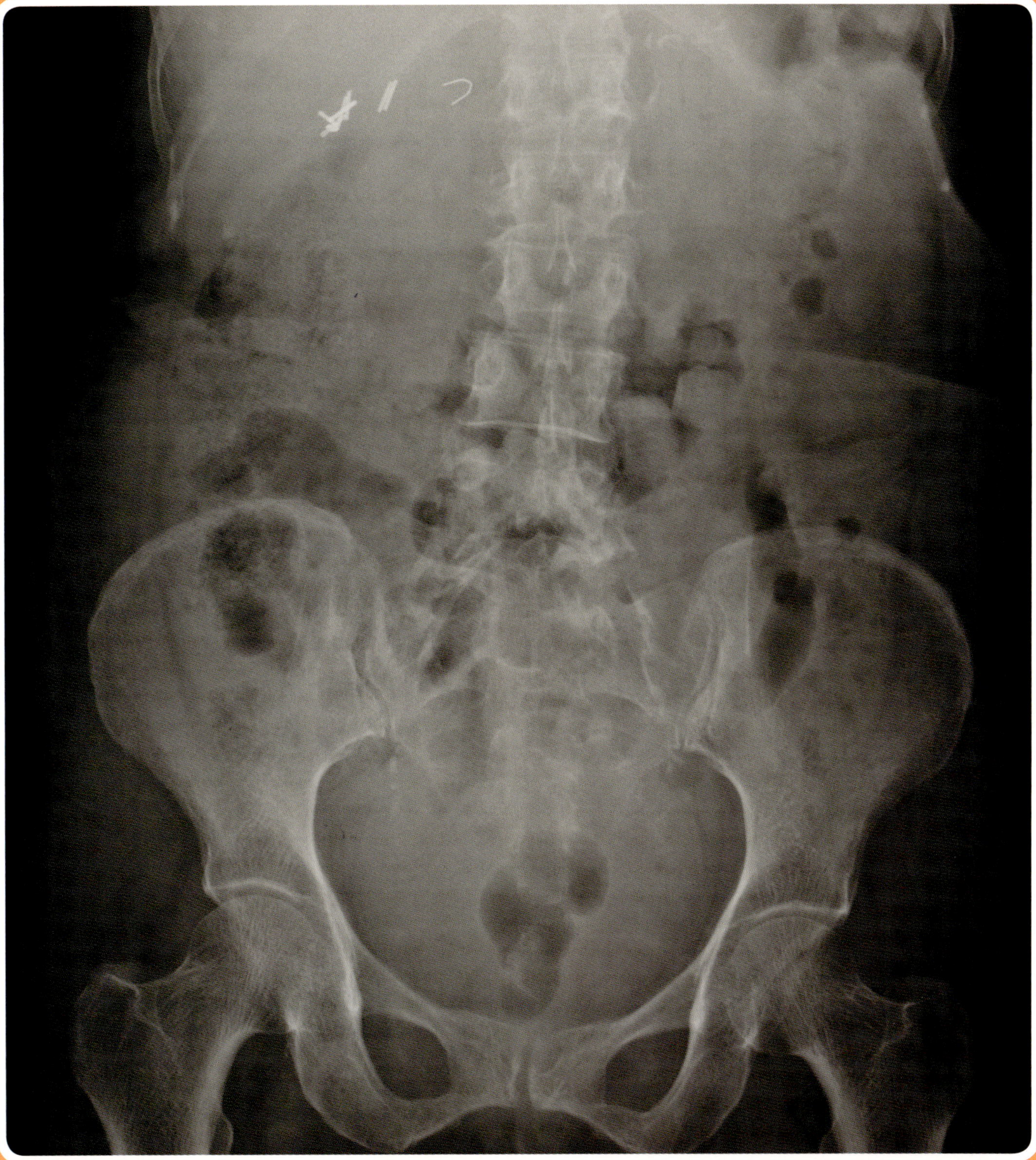

REPORT
Patient ID: Anonymous.
Projection: AP supine.
Rotation: Adequate.
Penetration: Adequate – the spinous processes are visible.
Coverage: Adequate – the anterior ribs are visible superiorly and the pubic rami are visible inferiorly.

BOWEL GAS PATTERN
The bowel gas pattern is normal.

There is a moderate volume of faecal residue present throughout the ascending colon with hard faeces within the transverse colon.

BOWEL WALL
There is no evidence of mural thickening or intramural gas within the large or small bowel.

PNEUMOPERITONEUM
There is no evidence of free intra-abdominal gas.

SOLID ORGANS
The solid organ contours are within normal limits with no solid organ calcification.

VASCULAR
There is mild calcification of the right common iliac artery.

BONES
There are moderate degenerative changes seen within the imaged lumbar spine, particularly at the L5/S1 level. There is mild scoliosis convex to the left in the lumbar spine. No fractures or destructive bone lesions are visible in the imaged skeleton.

SOFT TISSUES
The psoas muscle outline is visible bilaterally.

The extra-abdominal soft tissues are unremarkable.

OTHER
There are radiopaque surgical clips seen projected over the region of the inferior aspect of the liver, in keeping with cholecystectomy clips.

There are no vascular lines or drains.

REVIEW AREAS
Gallstones / Renal calculi: No radiopaque calculi.
Lung bases: Not fully included.
Spine: Moderate degenerative changes particularly at L5/S1 level.
Femoral heads: Normal.

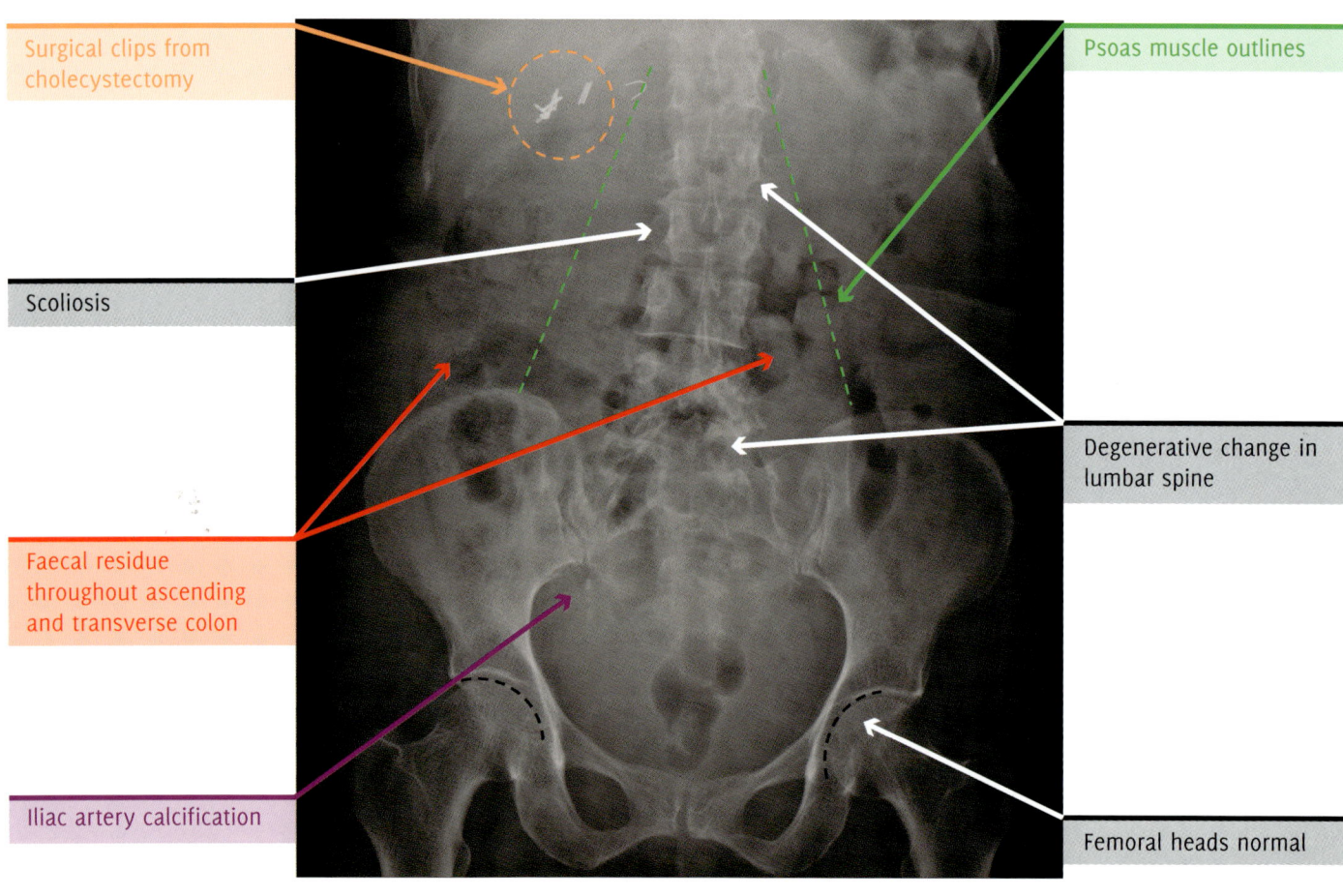

Surgical clips from cholecystectomy

Psoas muscle outlines

Scoliosis

Faecal residue throughout ascending and transverse colon

Degenerative change in lumbar spine

Iliac artery calcification

Femoral heads normal

SUMMARY
This X-ray demonstrates no evidence of bowel obstruction. There is moderate faecal loading throughout the ascending and transverse colon with hard faeces present. The cholecystectomy surgical clips, spinal degenerative changes and mild lumbar scoliosis convex to the left are incidental findings.

INVESTIGATIONS AND MANAGEMENT
Adequate analgesia and hydration should be provided.

If the patient is clinically constipated, current medications should be reviewed and laxatives considered. Advice should be given regarding lifestyle adjustments, including adequate fluid intake, sufficient dietary fibre and exercise if clinically appropriate.

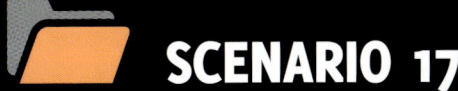

A 5 year old male presents to ED with worsening abdominal distension, nausea and vomiting. He has not opened his bowels for the past 24 hours. He has no significant past medical history. On examination, he has saturations of 99% in room air and a temperature of 36.8°C. His HR is 150 bpm, RR is 32 and blood pressure is 95/50 mmHg. The abdomen is rigid and there is generalised tenderness with tinkling bowel sounds. Urine dipstick is unremarkable.

An abdominal X-ray is requested to assess for possible obstruction.

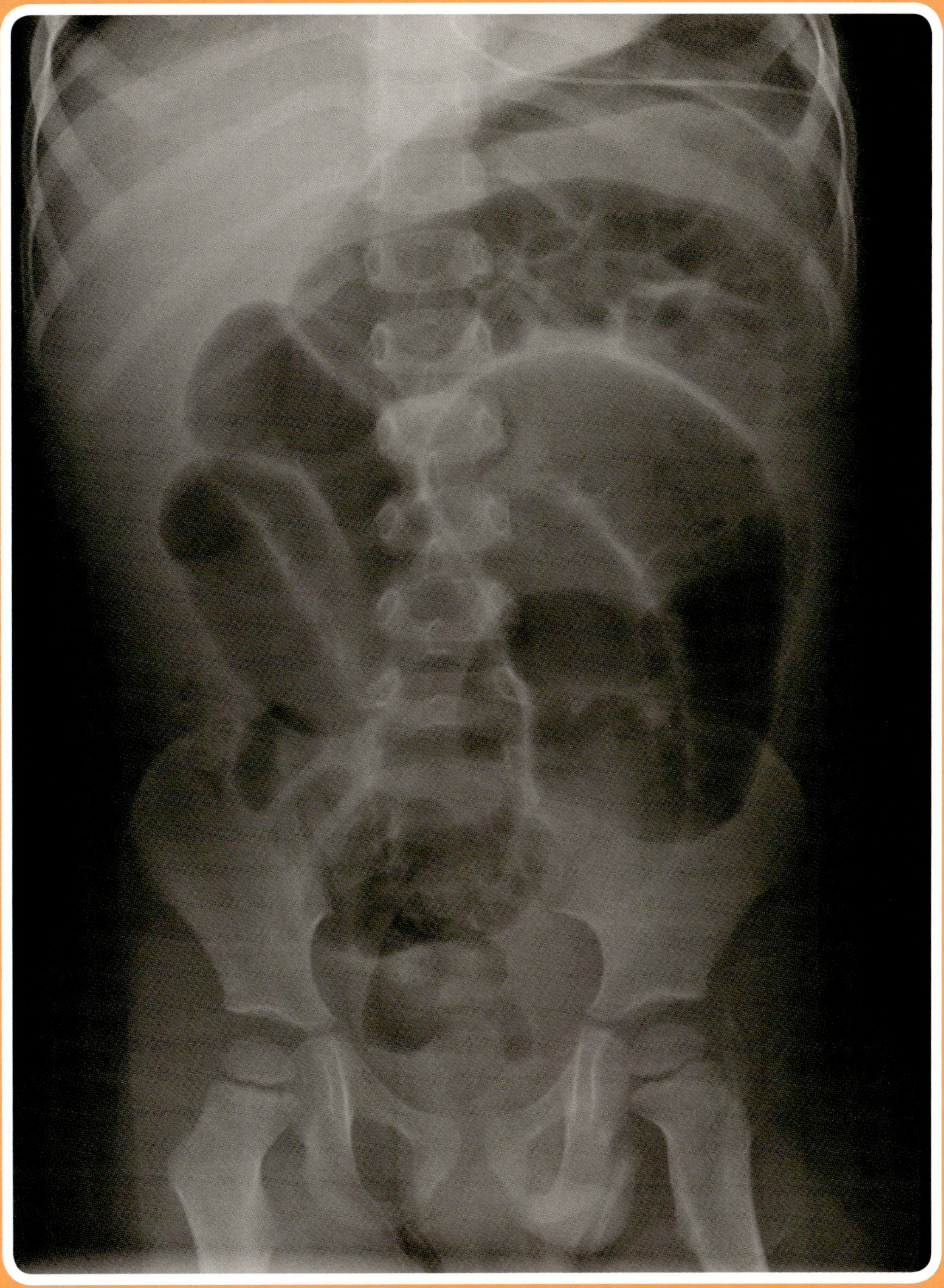

REPORT – SMALL BOWEL OBSTRUCTION

REPORT
Patient ID: Anonymous.
Projection: AP supine.
Rotation: Adequate.
Penetration: Adequate – the spinous processes are visible.
Coverage: Adequate – the anterior ribs are visible superiorly and the inferior pubic rami are visible.

BOWEL GAS PATTERN
There are multiple loops of dilated bowel seen centrally in the abdomen, in keeping with small bowel obstruction. The normal pattern of valvulae conniventes has been lost in several (but not all) dilated small bowel loops.

BOWEL WALL
There is no evidence of mural thickening or intramural gas within the large or small bowel.

PNEUMOPERITONEUM
There is no evidence of free intra-abdominal gas.

SOLID ORGANS
The solid organ contours are within normal limits with no solid organ calcification.

VASCULAR
No abnormal vascular calcification.

BONES
There are no abnormalities of the imaged thoracic and lumbar spine, or within the pelvis.

There are growth plates at the femoral head and acetabulum as the ossification centres have not yet fused, which is a normal finding in a child of this age.

SOFT TISSUES
The psoas muscle outline is not visible bilaterally, which is non-specific, particularly in a child of this age.

The extra-abdominal soft tissues are unremarkable.

OTHER
There is an NG tube in situ, with its tip projecting in the left upper quadrant, in the stomach.

There are no vascular lines, drains or surgical clips.

REVIEW AREAS
Gallstones / Renal calculi: No radiopaque calculi.
Lung bases: Not fully included.
Spine: Normal.
Femoral heads: Normal – growth plates present.

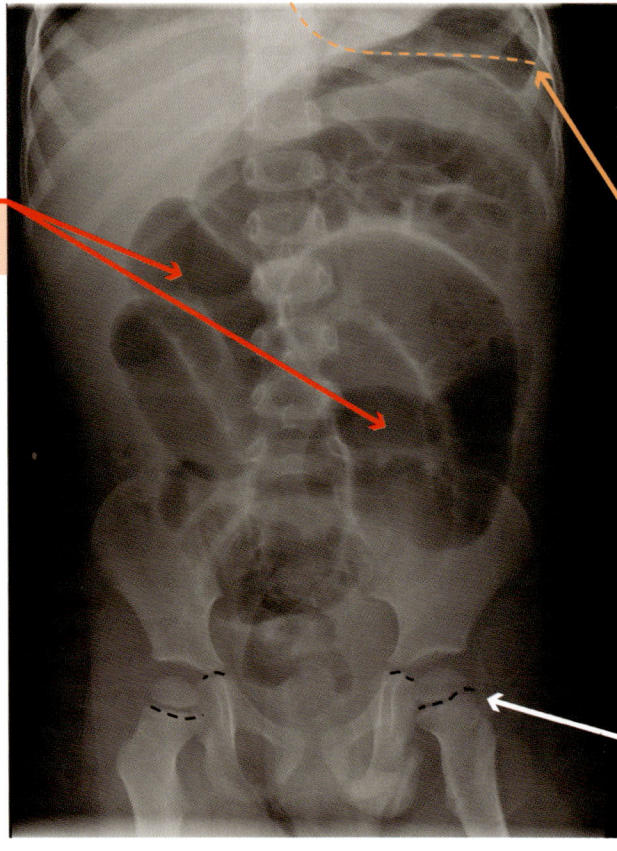

Small bowel dilatation with loss of valvulae conniventes

NG tube

Growth plates

SUMMARY
This X-ray demonstrates multiple loops of dilated bowel seen centrally in the abdomen, with loss of some of the normal valvulae conniventes, in keeping with small bowel obstruction, although no cause is obvious on the radiograph. There is an NG tube in situ with its tip in the stomach.

INVESTIGATIONS AND MANAGEMENT
The patient should be resuscitated using an ABCDE approach.

Adequate analgesia and hydration should be provided.

The patient should be kept NBM, have the NG tube put on free drainage, and be started on IV fluids.

Urgent bloods should be taken, including FBC, U&Es, CRP, LFTs, coagulation, blood gas, and group and save.

The paediatric surgical team should be contacted urgently and further radiological imaging of the abdomen and pelvis should be considered for better visualisation of the anatomy and further assessment.

SCENARIO 18

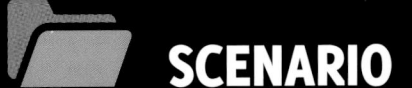

A 4 year old male presents to ED with worsening abdominal pain and distension. He has no significant past medical history. On examination, he has saturations of 97% in room air and a temperature of 37.3°C. His HR is 152 bpm, RR is 36 and blood pressure is 120/75 mmHg. The abdomen is rigid and there is generalised tenderness with tinkling bowel sounds. Urine dipstick is unremarkable.

An abdominal X-ray is requested to assess for possible obstruction.

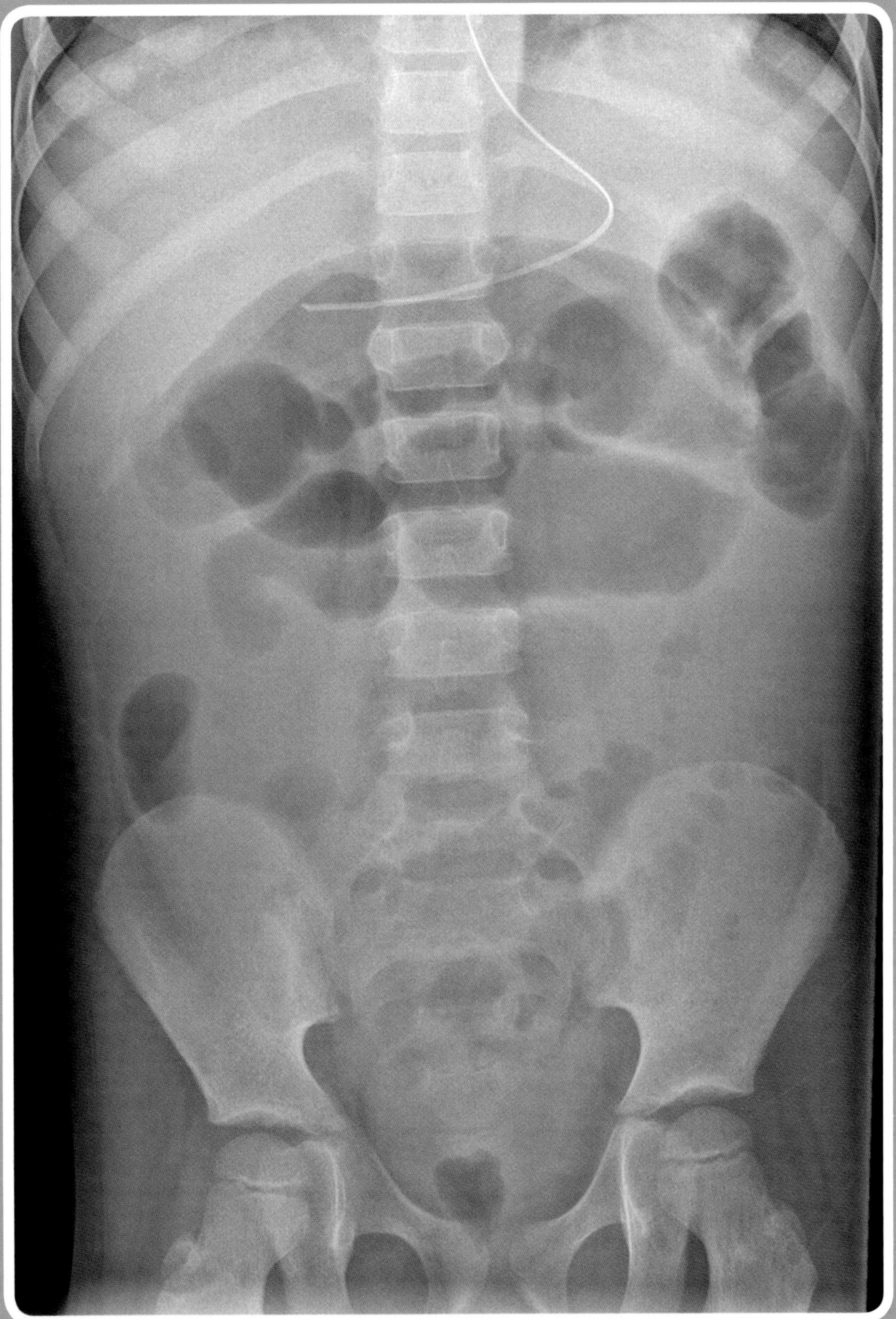

REPORT
Patient ID: Anonymous.
Projection: AP supine.
Rotation: Adequate.
Penetration: Adequate – the spinous processes are visible.
Coverage: Adequate – the anterior ribs are visible superiorly and the pubic rami are visible inferiorly.

BOWEL GAS PATTERN
There are multiple loops of dilated bowel seen centrally in the abdomen, suggestive of bowel obstruction.

BOWEL WALL
There is no evidence of mural thickening or intramural gas within the large or small bowel.

PNEUMOPERITONEUM
There is no evidence of free intra-abdominal gas.

SOLID ORGANS
The solid organ contours are within normal limits with no solid organ calcification.

VASCULAR
No abnormal vascular calcification.

BONES
There are no abnormalities of the imaged thoracic and lumbar spine, or within the pelvis.

There are growth plates at the femoral head and acetabulum as the ossification centres have not yet fused, which is a normal finding in a child of this age.

SOFT TISSUES
The psoas muscle outline is visible bilaterally.

The extra-abdominal soft tissues are unremarkable.

OTHER
There is an NG tube in situ, with its tip projected over the right upper quadrant of the abdomen, within the antrum of the stomach.

There are no vascular lines, drains or surgical clips.

REVIEW AREAS
Gallstones / Renal calculi: No radiopaque calculi.
Lung bases: There is a radiopacity projecting within the right lung base of indeterminate significance.
Spine: Normal.
Femoral heads: Normal – growth plates present.

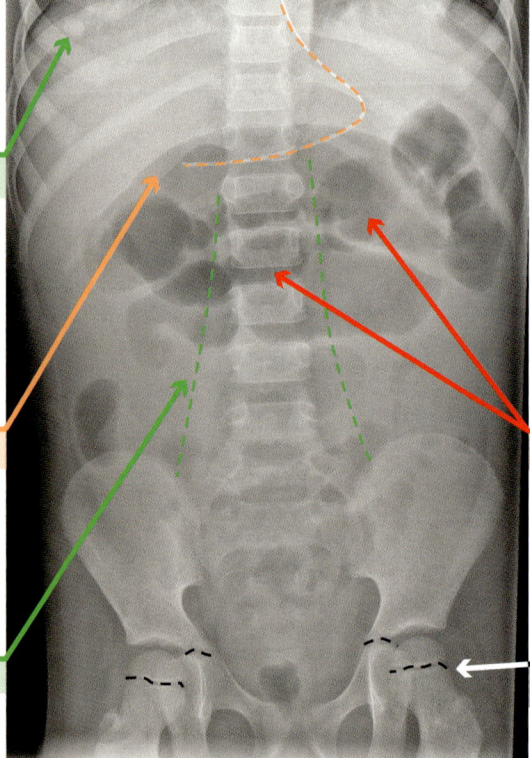

Right basal opacity

NG tube

Psoas muscle outlines

Bowel dilatation

Growth plates

SUMMARY
This X-ray demonstrates multiple loops of dilated bowel seen centrally within the abdomen, in keeping with likely small bowel obstruction, although no cause is visible on X-ray. There is an NG tube in situ which could be pulled back slightly. The right lung base radiopacity is of indeterminate significance and is an incidental finding,

INVESTIGATIONS AND MANAGEMENT
The patient should be resuscitated using an ABCDE approach.

Adequate analgesia and hydration should be provided.

The patient should be kept NBM, have their NG tube put on free drainage, and started on IV fluids.

Urgent bloods should be taken, including FBC, U&Es, CRP, LFTs, coagulation, blood gas, and group and save. Assuming this is a new finding, a chest X-ray should be performed to further assess the radiopacity projecting over the right lung base.

The paediatric surgical team should be contacted urgently and further radiological imaging of the abdomen and pelvis should be considered for better visualisation of the anatomy and further assessment.

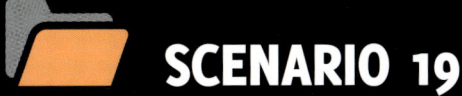

SCENARIO 19

A 21 year old female presents to ED with a 2 day history of generalised, worsening abdominal pain. She has not opened her bowels in that time and feels nauseated but has not vomited. Her past medical history is significant for cystic fibrosis, which is well controlled and she is not on laxatives. She is a non-smoker. On examination, she has saturations of 97% in room air and a temperature of 37.2°C. Her HR is 75 bpm, RR is 12 and blood pressure is 115/65 mmHg. The chest is resonant throughout and breath sounds are clear. The abdomen is mildly distended with generalised abdominal tenderness and voluntary guarding. Bowel sounds are normal. Urine dipstick is unremarkable and a pregnancy test is negative.

An abdominal X-ray is requested to assess for possible bowel obstruction.

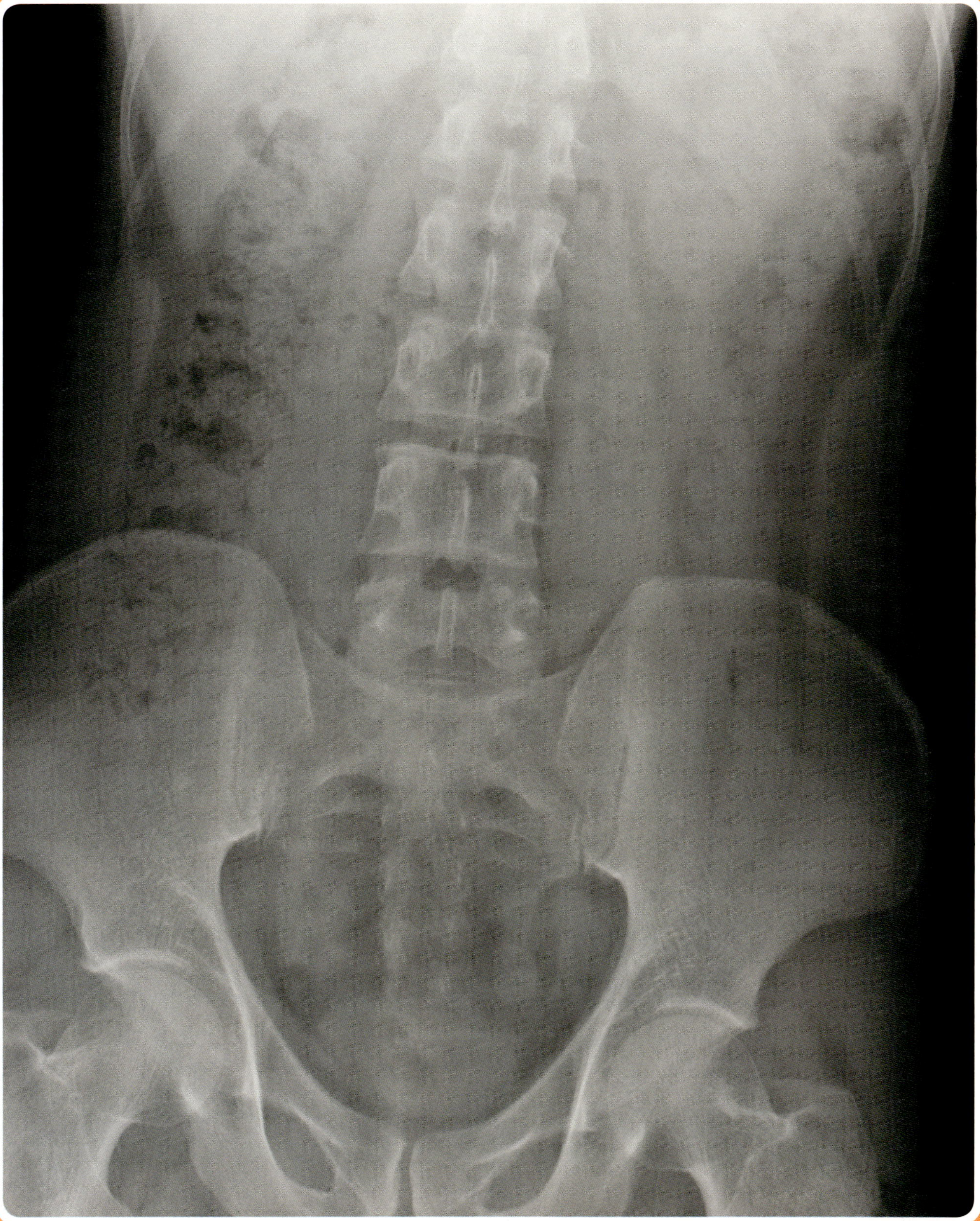

REPORT

Patient ID: Anonymous.
Projection: AP supine.
Rotation: Adequate.
Penetration: Adequate – the spinous processes are visible.
Coverage: Adequate – the anterior ribs are visible superiorly and the inferior pubic rami are visible.

BOWEL GAS PATTERN

There is a paucity of bowel gas but no bowel dilatation is visible.

There is a moderate amount of faecal residue present predominantly in the ascending colon and also throughout the visualised transverse and descending colon. The rectum is relatively empty.

BOWEL WALL

There is no evidence of mural thickening or intramural gas within the large or small bowel.

PNEUMOPERITONEUM

There is no evidence of free intra-abdominal gas.

SOLID ORGANS

The solid organ contours are within normal limits with no solid organ calcification.

VASCULAR

No abnormal vascular calcification.

BONES

There are no abnormalities of the imaged thoracic and lumbar spine, or within the pelvis.

SOFT TISSUES

The psoas muscle outline is visible bilaterally.

The extra-abdominal soft tissues are unremarkable.

OTHER

There are no radiopaque foreign bodies.

There are no vascular lines, drains or surgical clips.

REVIEW AREAS

Gallstones / Renal calculi: No radiopaque calculi.
Lung bases: Normal.
Spine: Normal.
Femoral heads: Normal.

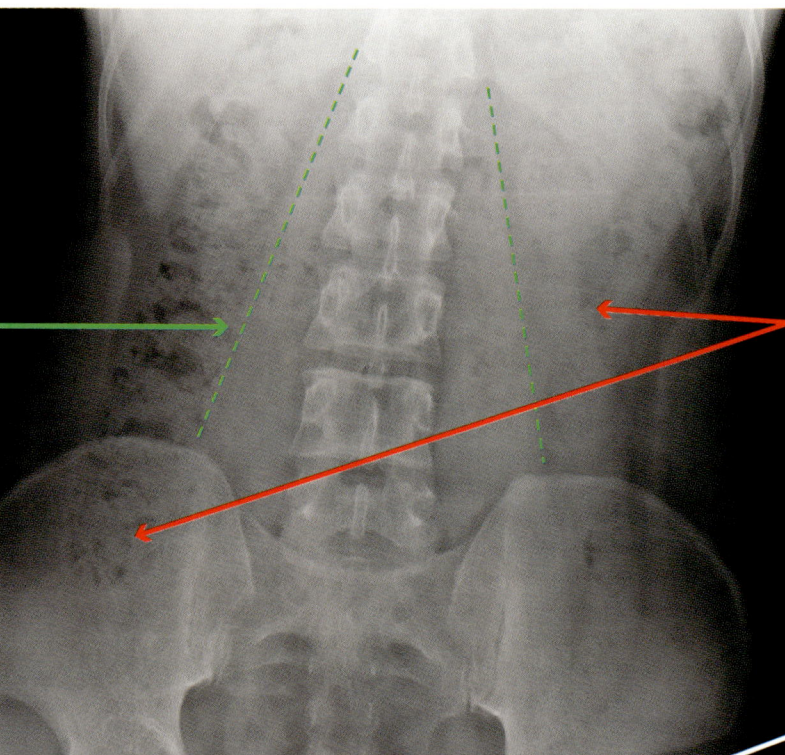

Psoas muscle outlines

Faecal residue from caecum to descending colon

Femoral heads normal

SUMMARY

This X-ray demonstrates a moderate volume of faecal residue predominantly in the ascending colon, and also in the visualised transverse and descending colon. There is no evidence of bowel obstruction or pneumoperitoneum.

INVESTIGATIONS AND MANAGEMENT

If the patient is clinically constipated, current medications should be reviewed and laxatives considered. Advice should be given regarding lifestyle adjustments, including adequate fluid intake, sufficient dietary fibre and exercise if clinically appropriate.

If the patient is otherwise well, no further investigation or imaging is required.

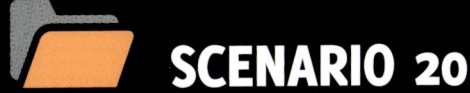
A 30 year old female presents to ED with right-sided pain radiating from her loin to her groin. She has no significant past medical history and is a non-smoker. On examination, she has saturations of 99% in room air and a temperature of 37.1°C. Her HR is 90 bpm, RR is 18 and blood pressure is 120/80 mmHg. The abdomen is soft and there is tenderness in the right flank with normal bowel sounds. Urine dipstick shows blood +++ and a pregnancy test is negative.

An abdominal X-ray is requested to assess for possible renal calculi.

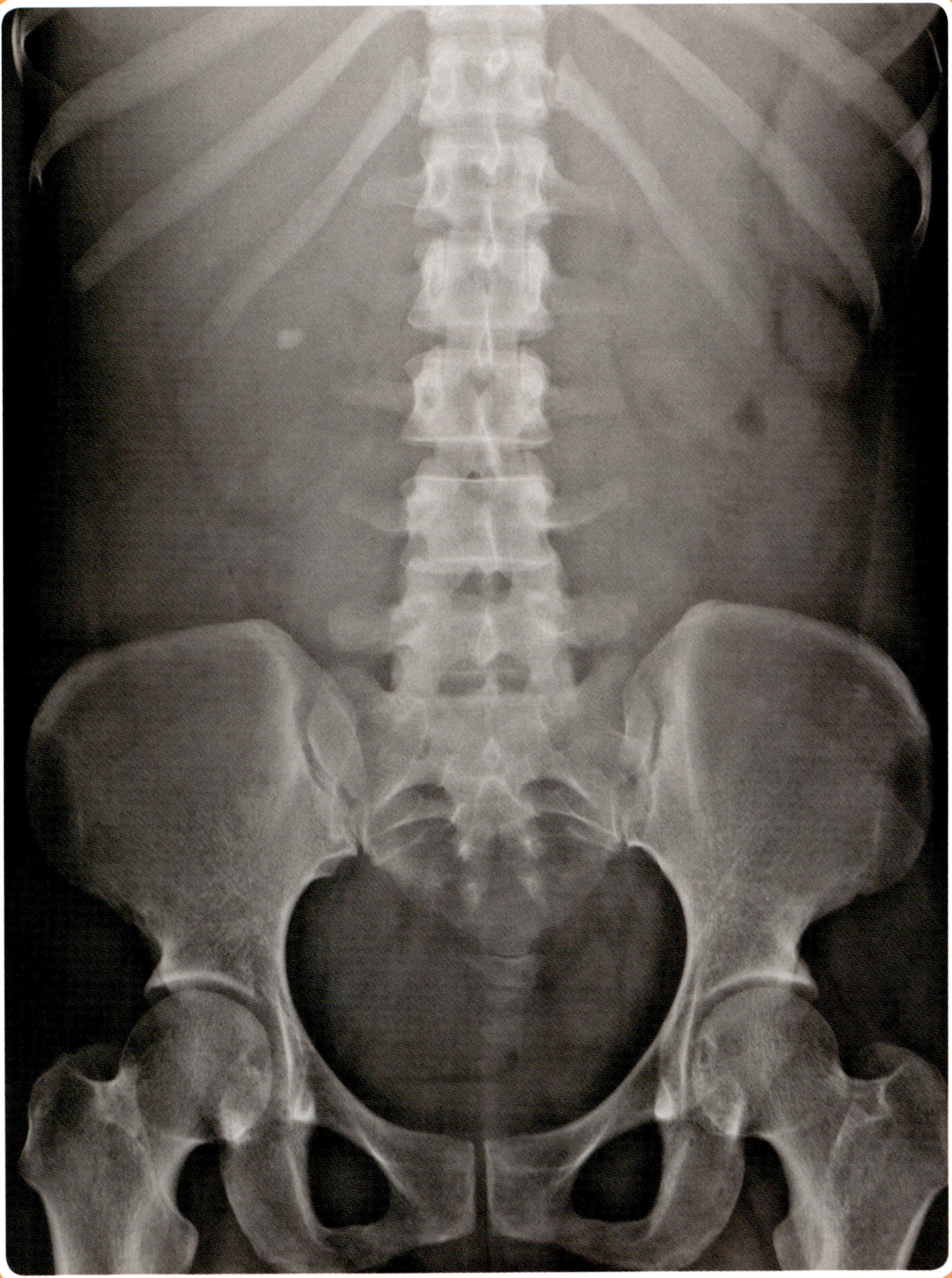

REPORT
Patient ID: Anonymous.
Projection: AP supine.
Rotation: Adequate.
Penetration: Adequate – the spinous processes are visible.
Coverage: Adequate – the anterior ribs are visible superiorly and the inferior pubic rami are visible.

BOWEL GAS PATTERN
There is a paucity of bowel gas, which is non-specific.

BOWEL WALL
There is no evidence of mural thickening or intramural gas within the large or small bowel.

PNEUMOPERITONEUM
There is no evidence of free intra-abdominal gas.

SOLID ORGANS
There is a well-defined radiopaque density projected over the upper pole of the right kidney, in keeping with a renal calculus.

VASCULAR
No abnormal vascular calcification.

BONES
There are no abnormalities of the imaged thoracic and lumbar spine, or within the pelvis.

SOFT TISSUES
The psoas muscle outline is visible bilaterally.

The extra-abdominal soft tissues are unremarkable.

OTHER
There are no radiopaque foreign bodies.

There are no vascular lines, drains or surgical clips.

REVIEW AREAS
Gallstones / Renal calculi: Likely renal calculus in the upper pole of the right kidney.
Lung bases: Not fully included.
Spine: Normal.
Femoral heads: Normal.

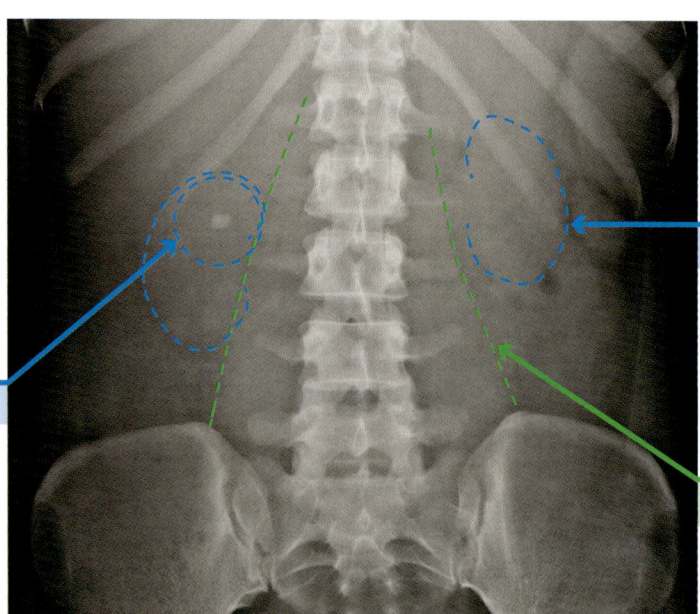

Renal calculus

Renal contours

Psoas muscle outlines

Femoral heads normal

SUMMARY
This X-ray demonstrates a well-defined radiopaque density projecting over the upper pole of the right kidney. Given the clinical history, the most likely diagnosis is a renal calculus. Other differentials include calcification of an artery, lymph node or a radiopaque gallstone within a distended gallbladder. There is a paucity of bowel gas, which is non-specific.

INVESTIGATIONS AND MANAGEMENT
The patient should be resuscitated using an ABCDE approach.

Adequate analgesia and hydration should be provided.

Urgent bloods should be taken, including FBC, U&Es, CRP, LFTs, blood gas, and bone profile.

The patient should be assessed for acute kidney injury, and if present, an ultrasound of the urinary tract in the first instance would be beneficial in assessing for hydronephrosis.

Smaller stones may pass spontaneously, but the patient should be referred to urology for possible further intervention and follow up. A CT scan of the kidneys, ureters and bladder may be useful for better visualisation of the anatomy.

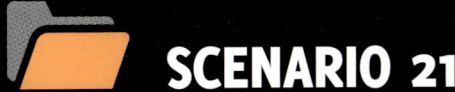
A 35 year old female presents to ED with colicky abdominal pain. Her past medical history is significant for Crohn's disease and she is a non-smoker. On examination, she has saturations of 99% in room air and a temperature of 36.6°C. Her HR is 85 bpm, RR is 18 and blood pressure is 118/66 mmHg. The abdomen is soft and there is generalised mild tenderness with normal bowel sounds. An ileostomy is present which appears healthy on examination with normal bag contents. Urine dipstick is unremarkable and a pregnancy test is negative.

An abdominal X-ray is requested to assess for possible bowel obstruction.

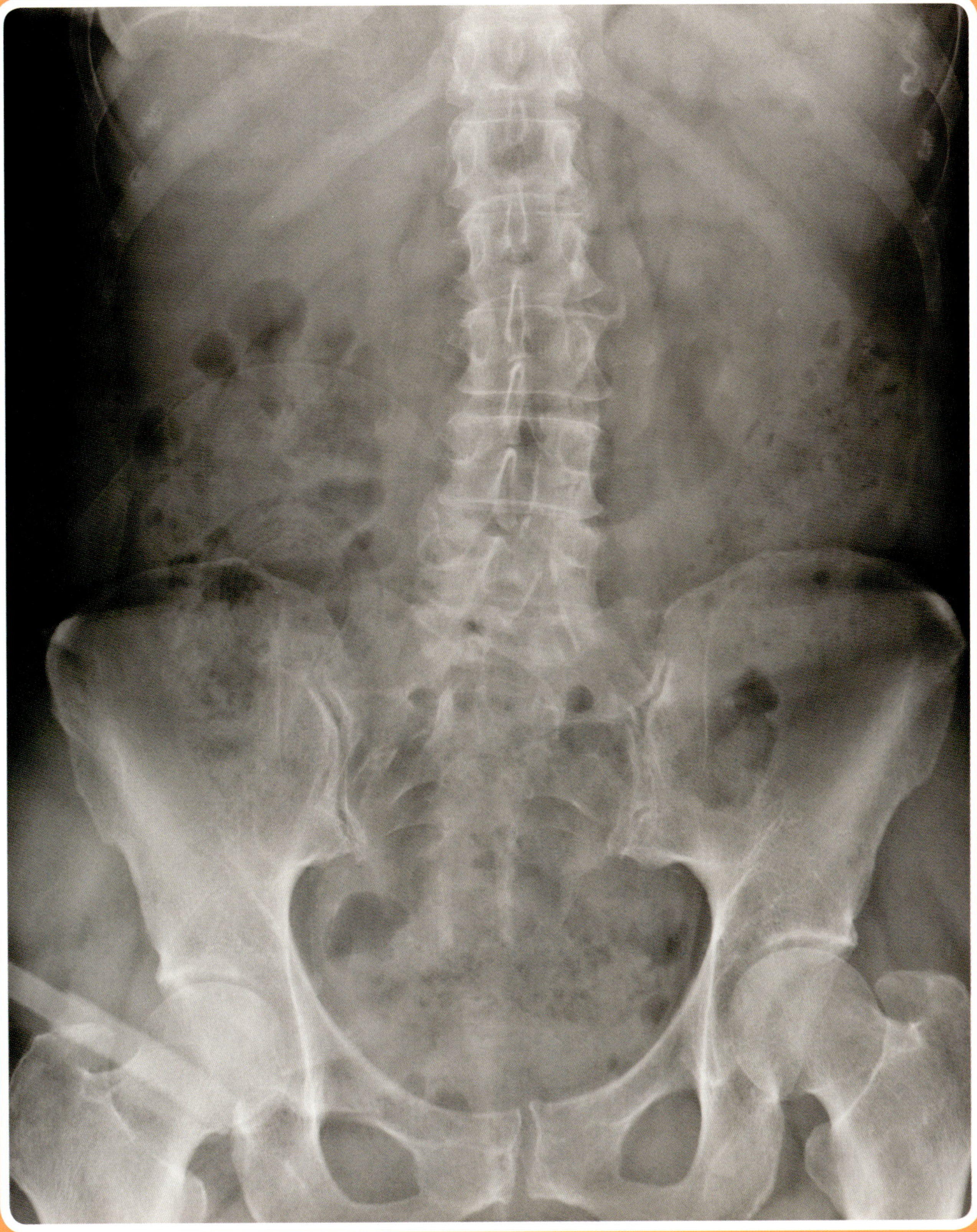

REPORT
Patient ID: Anonymous.
Projection: AP supine.
Rotation: Adequate.
Penetration: Adequate – the spinous processes are visible.
Coverage: Adequate – the anterior ribs are visible superiorly and the inferior pubic rami are visible.

BOWEL GAS PATTERN
The bowel gas pattern is normal.

There is a mild to moderate volume of faecal residue present throughout the large bowel.

BOWEL WALL
There is no evidence of mural thickening or intramural gas within the large or small bowel.

PNEUMOPERITONEUM
There is no evidence of free intra-abdominal gas.

SOLID ORGANS
The solid organ contours are within normal limits with no solid organ calcification.

VASCULAR
No abnormal vascular calcification.

BONES
There is mild lumbar scoliosis seen convex to the left, centred at the L2/L3 level.

No fractures or destructive bone lesions are visible in the imaged skeleton.

SOFT TISSUES
The psoas muscle outline is visible bilaterally.

The extra-abdominal soft tissues are unremarkable.

OTHER
There is a rounded radiopaque density projected over the right iliac fossa, in keeping with an ileostomy. Superior to this, there is a curvilinear radiopaque density in keeping with an ileostomy bag external to the patient.

There is a radiopaque density in the lower right region of the X-ray, representing an external artefact.

REVIEW AREAS
Gallstones / Renal calculi: No radiopaque calculi.
Lung bases: Not fully included.
Spine: Lumbar scoliosis seen convex to the left, centred at the L2/3 level.
Femoral heads: Normal.

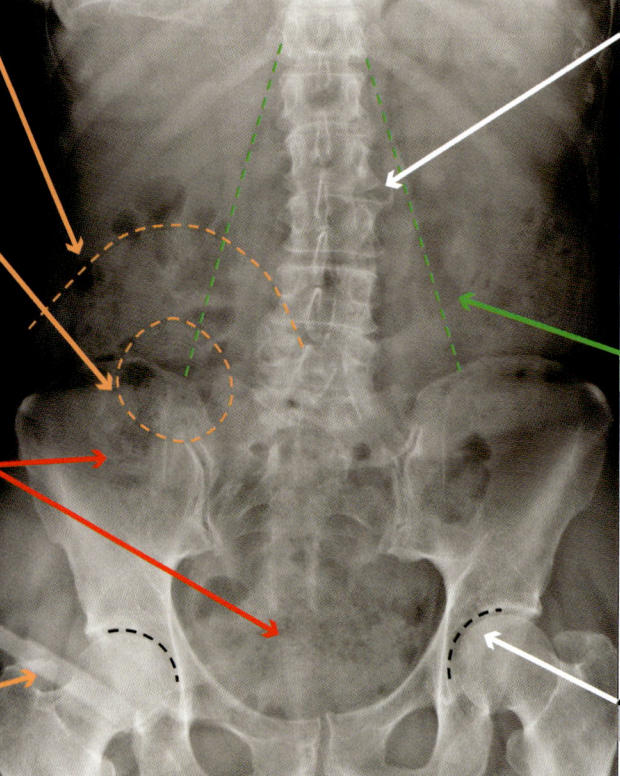

Ileostomy bag

Ileostomy

Faecal residue throughout colon

External artefact

Scoliosis

Psoas muscle outlines

Femoral heads normal

SUMMARY
This X-ray demonstrates an ileostomy. It also demonstrates a mild to moderate volume of faecal residue throughout the large bowel. There is no evidence of bowel obstruction. The scoliosis seen at the L3 vertebral body is an incidental finding.

INVESTIGATIONS AND MANAGEMENT
Adequate analgesia and hydration should be provided.

Urgent bloods should be taken, including FBC, U&Es, CRP, LFTs, amylase, blood gas, and bone profile.

This may represent a flare up of her Crohn's disease, warranting further investigation. A CT scan of the abdomen/pelvis with IV contrast may be considered for further evaluation of the abdomen and surgical/gastroenterology input should be considered.

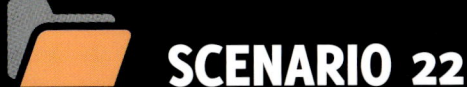

A 55 year old male presents to ED with a 4 day history of left iliac fossa pain that is worse on straining. He has no significant past medical history and is a non-smoker. On examination, he has saturations of 99% in room air and a temperature of 37.1°C. His HR is 80 bpm, RR is 15 and blood pressure is 120/65 mmHg. The abdomen is soft and there is tenderness in the left iliac fossa with normal bowel sounds. Urine dipstick is unremarkable.

An abdominal X-ray is requested to look for possible bowel obstruction.

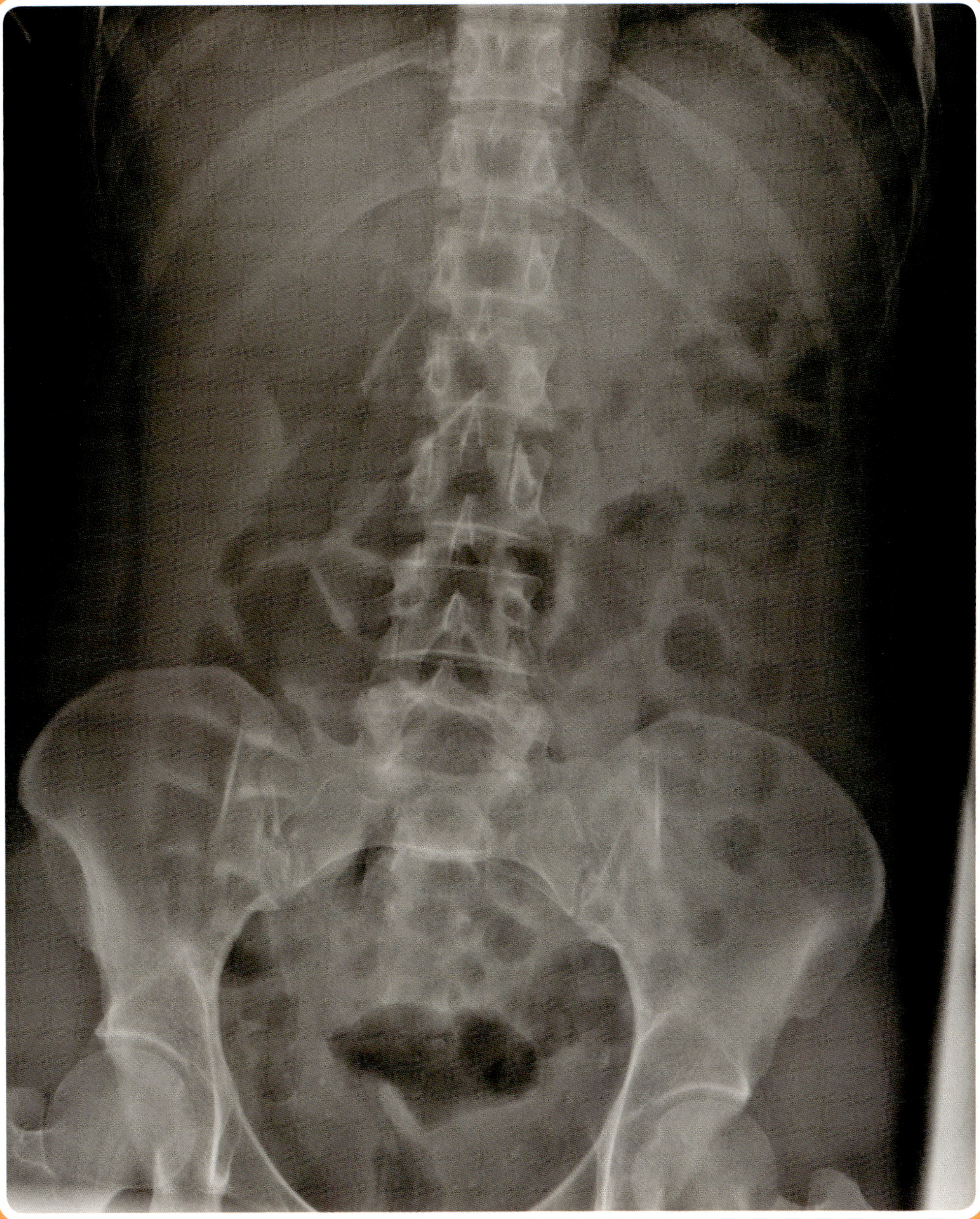

REPORT
Patient ID: Anonymous.
Projection: AP supine.
Rotation: Adequate
Penetration: Adequate – the spinous processes are visible.
Coverage: Inadequate – the inferior pubic rami have not been included.

BOWEL GAS PATTERN
The bowel gas pattern is normal.

BOWEL WALL
There is no evidence of mural thickening or intramural gas within the large or small bowel.

PNEUMOPERITONEUM
There is no evidence of free intra-abdominal gas.

SOLID ORGANS
The solid organ contours are within normal limits with no solid organ calcification.

VASCULAR
No abnormal vascular calcification.

BONES
There are no abnormalities of the imaged thoracic and lumbar spine, or within the pelvis.

SOFT TISSUES
The psoas muscle outline is preserved.

The extra-abdominal soft tissues are unremarkable.

OTHER
There are no radiopaque foreign bodies.

There are no vascular lines, drains or surgical clips.

REVIEW AREAS
Gallstones / Renal calculi: No radiopaque calculi.
Lung bases: Not fully included.
Spine: Normal.
Femoral heads: Normal.

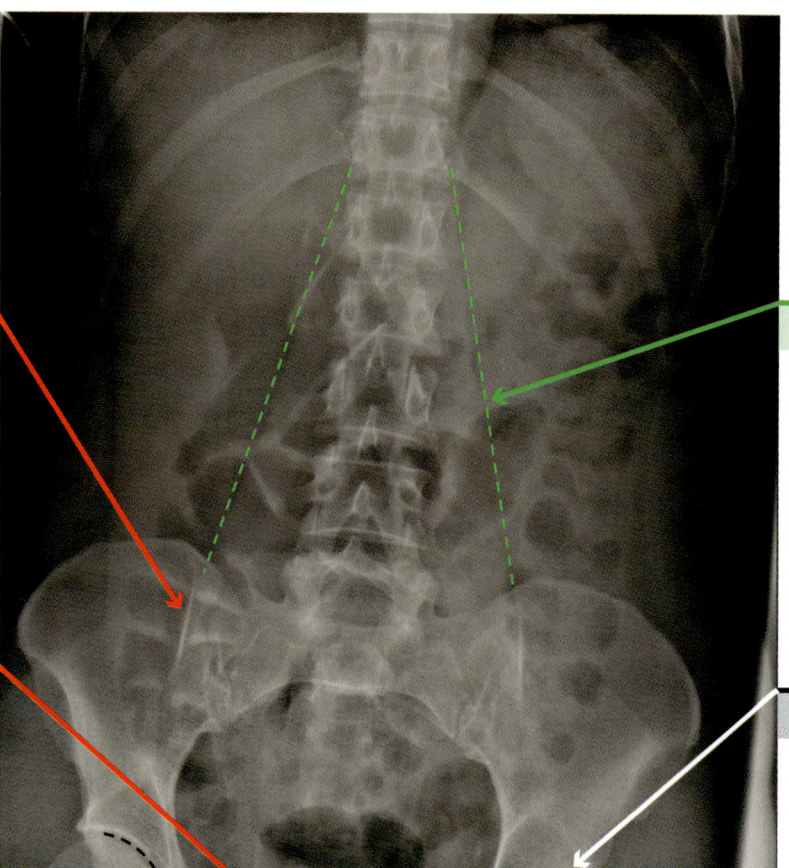

Normal bowel gas pattern

Gas in rectum

Psoas muscle outlines

Femoral heads normal

SUMMARY
This X-ray demonstrates a normal appearance with no evidence of bowel obstruction.

INVESTIGATIONS AND MANAGEMENT
Adequate analgesia and hydration should be provided.

Bloods should be taken, including FBC, U&Es, LFTs, amylase, bone profile, blood gas, and CRP.

There are no clear findings on the abdominal X-ray to explain the patient's clinical presentation. Surgical input should be sought, and a CT abdomen/pelvis with IV contrast or a sigmoidoscopy considered.

SCENARIO 23

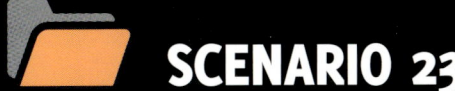

A 20 year old male presents to his doctor with a 3 week history of generalised abdominal pain. He has no significant past medical history and is a non-smoker. On examination, he has saturations of 98% in room air and a temperature of 36.6°C. His HR is 65 bpm, RR is 14 and blood pressure is 120/72 mmHg. The abdomen is rigid and there is generalised tenderness with normal bowel sounds. Urine dipstick is unremarkable.

An abdominal X-ray is requested to assess for possible bowel obstruction.

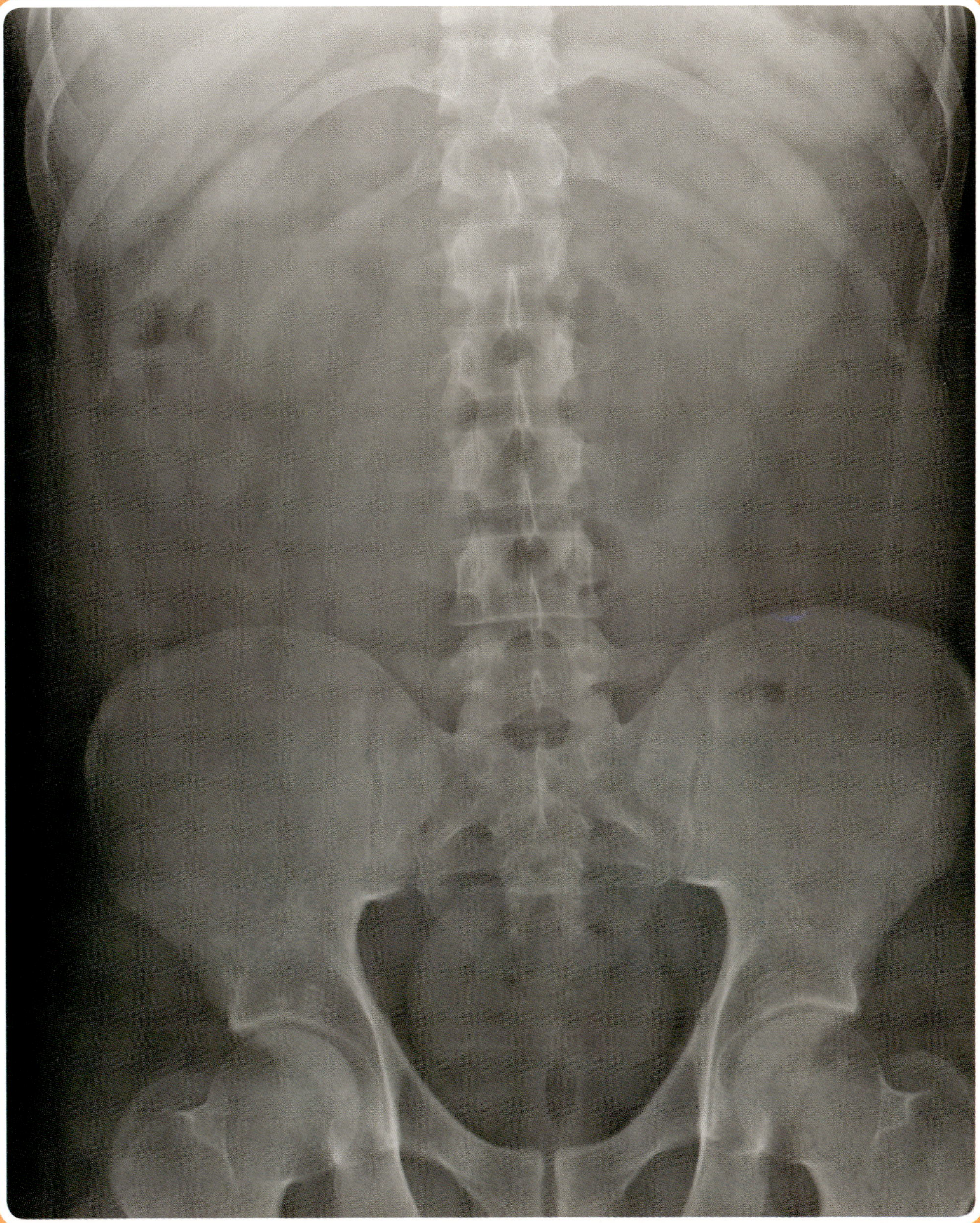

REPORT
Patient ID: Anonymous.
Projection: AP supine.
Rotation: Adequate.
Penetration: Adequate – the spinous processes are visible.
Coverage: Inadequate – the pubic symphysis and inferior pubic rami have not been included.

BOWEL GAS PATTERN
The bowel gas pattern is normal.

BOWEL WALL
There is no evidence of mural thickening or intramural gas within the large or small bowel.

PNEUMOPERITONEUM
There is no evidence of free intra-abdominal gas.

SOLID ORGANS
The solid organ contours are within normal limits with no solid organ calcification.

VASCULAR
No abnormal vascular calcification.

BONES
There are no abnormalities of the imaged thoracic and lumbar spine, or within the pelvis.

SOFT TISSUES
The psoas muscle outline is visible bilaterally.

The extra-abdominal soft tissues are unremarkable.

OTHER
There are no radiopaque foreign bodies.

There are no vascular lines, drains or surgical clips.

REVIEW AREAS
Gallstones / Renal calculi: No radiopaque calculi.
Lung bases: Normal (right lung base not well visualised).
Spine: Normal.
Femoral heads: Normal.

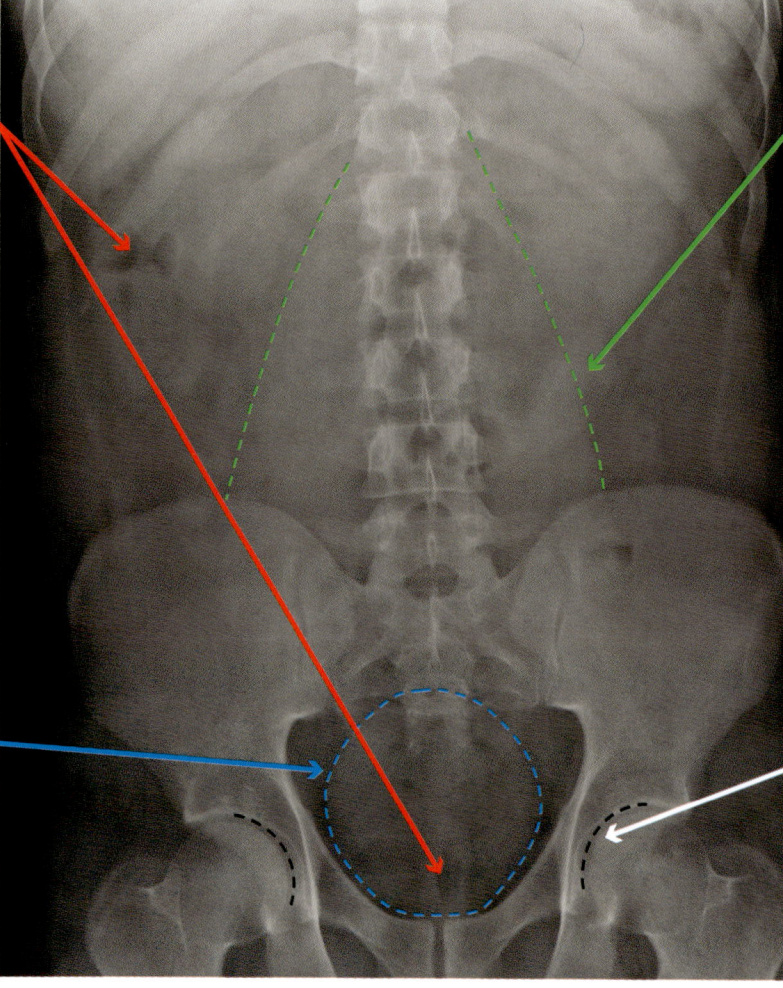

Normal bowel gas pattern

Psoas muscle outlines

Urinary bladder

Femoral heads normal

SUMMARY
This X-ray demonstrates normal appearances with no evidence of bowel obstruction.

INVESTIGATIONS AND MANAGEMENT
Adequate analgesia and hydration should be provided.

Bloods should be taken, including FBC, U&Es, LFTs, amylase, bone profile, blood gas, and CRP.

There are no clear findings on the abdominal X-ray to explain the patient's clinical presentation. A CT scan of the abdomen/pelvis with IV contrast may be considered for further evaluation of the abdomen and surgical input should be sought.

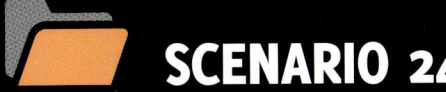

SCENARIO 24

A 17 year old female presents to her doctor with mild, intermittent left sided abdominal pain. She has also recently noticed some spotting on her underwear. She has no significant past medical history and is a non-smoker. She is currently sexually active and has an IUCD in situ. On examination, she has saturations of 99% in room air and a temperature of 36.8°C. Her HR is 70 bpm, RR is 14 and blood pressure is 115/62 mmHg. The abdomen is soft and there is mild generalised tenderness with normal bowel sounds. Urine dipstick is unremarkable and a pregnancy test is negative.

An abdominal X-ray is requested to assess for possible bowel obstruction.

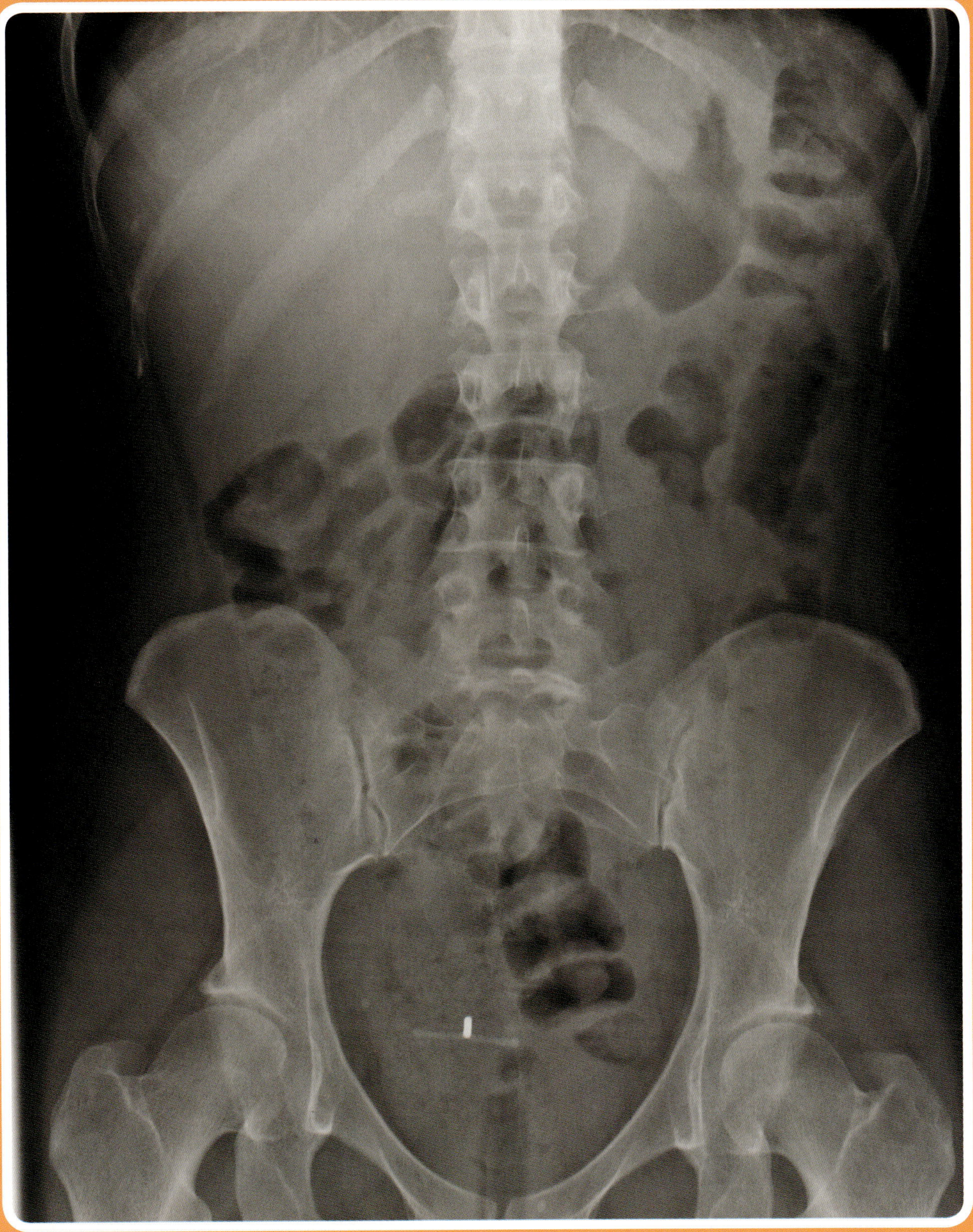

REPORT
Patient ID: Anonymous.
Projection: AP supine.
Rotation: Adequate.
Penetration: Adequate – the spinous processes are visible.
Coverage: Inadequate – the pubic symphysis and inferior pubic rami have not been included.

BOWEL GAS PATTERN
The bowel gas pattern is normal.

BOWEL WALL
There is no evidence of mural thickening or intramural gas within the large or small bowel.

PNEUMOPERITONEUM
There is no evidence of free intra-abdominal gas.

SOLID ORGANS
The solid organ contours are within normal limits with no solid organ calcification.

VASCULAR
No abnormal vascular calcification.

BONES
There are no abnormalities of the imaged thoracic and lumbar spine, or within the pelvis.

SOFT TISSUES
The psoas muscle outline is visible bilaterally.

The extra-abdominal soft tissues are unremarkable.

OTHER
There is a radiopaque density projected over the region of the pelvis, in keeping with an IUCD. There is a lucency projecting over the region of the lower pelvis in keeping with a tampon in the vagina.

There are no vascular lines, drains or surgical clips.

REVIEW AREAS
Gallstones / Renal calculi: No radiopaque calculi.
Lung bases: Normal.
Spine: Normal.
Femoral heads: Normal.

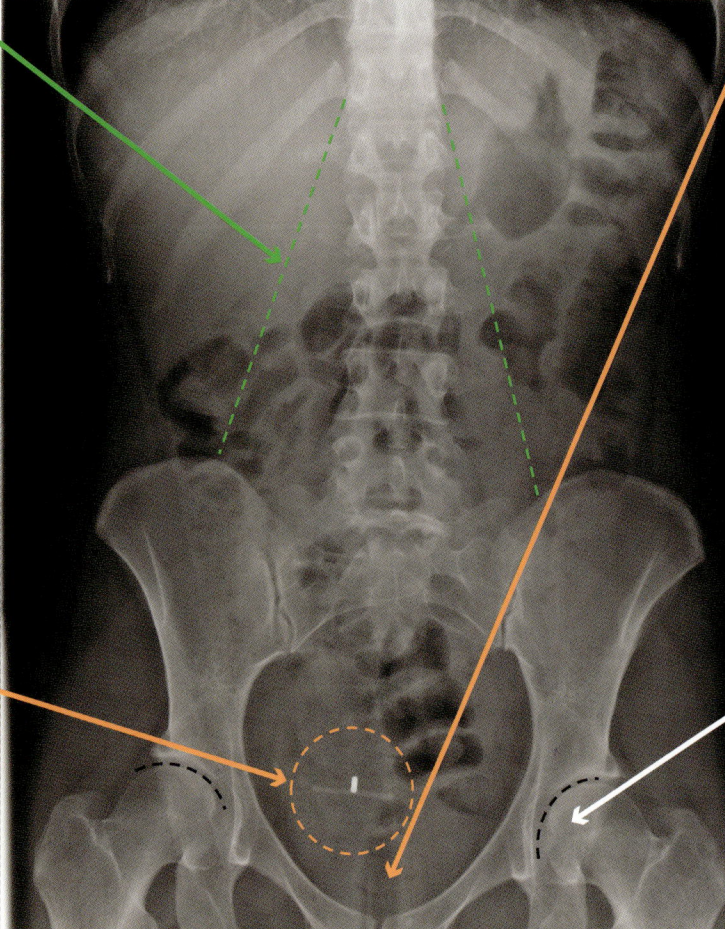

Psoas muscle outlines

Tampon

Intrauterine contraceptive device

Femoral heads normal

SUMMARY
This X-ray demonstrates a normal abdominal appearance with no evidence of bowel obstruction. The IUCD is projecting within the pelvis. Incidental note is made of a vaginal tampon.

INVESTIGATIONS AND MANAGEMENT
Adequate analgesia and hydration should be provided.

Bloods should be taken, including FBC, U&Es, LFTs, bone profile, amylase, blood gas, and CRP.

There are no clear findings on the abdominal X-ray to explain the patient's clinical presentation.

If the patient is otherwise well, and the blood tests are reassuring, the patient should continue to be monitored in the community to assess progression of symptoms.

If the IUCD in situ is a Mirena coil, spotting may be related to this.

An ultrasound scan of the pelvis including a trans-vaginal scan should be considered if the patient's symptoms fail to resolve. Triple swabs of the vagina should also be considered to further assess for possible pelvic inflammatory disease.

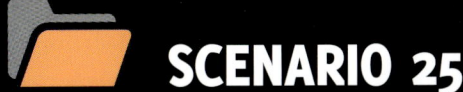

A 28 year old female presents to the renal outpatient clinic with worsening right sided abdominal pain. Her past medical history is significant for renal failure, and she undergoes peritoneal dialysis. She is a non-smoker. On examination, she has saturations of 97% in room air and a temperature of 39°C. Her HR is 109 bpm, RR is 22 and blood pressure is 120/68 mmHg. The abdomen is rigid and there is generalised tenderness with normal bowel sounds. Urine dipstick is unremarkable and a pregnancy test is negative.

An abdominal X-ray is requested to assess for possible bowel obstruction.

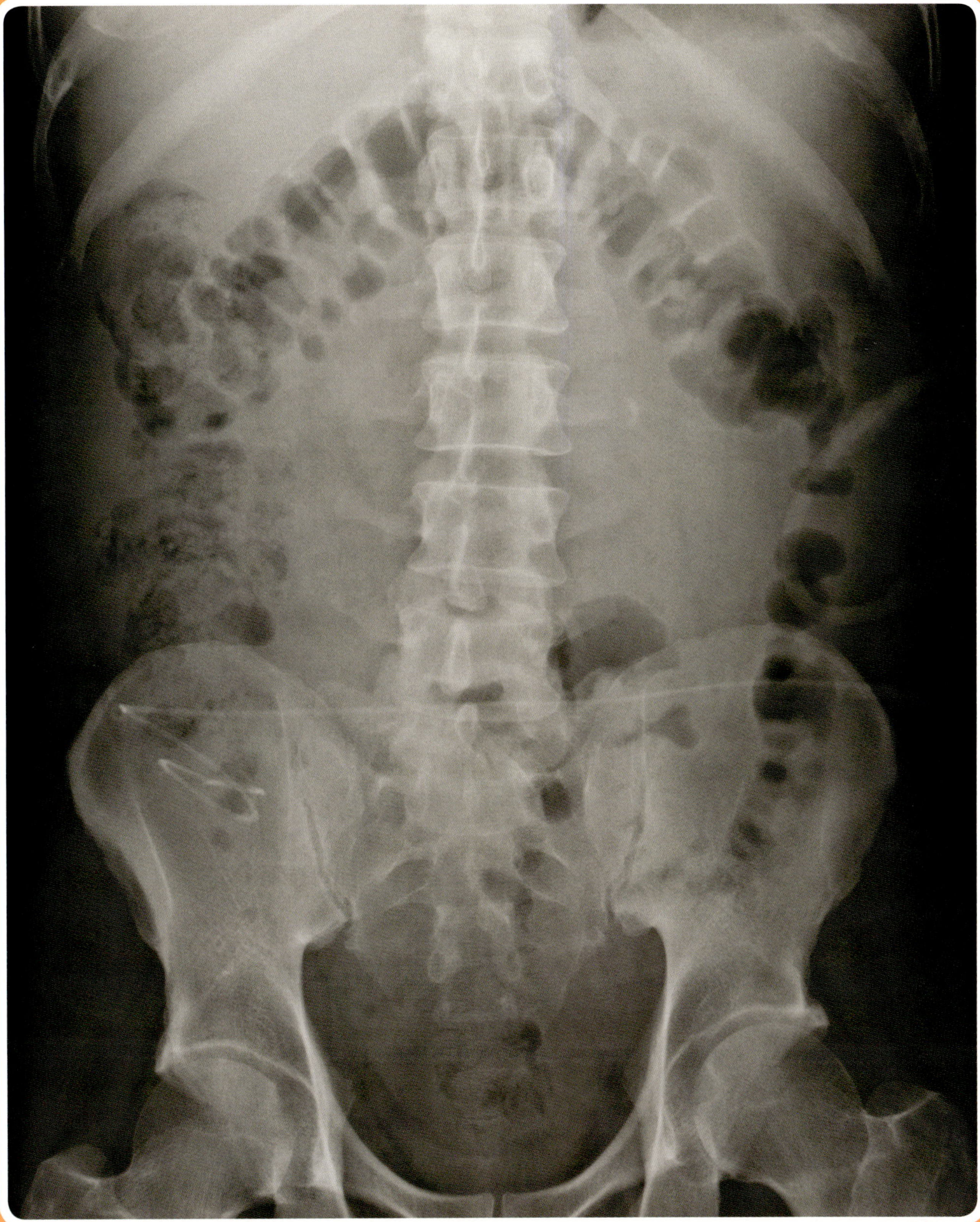

REPORT

Patient ID: Anonymous.
Projection: AP supine.
Rotation: Adequate.
Penetration: Adequate – the spinous processes are visible.
Coverage: Inadequate – the pubic symphysis and inferior pubic rami have not been included.

BOWEL GAS PATTERN

The bowel gas pattern is normal.

There is a mild volume of faecal residue present throughout the ascending colon and within the rectum.

BOWEL WALL

There is no evidence of mural thickening or intramural gas within the large or small bowel.

PNEUMOPERITONEUM

There is no evidence of free intra-abdominal gas.

SOLID ORGANS

The solid organ contours are within normal limits with no solid organ calcification.

VASCULAR

No abnormal vascular calcification.

BONES

There are no abnormalities of the imaged thoracic and lumbar spine, or within the pelvis.

SOFT TISSUES

The psoas muscle outline is visible bilaterally.

The extra-abdominal soft tissues are unremarkable.

OTHER

There is a radiopaque line projected horizontally across the abdomen from the left side with its tip projecting within the right iliac fossa, in keeping with the known peritoneal dialysis catheter. The continuity of the peritoneal dialysis catheter is interrupted due to being outside the field of view.

There are no vascular lines, drains or surgical clips.

REVIEW AREAS

Gallstones / Renal calculi: No radiopaque calculi.
Lung bases: Not fully included.
Spine: Normal.
Femoral heads: Normal.

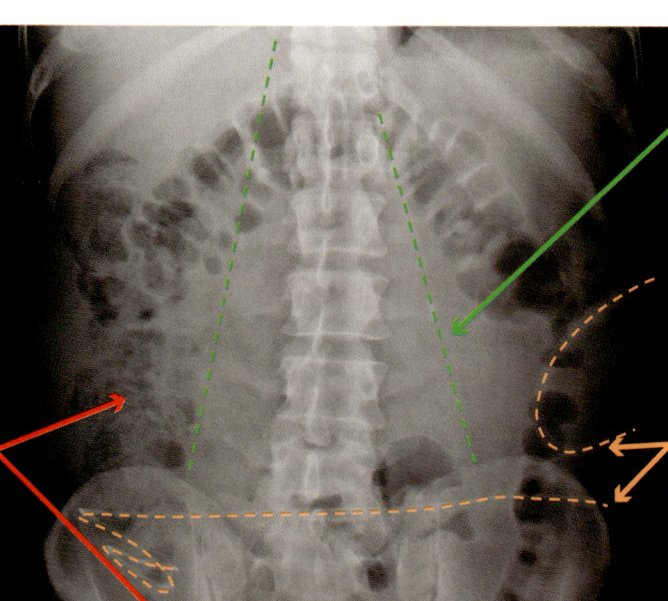

Psoas muscle outlines

Faecal residue throughout ascending colon and rectum

Peritoneal dialysis catheter

Femoral heads normal

SUMMARY

This X-ray demonstrates a peritoneal dialysis catheter with its tip projecting within the right iliac fossa. There is no evidence of pneumoperitoneum.

INVESTIGATIONS AND MANAGEMENT

The patient should be admitted to hospital and resuscitated using an ABCDE approach.

Adequate analgesia and hydration should be provided.

Urgent bloods should be taken including FBC, U&Es, LFTs, amylase, bone profile, blood culture, blood gas, and CRP. Culture of peritoneal fluid should also be sent.

The patient should be made NBM and started on IV fluids and broad-spectrum antibiotics.

There are no clear findings on the abdominal X-ray to explain the patient's clinical presentation. The general surgical team should be involved. The renal team also need to be involved to optimise management of the patient's dialysis.

SCENARIO 26

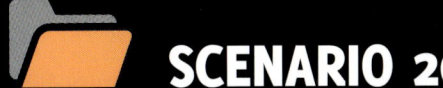

A 13 month old boy presents to ED with worsening abdominal pain and a 2 day history of diarrhoea and vomiting. He has no significant past medical history. On examination, he has saturations of 98% in room air and a temperature of 38.3°C. His HR is 150 bpm and RR is 35. The abdomen is soft and there is generalised tenderness with normal bowel sounds. Urine dipstick is unremarkable.

An abdominal X-ray is requested to assess for possible bowel obstruction.

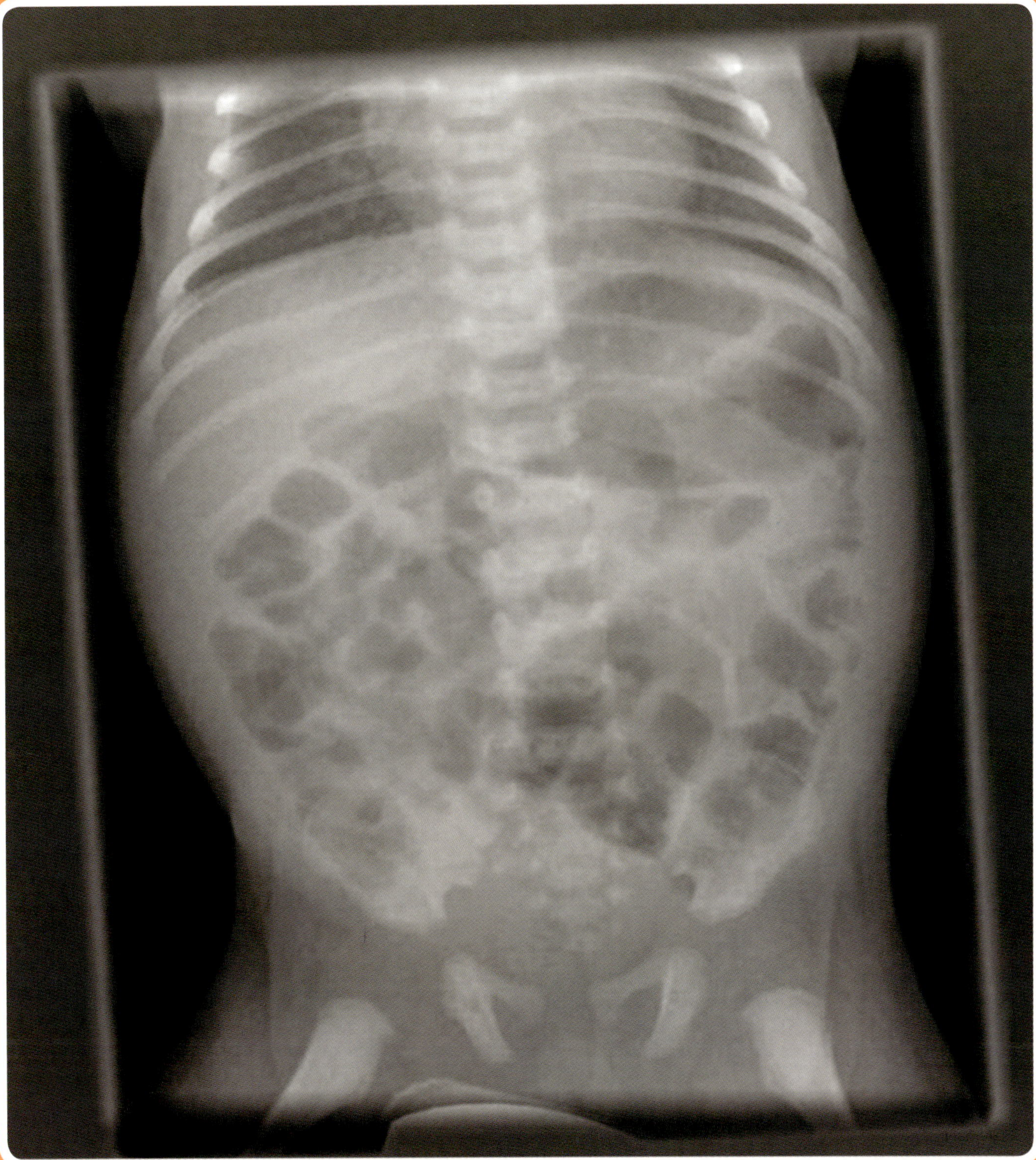

REPORT
Patient ID: Anonymous.
Projection: AP supine.
Rotation: Adequate.
Penetration: Adequate – the spine is visible.
Coverage: Adequate – the anterior ribs are visible superiorly and the inferior pubic rami are visible.

BOWEL GAS PATTERN
The bowel gas pattern is normal.

BOWEL WALL
There is no evidence of mural thickening or intramural gas within the large or small bowel.

PNEUMOPERITONEUM
There is no evidence of free intra-abdominal gas.

SOLID ORGANS
The solid organ contours are within normal limits with no solid organ calcification.

VASCULAR
No abnormal vascular calcification.

BONES
There are no abnormalities of the imaged thoracic and lumbar spine, or within the pelvis.

SOFT TISSUES
The psoas muscle outline is not visible bilaterally, which is non-specific, particularly in a child of this age.

The extra-abdominal soft tissues are unremarkable.

OTHER
There is a gonadal shield in situ.

There are no vascular lines, drains or surgical clips.

REVIEW AREAS
Gallstones / Renal calculi: No radiopaque calculi.
Lung bases: Normal.
Spine: Normal – cartilage between vertebrae.
Femoral heads: Normal – growth plates present.

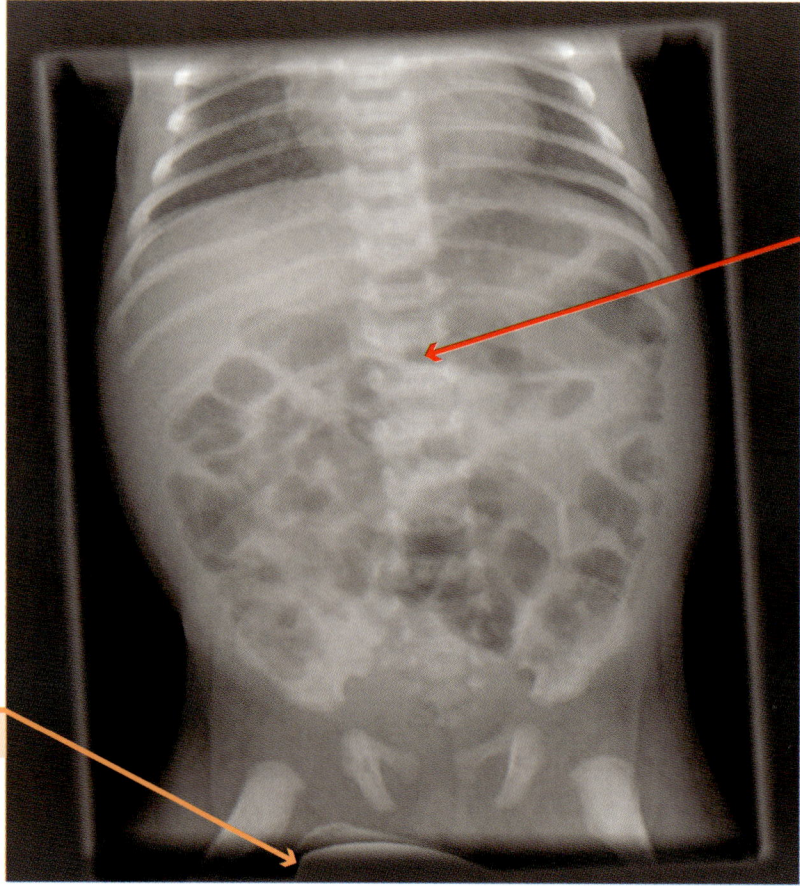

Normal bowel gas pattern

Gonadal shield

SUMMARY
This X-ray demonstrates a normal abdominal appearance with no evidence of bowel obstruction.

INVESTIGATIONS AND MANAGEMENT
The child should be resuscitated using an ABCDE approach.

Adequate analgesia and hydration should be provided.

Urgent bloods should be taken, including FBC, U&Es, CRP, and blood gas.

The most likely diagnosis is gastroenteritis, given the pyrexia, that the child is otherwise well, and the history of diarrhoea and vomiting. Treatment for this would include rehydration (either orally, by NG tube or by IV fluids depending on the clinical picture) and management of the pyrexia if symptomatic.

SCENARIO 27

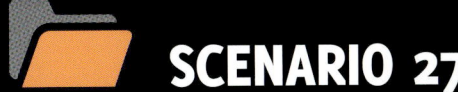

A 40 year old male presents to ED with worsening abdominal pain. He has no significant past medical history and is a non-smoker. On examination, he has saturations of 96% in room air and a temperature of 37.4°C. His HR is 88 bpm, RR is 28 and blood pressure is 128/76 mmHg. The abdomen is rigid and there is generalised tenderness with normal bowel sounds. Urine dipstick is unremarkable.

An abdominal X-ray is requested to assess for possible bowel obstruction.

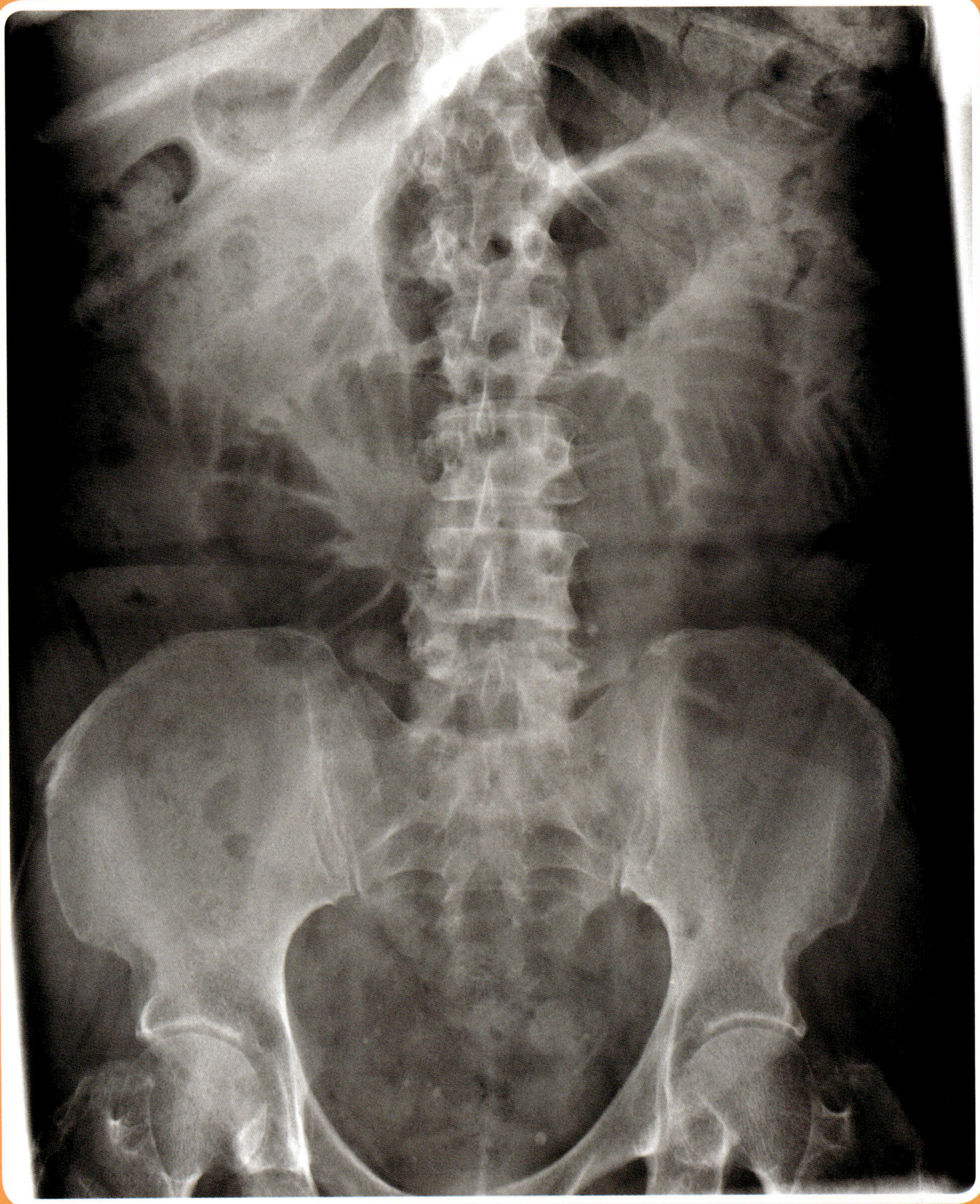

REPORT
Patient ID: Anonymous.
Projection: AP supine.
Rotation: Adequate.
Penetration: Adequate – the spinous processes are visible.
Coverage: Inadequate – the pubic symphysis and inferior pubic rami have not been included.

BOWEL GAS PATTERN
There are multiple loops of dilated bowel seen centrally and in the left upper quadrant within the abdomen demonstrating valvulae conniventes in keeping with small bowel obstruction.

BOWEL WALL
There is no evidence of mural thickening or intramural gas within the large or small bowel.

PNEUMOPERITONEUM
There is no evidence of free intra-abdominal gas.

SOLID ORGANS
The solid organ contours are within normal limits with no solid organ calcification.

VASCULAR
No abnormal vascular calcification.

BONES
There is mild degenerative change with osteophyte formation in the lower spine.

SOFT TISSUES
The psoas muscle outline is visible bilaterally.

The extra-abdominal soft tissues are unremarkable.

OTHER
There are multiple rounded radiopaque densities projected over the region of the pelvis in keeping with phleboliths.

There are no radiopaque foreign bodies.

There are no vascular lines, drains or surgical clips.

REVIEW AREAS
Gallstones / Renal calculi: No radiopaque calculi.
Lung bases: Not fully included.
Spine: Mild degenerative change.
Femoral heads: Normal.

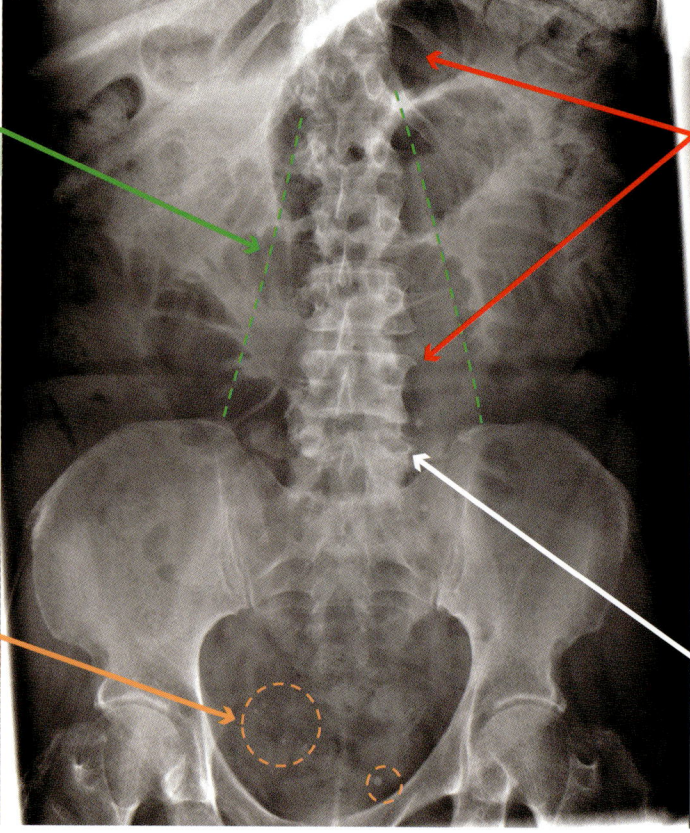

Psoas muscle outlines

Small bowel dilatation with valvulae conniventes

Phleboliths

Degenerative change in the spine

SUMMARY
This X-ray demonstrates multiple loops of dilated bowel centrally and in the left upper quadrant within the abdomen demonstrating valvulae conniventes, in keeping with small bowel obstruction, although the cause of this is not visible on the X-ray. The mild degenerative change in the spine and pelvic phleboliths are incidental findings.

INVESTIGATIONS AND MANAGEMENT
The patient should be resuscitated using an ABCDE approach.

Adequate analgesia and hydration should be provided.

The patient should be kept NBM and have an NG tube inserted on free drainage to relieve the pressure in the small bowel. IV fluids should be commenced.

Urgent bloods should be taken, including FBC, U&Es, CRP, LFTs, coagulation, blood gas, and group and save.

The general surgical team should be contacted urgently and a CT scan of the abdomen/pelvis with IV contrast should be considered for better visualisation of the anatomy and further assessment.

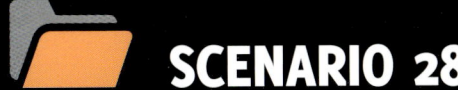
A 34 year old female presents to ED with acute generalised abdominal pain. Over the past 3 days she has been experiencing nausea with worsening vomiting which appears bile stained. Her past medical history is significant for an appendicectomy 6 months ago and she is a non-smoker. On examination, she has saturations of 99% in room air and a temperature of 36.8°C. Her HR is 94 bpm, RR is 24 and blood pressure is 120/68 mmHg. The abdomen is peritonitic with tinkling bowel sounds. Urine dipstick is unremarkable and a pregnancy test is negative.

An abdominal X-ray is requested to assess for possible bowel obstruction.

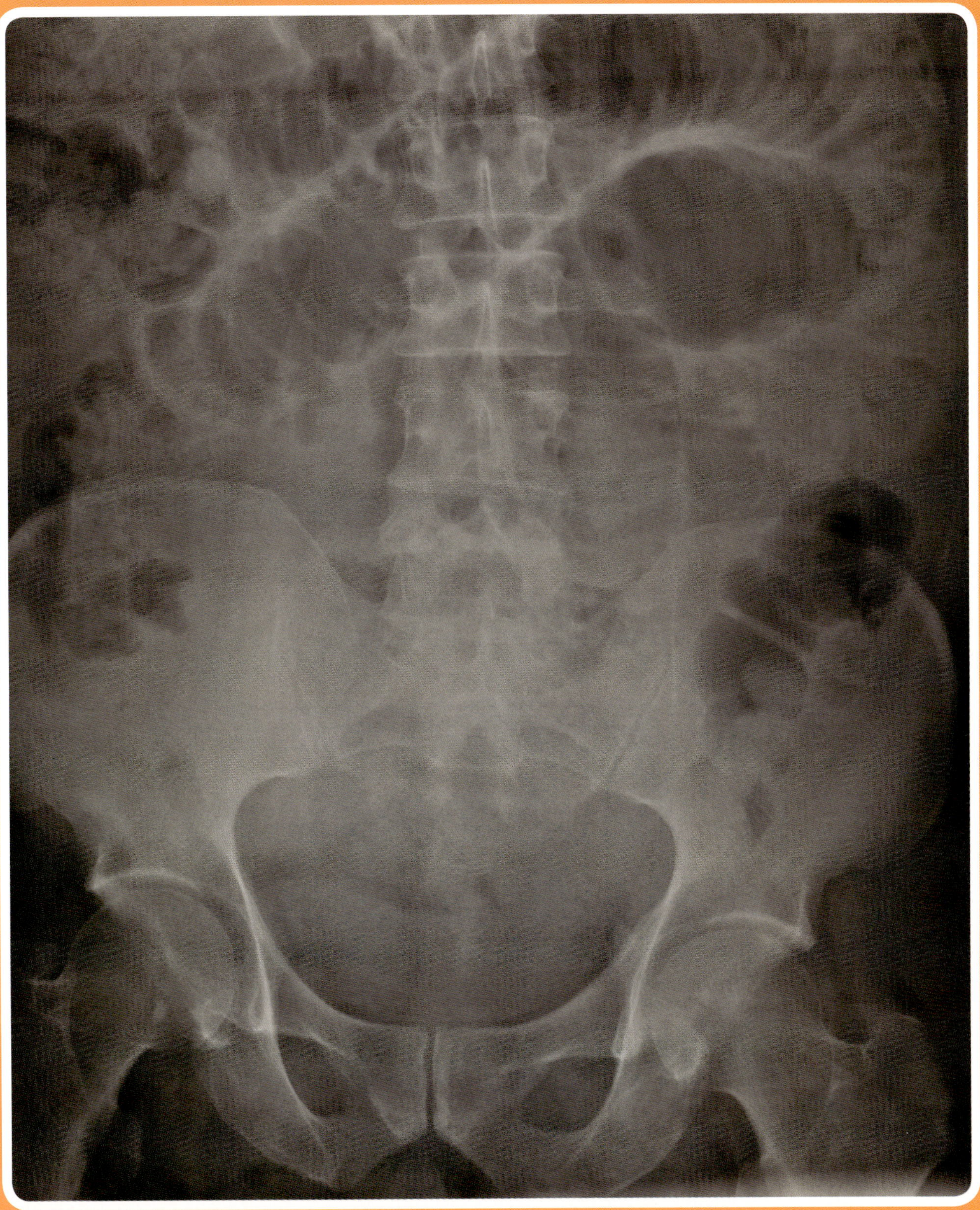

REPORT
Patient ID: Anonymous.
Projection: AP supine.
Rotation: Adequate.
Penetration: Adequate – the spinous processes are visible.
Coverage: Inadequate – the anterior ribs have not been included.

BOWEL GAS PATTERN
There are multiple loops of dilated bowel seen centrally in the abdomen demonstrating valvulae conniventes, in keeping with small bowel obstruction.

There is a small volume of faecal residue throughout the colon.

BOWEL WALL
There is no evidence of mural thickening or intramural gas within the large or small bowel.

PNEUMOPERITONEUM
There is no evidence of free intra-abdominal gas.

SOLID ORGANS
The solid organ contours are within normal limits with no solid organ calcification.

VASCULAR
No abnormal vascular calcification.

BONES
There is mild degenerative change seen in the lower lumbar spine.

There is a benign bone island in the right femoral head.

No fractures or destructive bone lesions are visible in the imaged skeleton.

SOFT TISSUES
The psoas muscle outline is visible bilaterally.

The extra-abdominal soft tissues are unremarkable.

OTHER
There are no radiopaque foreign bodies.

There are no vascular lines, drains or surgical clips.

REVIEW AREAS
Gallstones / Renal calculi: No radiopaque calculi.
Lung bases: Not fully included.
Spine: Mild degenerative change in lower lumbar spine.
Femoral heads: Normal.

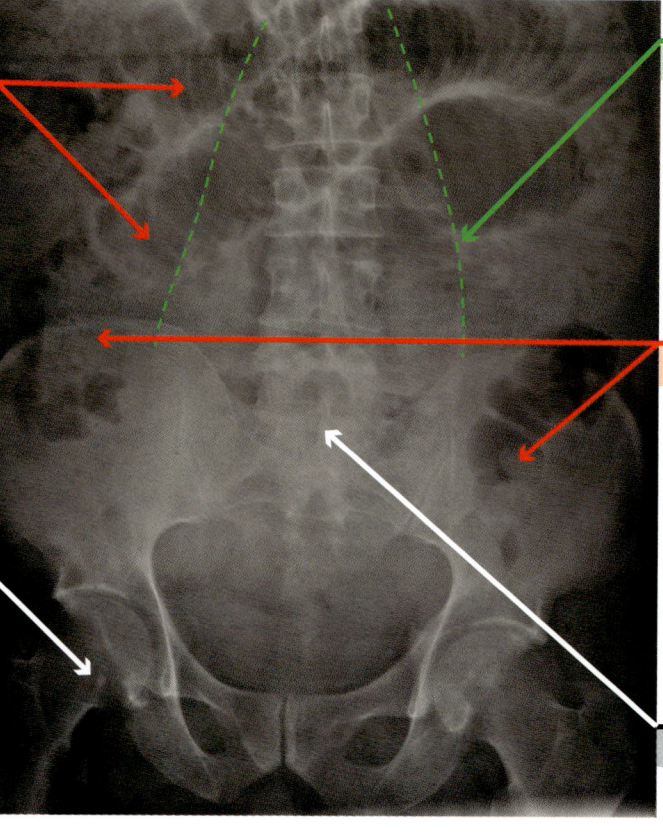

Small bowel dilatation with valvulae conniventes

Psoas muscle outlines

Faecal residue throughout colon

Bone island

Degenerative change

SUMMARY
This X-ray demonstrates multiple loops of dilated bowel seen centrally within the abdomen demonstrating valvulae conniventes, in keeping with small bowel obstruction. The cause of this is not visible on the X-ray, but it may be due to adhesions given the previous surgery. The mild degenerative change in the lower lumbar spine and right femoral head bone island are incidental findings.

INVESTIGATIONS AND MANAGEMENT
The patient should be resuscitated using an ABCDE approach.

Adequate analgesia and hydration should be provided.

The patient should be kept NBM and have an NG tube inserted on free drainage to relieve the pressure in the small bowel. IV fluids should be commenced.

Urgent bloods should be taken, including FBC, U&Es, bone profile, CRP, LFTs, coagulation, blood gas, and group and save.

The general surgical team should be contacted urgently and a CT scan of the abdomen/pelvis with IV contrast should be considered for better visualisation of the anatomy and further assessment.

Arthritic changes in the first instance should be managed with lifestyle changes and analgesia, if they are causing symptoms.

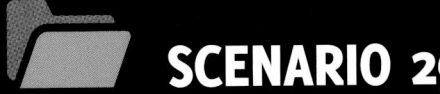

A 16 year old female presents to ED with abdominal and back pain. Her past medical history is significant for sciatica and she is a non-smoker. On examination, she has saturations of 97% in room air and a temperature of 36.6°C. Her HR is 84 bpm, RR is 20 and blood pressure is 110/62 mmHg. The abdomen is soft and there is mild generalised tenderness with normal bowel sounds. Urine dipstick is unremarkable and a pregnancy test is negative.

An abdominal X-ray is requested to assess for bowel obstruction.

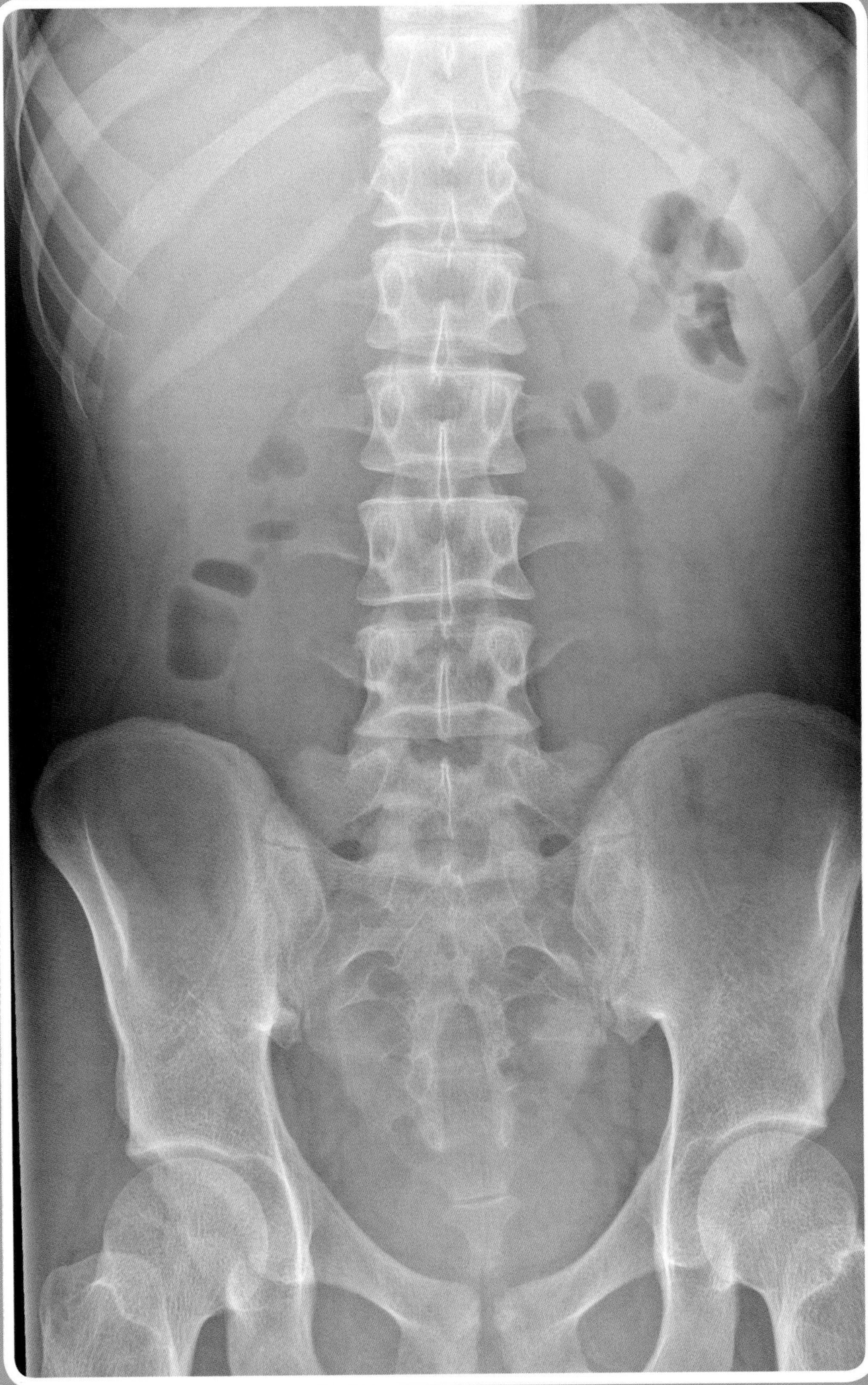

REPORT
Patient ID: Anonymous.
Projection: AP supine.
Rotation: Adequate.
Penetration: Adequate – the spinous processes are visible.
Coverage: Adequate – the anterior ribs are visible superiorly and the pubic rami are visible inferiorly.

BOWEL GAS PATTERN
The bowel gas pattern is normal.

BOWEL WALL
There is no evidence of mural thickening or intramural gas within the large or small bowel.

PNEUMOPERITONEUM
There is no evidence of free intra-abdominal gas.

SOLID ORGANS
The solid organ contours are within normal limits with no solid organ calcification.

VASCULAR
No abnormal vascular calcification.

BONES
There is sacralisation of the L5 vertebral body, which is a normal anatomical variant.

There are no abnormalities of the imaged thoracic spine.

SOFT TISSUES
The psoas muscle outline is visible bilaterally.

The extra-abdominal soft tissues are unremarkable.

OTHER
There are no radiopaque foreign bodies.

There are no vascular lines, drains or surgical clips.

REVIEW AREAS
Gallstones / Renal calculi: No radiopaque calculi.
Lung bases: Not fully included.
Spine: Sacralisation of the L5 vertebral body.
Femoral heads: Normal.

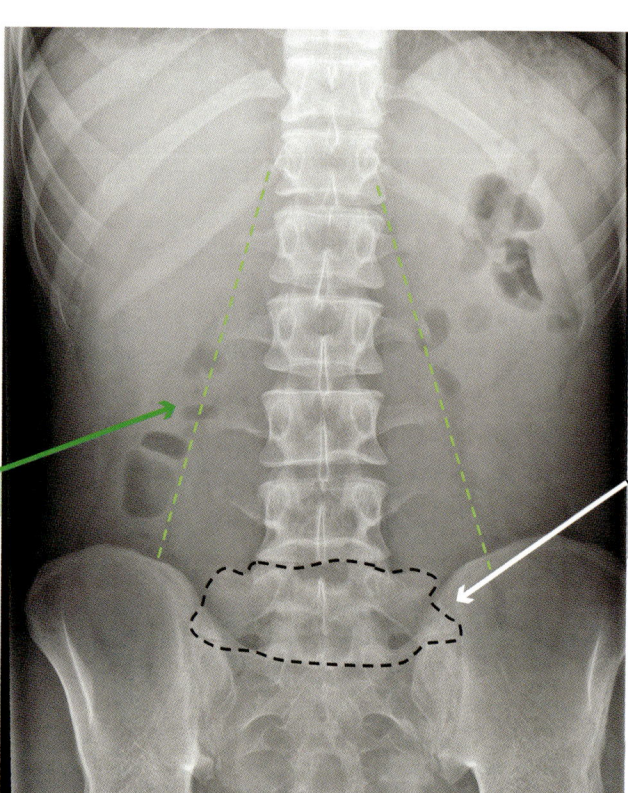

Psoas muscle outlines

Sacralisation of L5 vertebral body

Femoral heads normal

SUMMARY
This X-ray demonstrates no evidence of bowel obstruction with incidental sacralisation of the L5 vertebral body.

INVESTIGATIONS AND MANAGEMENT
Adequate analgesia and hydration should be provided.

Further investigation of back and abdominal pain is warranted if symptoms persist.

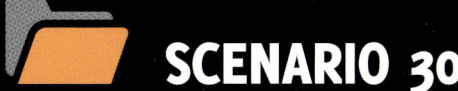

SCENARIO 30

A 30 year old male presents to ED with generalised abdominal pain and possible foreign body ingestion. His past medical history is significant for schizophrenia and he is a non-smoker. On examination, he has saturations of 97% in room air and a temperature of 37.0°C. His HR is 92 bpm, RR is 22 and blood pressure is 125/68 mmHg. The abdomen is soft and there is generalised tenderness with normal bowel sounds. Urine dipstick is unremarkable.

An abdominal X-ray is requested to assess for a possible foreign body.

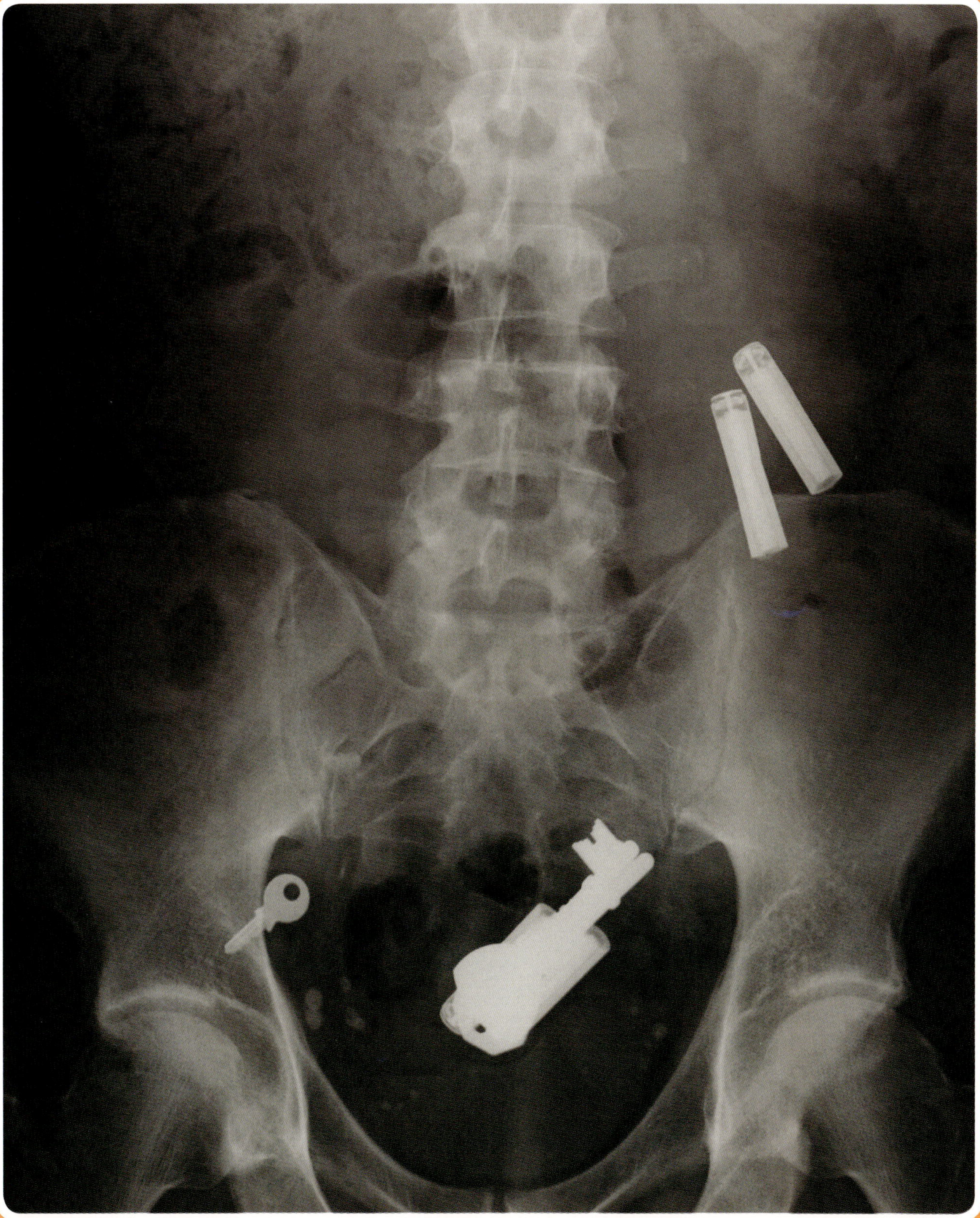

REPORT
Patient ID: Anonymous.
Projection: AP supine.
Rotation: Adequate.
Penetration: Adequate – the spinous processes are visible.
Coverage: Inadequate – the pubic symphysis and inferior pubic rami have not been fully included.

BOWEL GAS PATTERN
The bowel gas pattern is normal.

There is a moderate volume of faecal residue present throughout the ascending colon and hepatic flexure.

BOWEL WALL
There is no evidence of mural thickening or intramural gas within the large or small bowel.

PNEUMOPERITONEUM
There is no evidence of free intra-abdominal gas.

SOLID ORGANS
The solid organ contours are within normal limits with no solid organ calcification.

VASCULAR
No abnormal vascular calcification.

BONES
There are no abnormalities of the imaged thoracic and lumbar spine, or within the pelvis.

SOFT TISSUES
The psoas muscle outline is visible bilaterally.

The extra-abdominal soft tissues are unremarkable.

OTHER
There are two radiopaque foreign bodies resembling cylindrical cell batteries projected over the left side of the abdomen.

There are several radiopaque foreign bodies projected over the pelvis, resembling two keys, and there are also multiple phleboliths.

There are no vascular lines, drains or surgical clips.

REVIEW AREAS
Gallstones / Renal calculi: No radiopaque calculi.
Lung bases: Not fully included.
Spine: Normal.
Femoral heads: Normal.

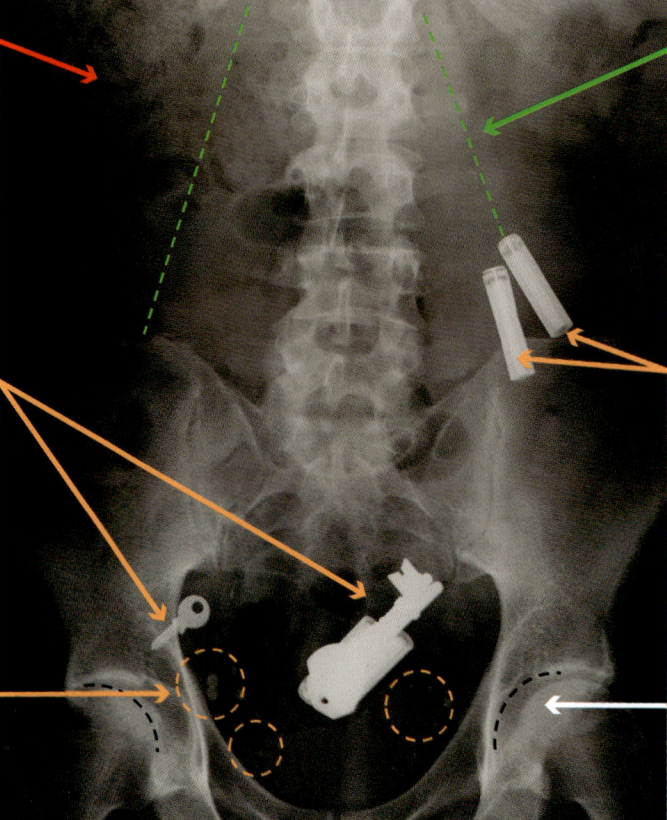

Faecal residue throughout ascending colon

Psoas muscle outlines

Ingested foreign bodies - keys

Ingested foreign bodies - batteries

Phleboliths

Femoral heads normal

SUMMARY
This X-ray demonstrates multiple radiopaque foreign bodies as described. There is no evidence of pneumoperitoneum. The moderate faecal loading in the ascending colon and hepatic flexure, and pelvic phleboliths are incidental findings.

INVESTIGATIONS AND MANAGEMENT
The patient should be resuscitated using an ABCDE approach.

Adequate analgesia and hydration should be provided.

Urgent bloods should be taken including FBC, U&Es, LFTs, coagulation, blood gas, and group and save.

The patient should be referred urgently to the surgical team, for consideration of removal of the foreign bodies. Removal depends on the location, size, shape and duration of ingestion.

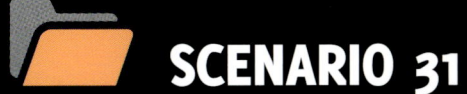

SCENARIO 31

A 16 year old male presents to ED with worsening abdominal distension and pain. He has not opened his bowels for more than 24 hours. He has no significant past medical history and is a non-smoker. On examination, he has saturations of 98% in room air and a temperature of 36.5°C. His HR is 68 bpm, RR is 16 and blood pressure is 115/65 mmHg. The abdomen is soft and there is generalised tenderness with normal bowel sounds. Urine dipstick is unremarkable.

An abdominal X-ray is requested to assess for possible obstruction.

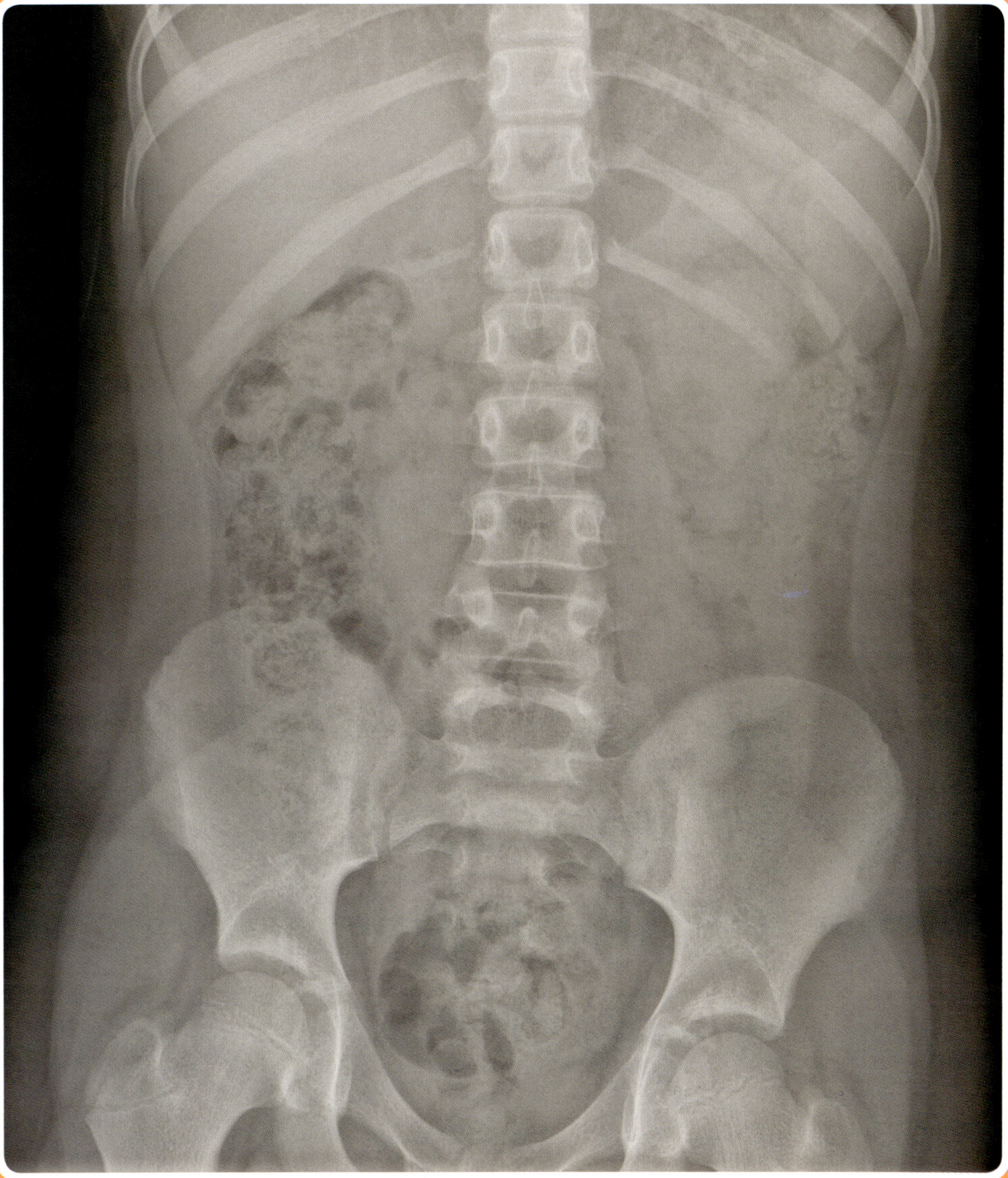

REPORT – FAECAL RESIDUE

REPORT
Patient ID: Anonymous.
Projection: AP supine.
Rotation: Adequate.
Penetration: Adequate – the spinous processes are visible.
Coverage: Inadequate – the pubic symphysis and inferior pubic rami have not been fully included.

BOWEL GAS PATTERN
The bowel gas pattern is normal.

There is a moderate volume of faecal residue present throughout the large bowel, from the ascending colon to rectum.

BOWEL WALL
There is no evidence of mural thickening or intramural gas within the large or small bowel.

PNEUMOPERITONEUM
There is no evidence of free intra-abdominal gas.

SOLID ORGANS
The solid organ contours are within normal limits with no solid organ calcification.

VASCULAR
No abnormal vascular calcification.

BONES
There are no abnormalities of the imaged thoracic and lumbar spine, or within the pelvis.

There are growth plates at the femoral head, greater trochanter and acetabulum as the ossification centres have not yet fused, which is a normal finding in a child of this age.

SOFT TISSUES
The psoas muscle outline is visible bilaterally.

The extra-abdominal soft tissues are unremarkable.

OTHER
There are no radiopaque foreign bodies.

There are no vascular lines, drains or surgical clips.

REVIEW AREAS
Gallstones / Renal calculi: No radiopaque calculi.
Lung bases: Not fully included.
Spine: Normal.
Femoral heads: Normal – growth plates present.

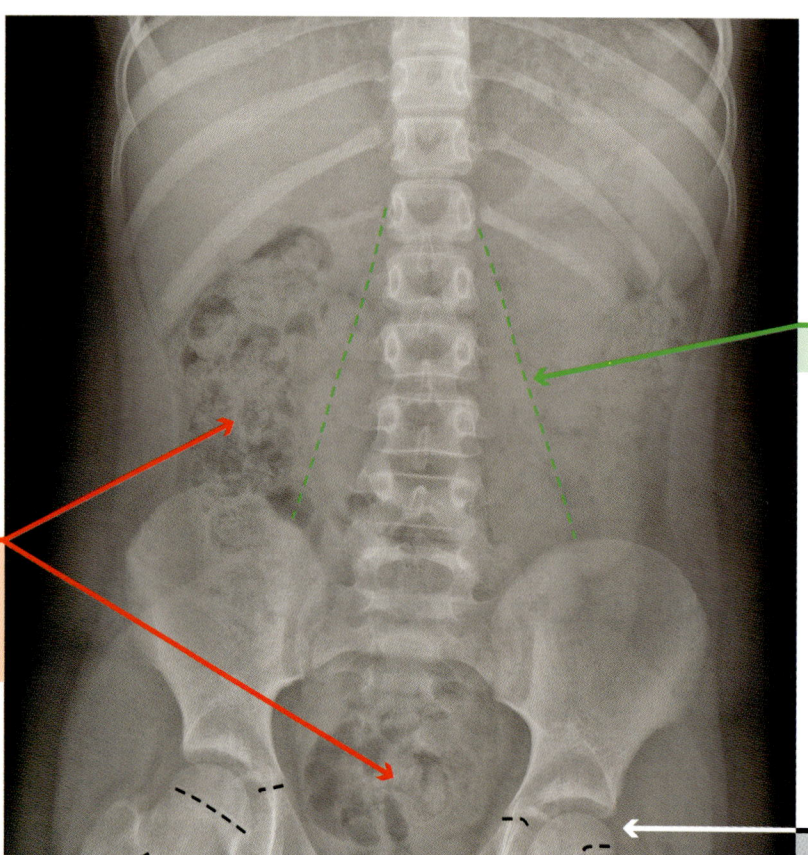

Faecal residue throughout large bowel from ascending colon to rectum

Psoas muscle outlines

Growth plates

SUMMARY
This X-ray demonstrates a moderate volume of faecal residue throughout the colon and rectum, which is likely within normal limits.

INVESTIGATIONS AND MANAGEMENT
If the patient is otherwise well, no further investigations or imaging is required.

If the patient is clinically constipated, current medications should be reviewed and laxatives considered. Advice should be given regarding lifestyle adjustments, including adequate fluid intake, sufficient dietary fibre and exercise if clinically appropriate.

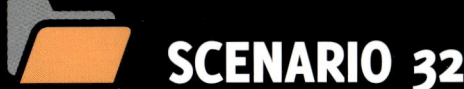

SCENARIO 32

A 2 year old male presents to ED having swallowed a foreign object. The parents are unsure of what the object is or how many he may have swallowed. He is completely well otherwise. He has no significant past medical history. On examination, he has saturations of 99% in room air and a temperature of 36.3°C. His HR is 110 bpm and RR is 24. The abdomen is soft and there is no tenderness with normal bowel sounds.

An abdominal X-ray is requested the assess the nature and position of the foreign object.

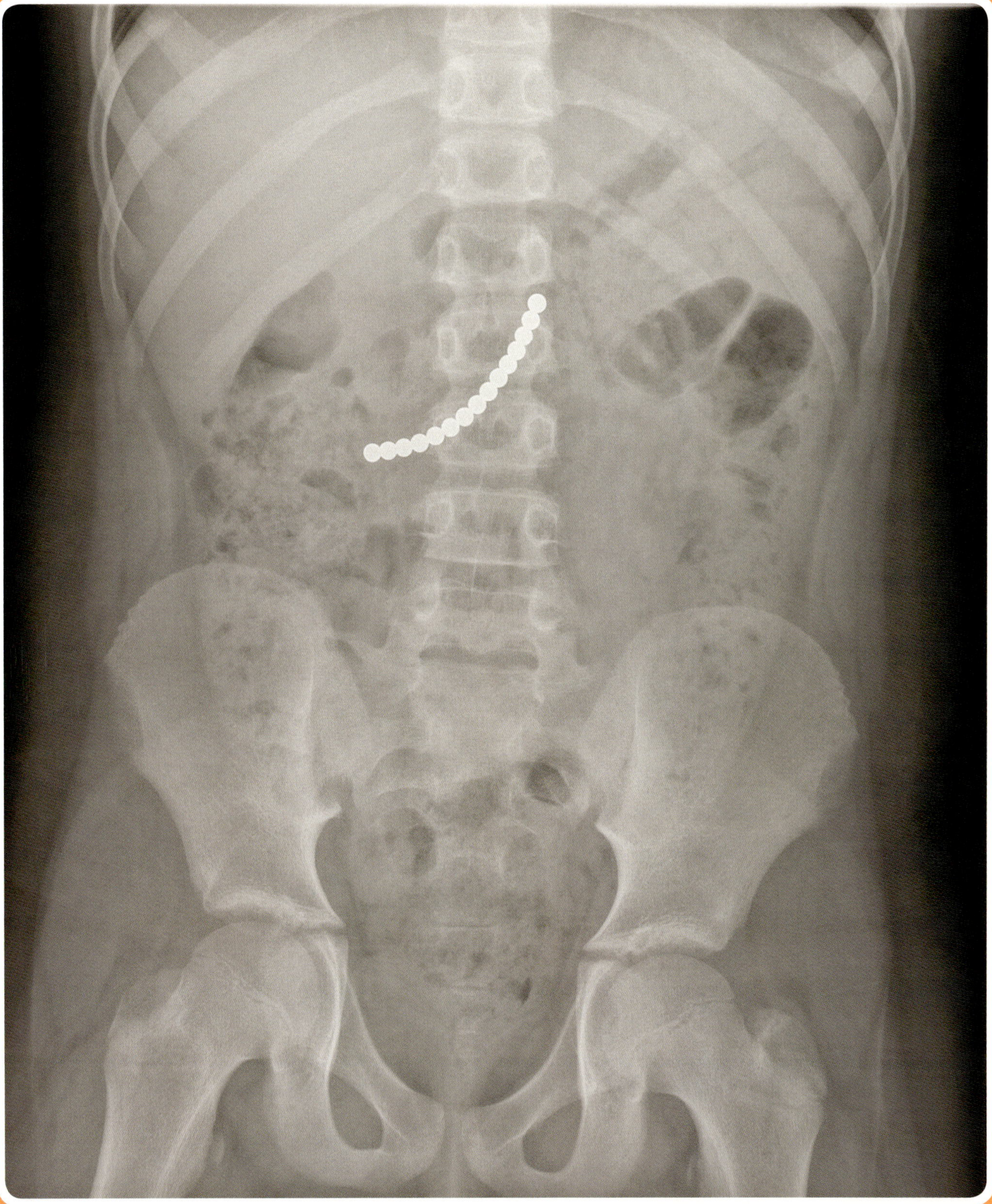

REPORT
Patient ID: Anonymous.
Projection: AP supine.
Rotation: Adequate.
Penetration: Adequate – the spinous processes are visible.
Coverage: Adequate – the anterior ribs are visible superiorly and the pubic rami are visible inferiorly.

BOWEL GAS PATTERN
The bowel gas pattern is normal.

There is a moderate volume of faecal residue present throughout the large bowel.

BOWEL WALL
There is no evidence of mural thickening or intramural gas within the large or small bowel.

PNEUMOPERITONEUM
There is no evidence of free intra-abdominal gas.

SOLID ORGANS
The solid organ contours are within normal limits with no solid organ calcification.

VASCULAR
No abnormal vascular calcification.

BONES
There are no abnormalities of the imaged thoracic and lumbar spine, or within the pelvis.

There are growth plates at the femoral head, greater trochanter and acetabulum as the ossification centres have not yet fused, which is a normal finding in a child of this age.

SOFT TISSUES
The right psoas muscle outline is not visible, which is non-specific.

The extra-abdominal soft tissues are unremarkable.

OTHER
There are multiple rounded radiopaque foreign bodies projected over the region of the epigastrium, likely within proximal small bowel, in keeping with ingested magnetic objects that have clumped together.

There are no vascular lines, drains or surgical clips.

REVIEW AREAS
Gallstones / Renal calculi: No radiopaque calculi.
Lung bases: Not fully included.
Spine: Normal.
Femoral heads: Normal – growth plates present.

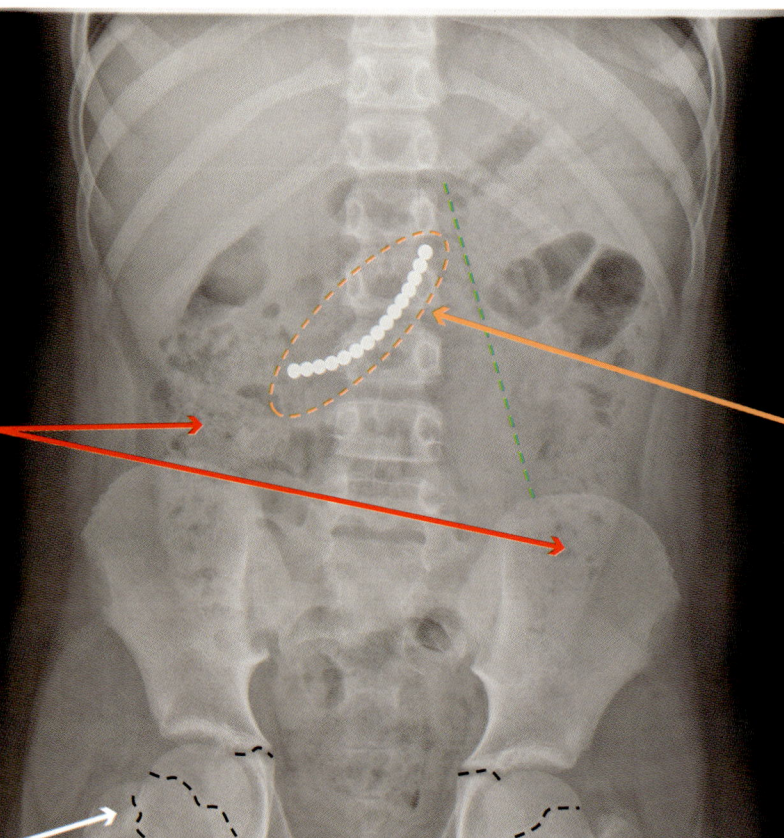

Faecal residue throughout large bowel

Ingested foreign bodies - magnetic objects

Growth plates

SUMMARY
This X-ray demonstrates multiple rounded radiopaque foreign bodies seen projected over the region of the epigastrium, likely within proximal small bowel, in keeping with ingested magnetic objects that have clumped together.

INVESTIGATIONS AND MANAGEMENT
As there are no signs of bowel perforation and the child appears well, observation with serial X-rays to monitor the progress of the foreign bodies may be appropriate. Laxatives should be considered. The paediatric gastroenterology and paediatric surgery teams should be involved and the patient should be monitored for signs of perforation or abdominal discomfort, in which case surgical intervention to retrieve the magnets will be required.

SCENARIO 33

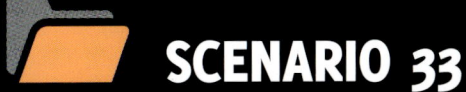

A 3 year old male presents to ED having swallowed an unknown foreign body. He has no significant past medical history. On examination, he has saturations of 99% in room air and a temperature of 36.7°C. His HR is 110 bpm and RR is 26. The abdomen is soft and there is no tenderness with normal bowel sounds.

An abdominal X-ray is requested to assess for a possible foreign body.

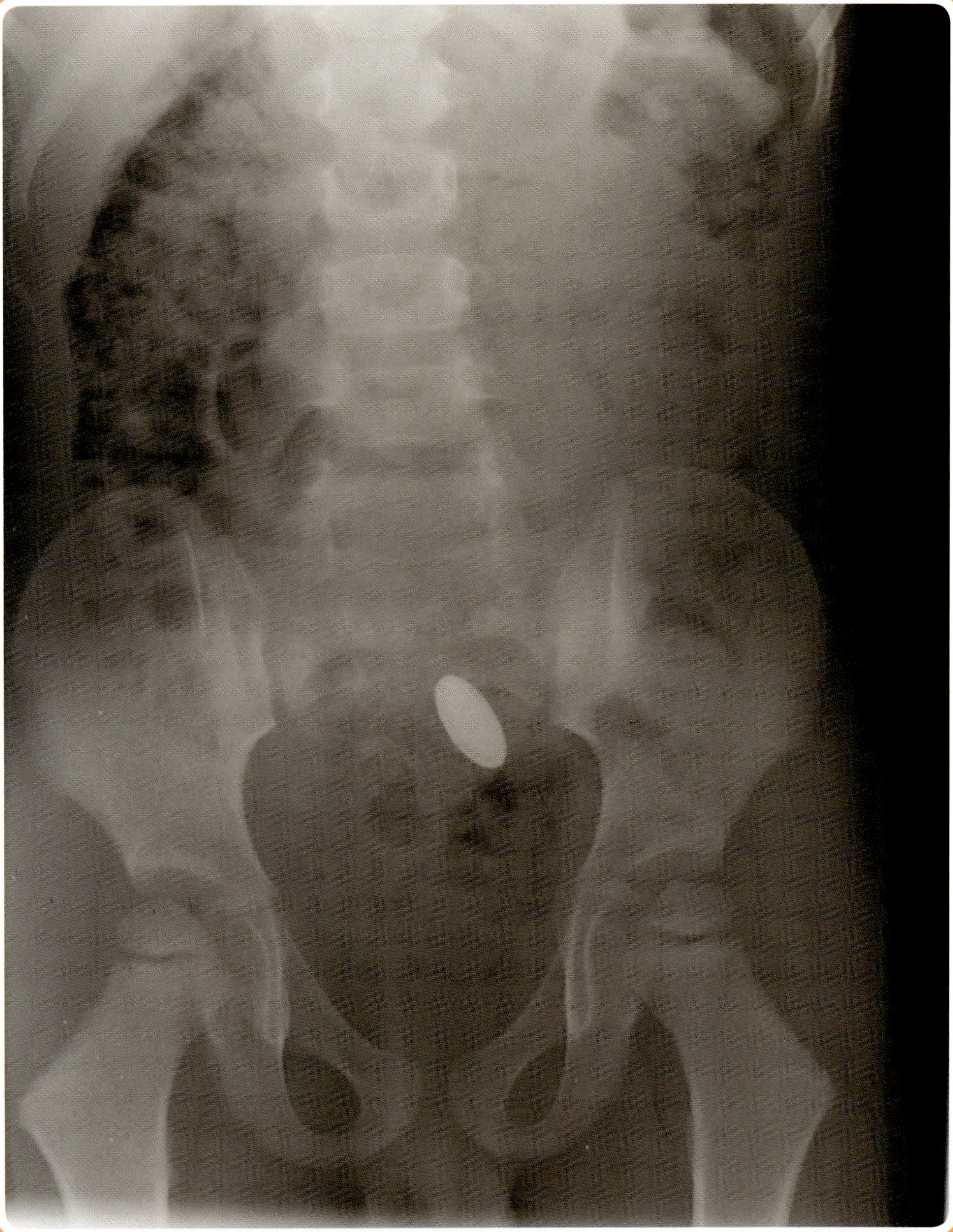

REPORT
Patient ID: Anonymous.
Projection: AP supine.
Rotation: Adequate.
Penetration: Adequate – the spine is visible.
Coverage: Inadequate – the hemidiaphragms have not been included.

BOWEL GAS PATTERN
The bowel gas pattern is normal. There is a moderate volume of faecal residue throughout the colon.

BOWEL WALL
There is no evidence of mural thickening or intramural gas within the large or small bowel.

PNEUMOPERITONEUM
There is no evidence of free intra-abdominal gas.

SOLID ORGANS
The solid organ contours are within normal limits with no solid organ calcification.

VASCULAR
No abnormal vascular calcification.

BONES
There are no abnormalities of the imaged thoracic and lumbar spine, or within the pelvis.

There is cartilage present between the pelvic bones and femurs as they have not yet fused which is a normal finding in a child of this age.

SOFT TISSUES
The psoas muscle outline is not visible bilaterally, which is non-specific, particularly in a child of this age.

The extra-abdominal soft tissues are unremarkable.

OTHER
There is a rounded radiopaque foreign body with a thin peripheral rim of reduced opacification (halo sign), resembling a button battery projecting over the region of the left hemipelvis, likely within distal small bowel or sigmoid colon.

There are no vascular lines, drains or surgical clips.

REVIEW AREAS
Gallstones / Renal calculi: No radiopaque calculi.
Lung bases: Not visualised.
Spine: Normal.
Femoral heads: Normal – growth plates present.

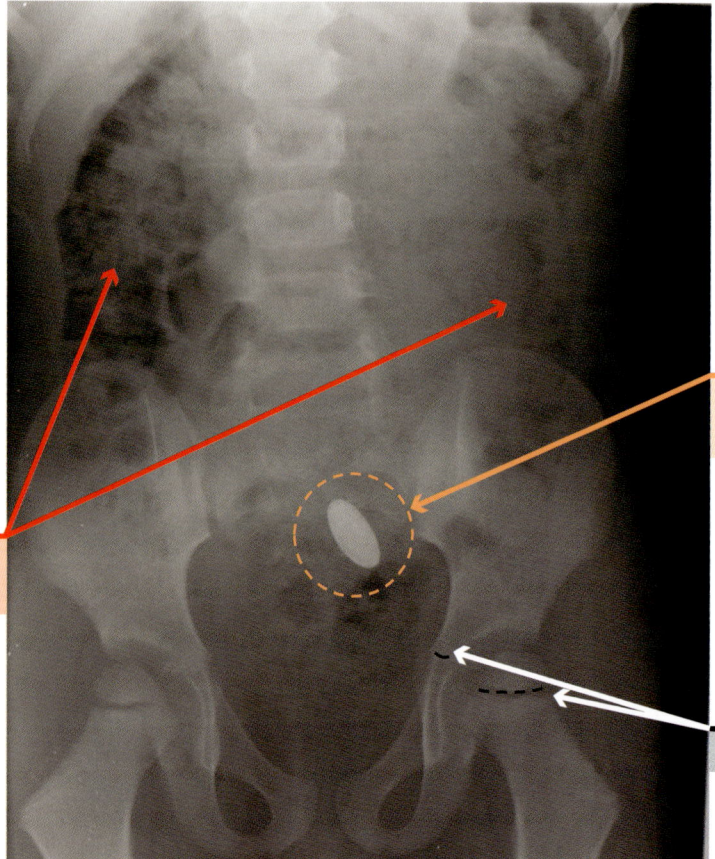

Faecal residue throughout the colon

Ingested foreign body resembling button battery

Growth plates

SUMMARY
This X-ray demonstrates a rounded radiopaque foreign body resembling a button battery projecting over the region of the left hemipelvis, likely within distal small bowel or sigmoid colon. The moderate volume of faecal residue throughout the colon is an incidental finding.

INVESTIGATIONS AND MANAGEMENT
Further history should be taken to try and confirm what the foreign body might be. Depending on the size, type and shape of the object, the symptoms, and length of time since ingestion, surgical removal may be required. Laxatives should be considered. If it is confirmed that a button battery may have been ingested, urgent surgical intervention is recommended as the patient is at risk from burn injuries to the bowel and resultant serious complications. Otherwise, the patient should have serial repeat abdominal X-rays to follow the foreign body through the gut into the rectum, and ensure that it is excreted.

INTERMEDIATE

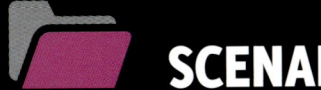

SCENARIO 34

A 75 year old female presents to ED with generalised abdominal pain and right-sided hip and groin pain radiating to the upper thigh. She is unable to move her right leg due to the pain. She has not opened her bowels in 1 week. Her past medical history is significant for multiple falls and she is a non-smoker. On examination, she has saturations of 97% in room air and a temperature of 36.9°C. Her HR is 90 bpm, RR is 20 and blood pressure is 115/65 mmHg. There is pain and bony instability on palpation of the right groin region. There is significant bruising of the groin region and upper thigh.

An abdominal X-ray is requested to assess for possible bowel obstruction.

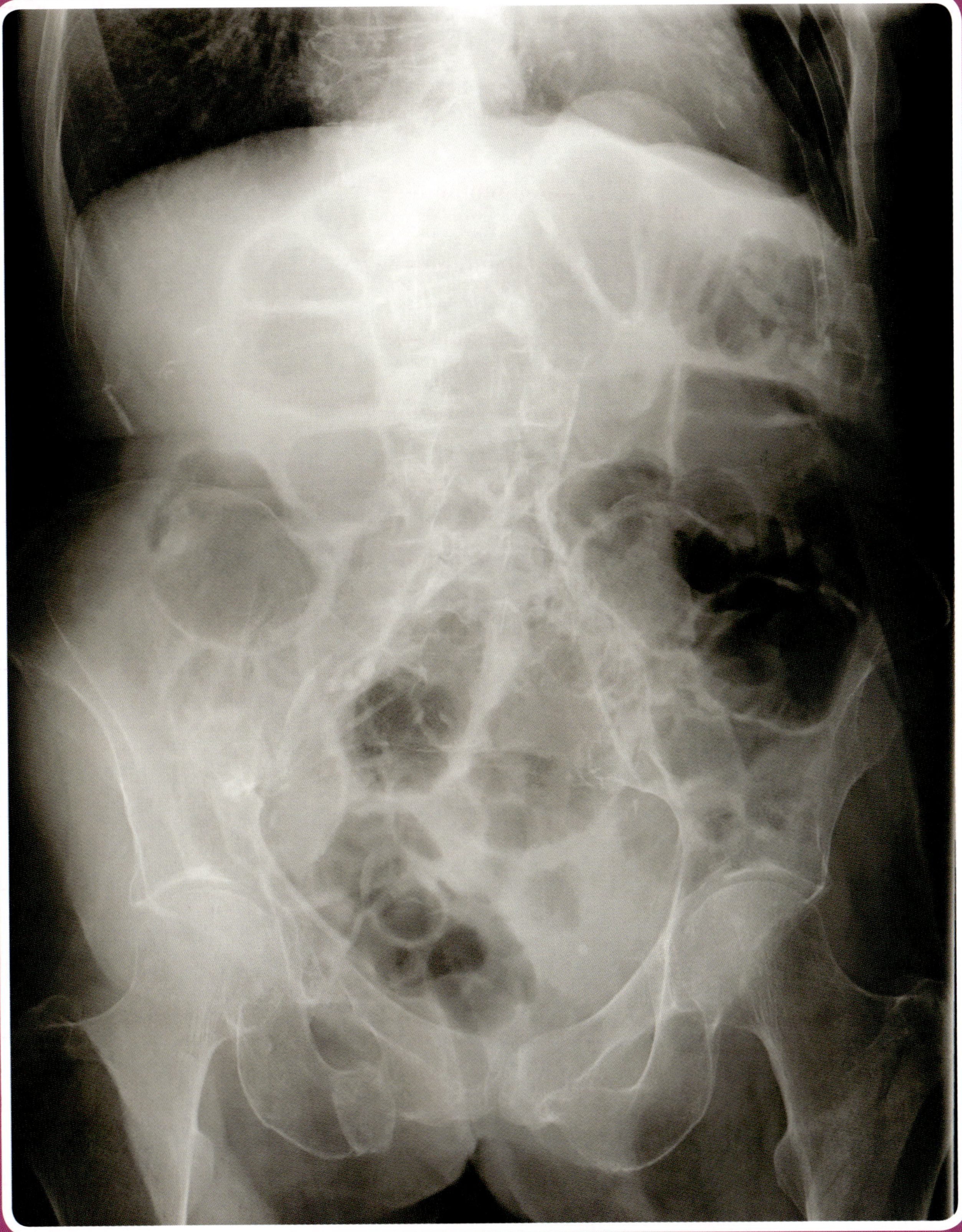

REPORT – MULTIPLE FRACTURES WITH VASCULAR CALCIFICATION

REPORT
Patient ID: Anonymous.
Projection: AP supine.
Rotation: Adequate.
Penetration: Underpenetrated – the spinous processes are not visible.
Coverage: Adequate – the anterior ribs are visible superiorly and the inferior pubic rami are visible.

BOWEL GAS PATTERN
There is a prominence of bowel loops throughout the abdomen, however no dilatation, which may represent a degree of ileus.

BOWEL WALL
There is no evidence of mural thickening or intramural gas within the large or small bowel.

PNEUMOPERITONEUM
There is no evidence of free intra-abdominal gas.

SOLID ORGANS
The solid organ contours are within normal limits with no solid organ calcification.

VASCULAR
The abdominal aorta is calcified.

There is calcification of the iliac arteries.

BONES
There are complete moderately displaced fractures of both the right-sided superior and inferior right pubic rami. The superior pubic ramus fracture appears acute. The inferior pubic ramus fracture is well-corticated and likely related to an old injury.

There is an area of sclerosis in the right ilium with adjacent disruption of the pelvic ring, which is suspicious for a further old fracture.

The thoracic and lumbar spine are not visible due to poor penetration.

There are no fractures of the femoral heads.

Bone density appears normal.

SOFT TISSUES
The psoas muscle outline is not visible bilaterally, which is non-specific.

The extra-abdominal soft tissues are unremarkable.

OTHER
There are no radiopaque foreign bodies.

There are no vascular lines, drains or surgical clips.

REVIEW AREAS
Gallstones / Renal calculi: No radiopaque calculi.
Lung bases: Normal.
Spine: Not visible due to underpenetration.
Femoral heads: Normal.

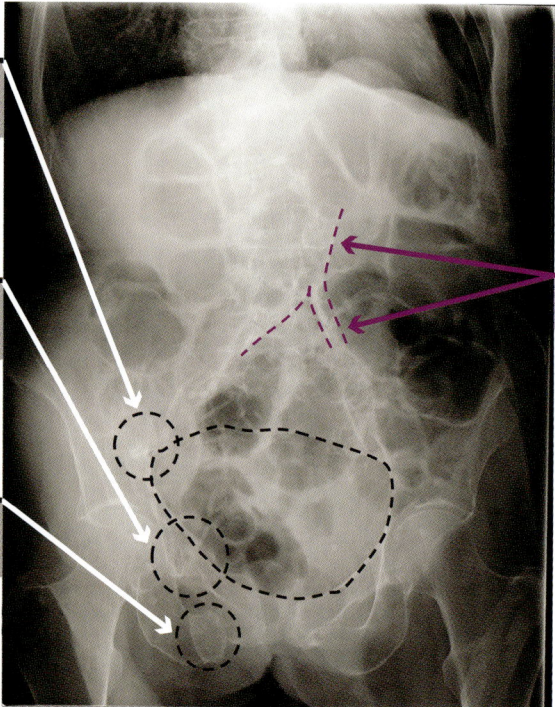

Right iliac fracture with disruption of pelvic ring

Fractured right superior pubic ramus

Fractured right inferior pubic ramus

Calcified aorta and iliac vessels

SUMMARY
This X-ray demonstrates prominent bowel loops throughout the abdomen, which may represent a degree of ileus, however no evidence of bowel obstruction. There is a probable acute fracture of the right superior pubic ramus and old fractures of the right ilium and the right inferior pubic ramus. The abdominal aorta is calcified. The iliac vessel calcification is an incidental finding.

INVESTIGATIONS AND MANAGEMENT
The patient should be resuscitated using an ABCDE approach.

Adequate analgesia and hydration should be provided.

Bloods should be taken, including FBC, U&Es, LFTs, bone profile, CRP, TFTs, blood gas, and group and save.

The patient should be referred urgently to the orthopaedic surgical team.

Depending on previous imaging, a CT of the pelvis should be considered to better assess the extent of injury, chronicity of injuries, for any potential operative planning and to assess for potential associated injuries (for example to the bladder).

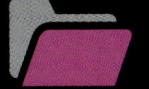

SCENARIO 35

A 32 year old male presents to ED with acute abdominal pain and a GCS of 13. He has no significant past medical history and is a non-smoker. On examination, he has saturations of 98% in room air and a temperature of 37.6°C. His HR is 75 bpm, RR is 25 and blood pressure is 115/65 mmHg. The abdomen is soft and there is generalised mild tenderness with normal bowel sounds. Urine dipstick is unremarkable.

An abdominal X-ray is requested to look for possible bowel obstruction.

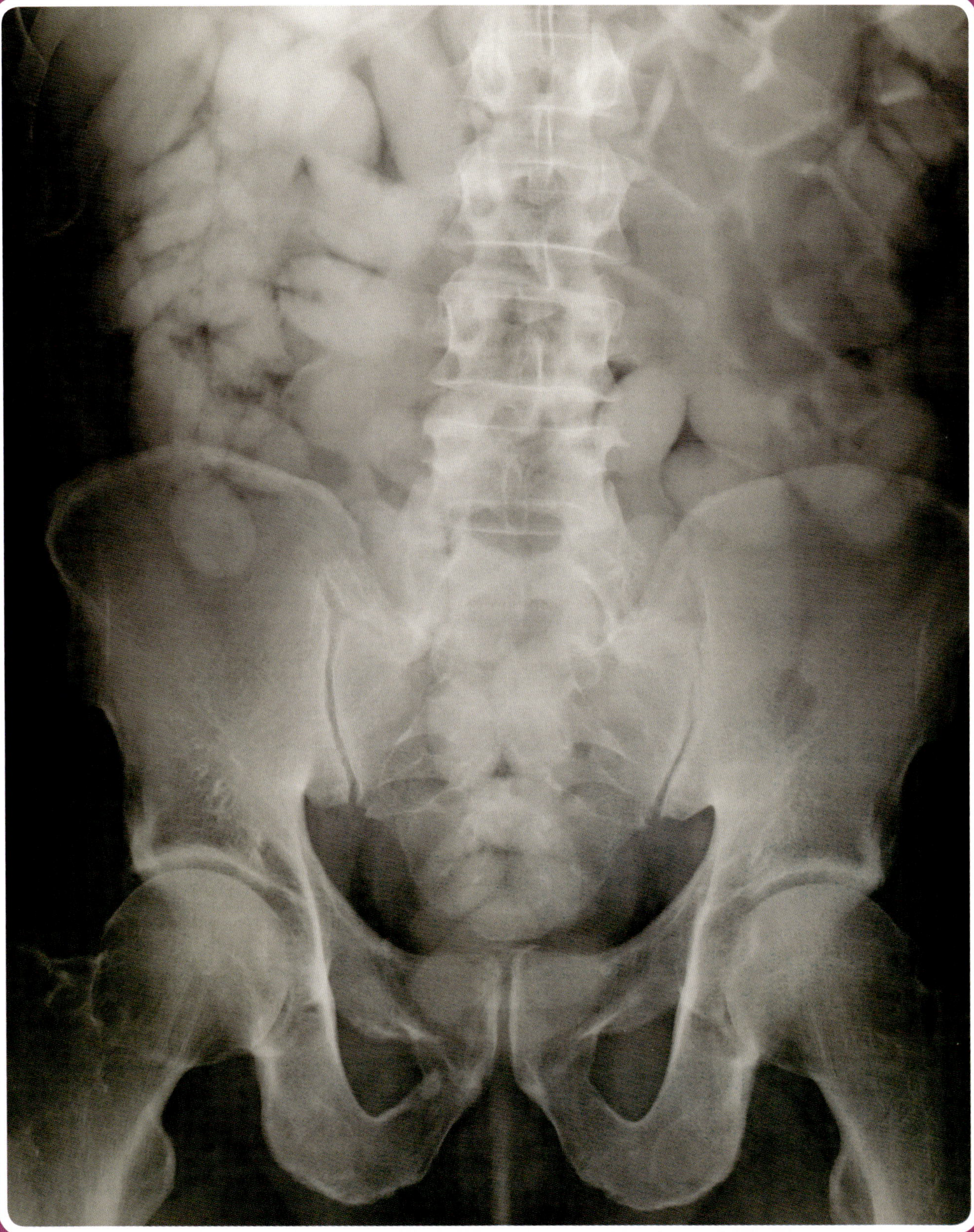

REPORT
Patient ID: Anonymous.
Projection: AP supine.
Rotation: Adequate.
Penetration: Adequate – the spinous processes are visible.
Coverage: Inadequate – the anterior ribs have not been included.

BOWEL GAS PATTERN
There is a prominence of bowel gas, however there is no bowel dilatation. The bowel gas pattern is partially obscured due to the presence of multiple ovoid radiopaque foreign bodies.

BOWEL WALL
There is no evidence of mural thickening or intramural gas within the large or small bowel.

PNEUMOPERITONEUM
There is no evidence of free intra-abdominal gas.

SOLID ORGANS
The solid organ contours are within normal limits with no solid organ calcification.

VASCULAR
No abnormal vascular calcification.

BONES
There is incidental sacralisation of L5.

There are no abnormalities of the imaged thoracic and lumbar spine, or within the pelvis.

SOFT TISSUES
The psoas muscle outline is visible bilaterally.

The extra-abdominal soft tissues are unremarkable.

OTHER
There are multiple radiopaque densities located predominantly throughout the large bowel and rectum, in keeping with bags of an unknown substance.

There are no vascular lines, drains or surgical clips.

REVIEW AREAS
Gallstones / Renal calculi: No radiopaque calculi.
Lung bases: Not fully included.
Spine: Normal.
Femoral heads: Normal.

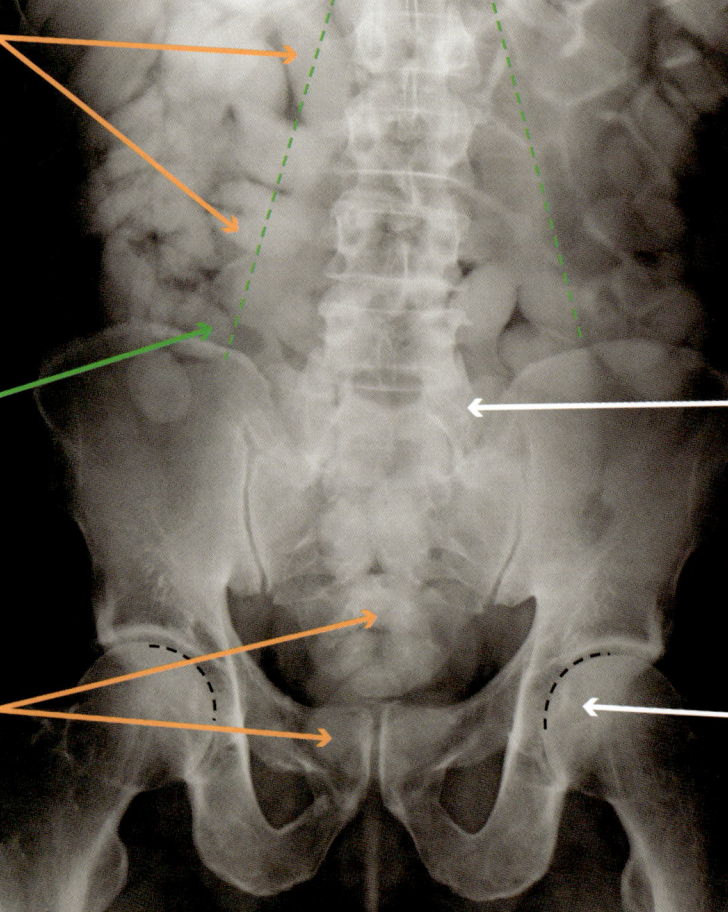

Ingested foreign bodies in stomach and small bowel

Psoas muscle outlines

Foreign bodies in rectum

Sacralisation of L5

Femoral heads normal

SUMMARY
This X-ray demonstrates multiple radiopaque densities located throughout the abdomen within the colon and rectum, in keeping with a drug mule who has ingested multiple bags of drugs. The sacralisation of L5 is an incidental finding.

INVESTIGATIONS AND MANAGEMENT
The patient should be resuscitated using an ABCDE approach.

Adequate analgesia and hydration should be provided.

Rupture of the drug capsules should be considered and reference to Toxbase for possible overdose management should be sought.

Early surgical referral should be considered, as a laparotomy may be needed.

As this may be associated with possible criminal activity, the police should be involved, although this should be secondary to providing care to the patient.

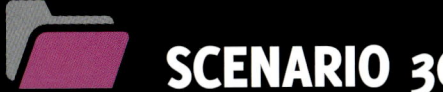
A 24 year old male presents to ED with worsening abdominal pain and 15 episodes of diarrhoea and passing mucus in the past 24 hours. He has no significant past medical history and is a non-smoker. On examination, he has saturations of 97% in room air and a temperature of 38.5°C. His HR is 94 bpm, RR is 22 and blood pressure is 115/65 mmHg. The abdomen is rigid and there is generalised tenderness with normal bowel sounds. Urine dipstick is unremarkable.

An abdominal X-ray is requested to assess for a possible colitis.

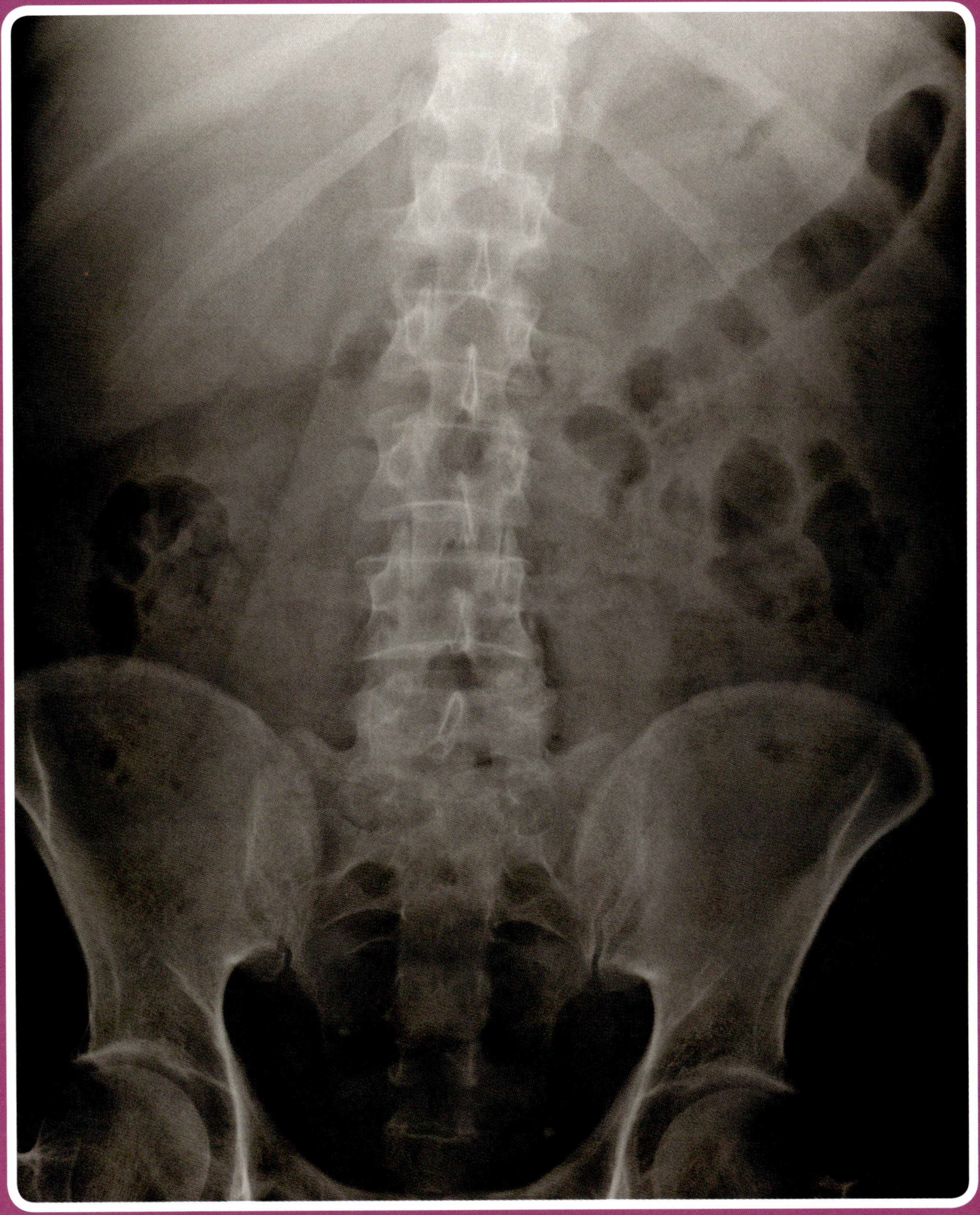

REPORT – COLITIS

REPORT
Patient ID: Anonymous.
Projection: AP supine.
Rotation: Adequate.
Penetration: Adequate – the spinous processes are visible.
Coverage: Inadequate – the pubic symphysis and inferior pubic rami have not been fully included.

BOWEL GAS PATTERN
The bowel gas pattern is normal.

BOWEL WALL
There is mural thickening of the distal transverse colon up to the splenic flexure in the left upper quadrant, which appears featureless with loss of the normal colonic haustral folds, in keeping with mural oedema. This is termed 'lead pipe colon'.

There is no evidence of intramural gas within the large or small bowel.

PNEUMOPERITONEUM
There is no evidence of free intra-abdominal gas.

SOLID ORGANS
The solid organ contours are within normal limits with no solid organ calcification.

VASCULAR
No abnormal vascular calcification.

BONES
There are no abnormalities of the imaged thoracic and lumbar spine, or within the pelvis.

SOFT TISSUES
The psoas muscle outline is visible bilaterally.

The extra-abdominal soft tissues are unremarkable.

OTHER
There are no radiopaque foreign bodies.

There are no vascular lines, drains or surgical clips.

There are several rounded radiopaque densities projected over the region of the pelvis in keeping with phleboliths.

REVIEW AREAS
Gallstones / Renal calculi: No radiopaque calculi.
Lung bases: Not fully included.
Spine: Normal.
Femoral heads: Normal.

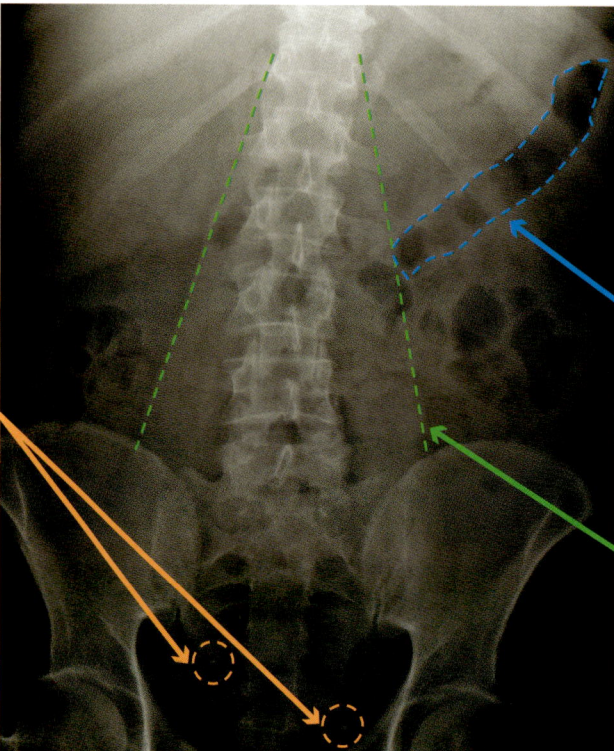

Phleboliths

Mural oedema of transverse colon with loss of haustral folds

Psoas muscle outlines

SUMMARY
This X-ray demonstrates mural oedema of the distal transverse colon up to the splenic flexure, which appears featureless with loss of the normal colonic haustral folds. Given the clinical history, this is suggestive of colitis, likely infective or inflammatory in nature. The pelvic phleboliths are an incidental finding.

INVESTIGATIONS AND MANAGEMENT
This patient should be resuscitated using an ABCDE approach.

Adequate analgesia and hydration should be provided.

Urgent bloods should be taken, including FBC, U&Es, LFTs, ESR, CRP, iron studies, folate, blood gas, and group and save. A stool sample should be sent.

Urgent referral to the gastroenterology team should be considered.

A CT scan of the abdomen/pelvis with IV contrast should be considered for better visualisation of the anatomy and to assess for complications such as pneumoperitoneum and abscess formation.

Treatment will depend on the results of further investigations, as well as the clinical state of the patient.

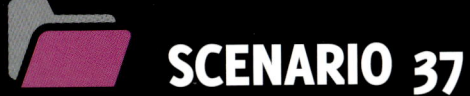
A 60 year old female is currently admitted on the surgical ward having just had an endovascular aortic stent insertion. Her past medical history is significant for abdominal aortic aneurysm and she is a smoker. On examination, she has saturations of 98% in room air and a temperature of 36.4°C. Her HR is 68 bpm, RR is 14 and blood pressure is 125/65 mmHg. The abdomen is soft and there is some tenderness centrally with normal bowel sounds. Urine dipstick is unremarkable.

You are asked to review the post-op abdominal X-ray and comment on the position of the stent.

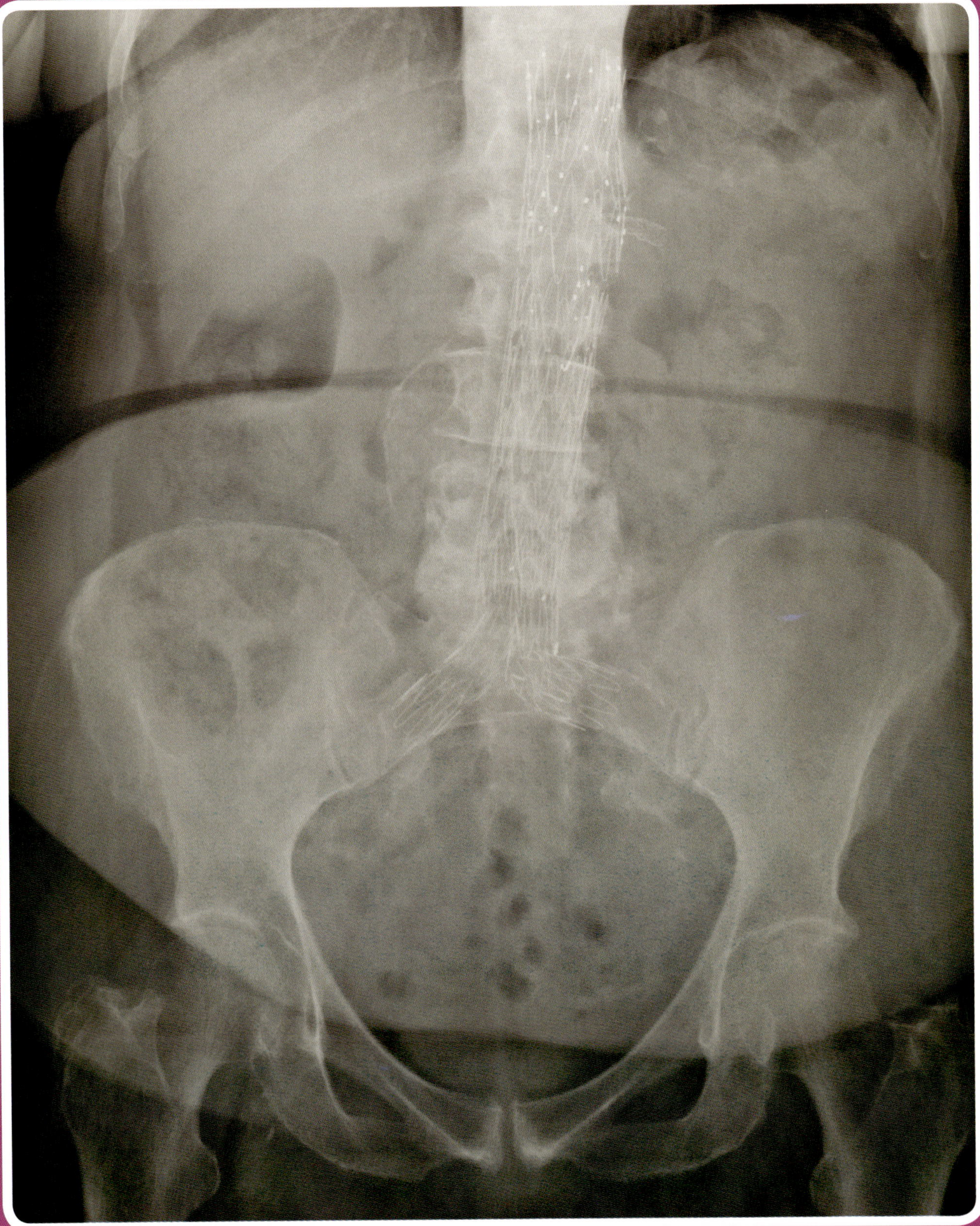

REPORT
Patient ID: Anonymous.
Projection: AP supine.
Rotation: Adequate.
Penetration: Adequate – the spinous processes are visible.
Coverage: Adequate – the anterior ribs are visible superiorly and the pubic rami are visible inferiorly.

BOWEL GAS PATTERN
The bowel gas pattern is normal.

BOWEL WALL
There is no evidence of mural thickening or intramural gas within the large or small bowel.

PNEUMOPERITONEUM
There is no evidence of free intra-abdominal gas.

SOLID ORGANS
The solid organ contours are within normal limits with no solid organ calcification.

VASCULAR
There is a fenestrated endovascular iliac branch aortic stent seen within the abdominal aorta, extending into the common iliac arteries bilaterally. There are separate renal artery stents in situ. A partially calcified infra-renal abdominal aortic aneurysm is visible.

BONES
There is minor bilateral degenerative change seen within the hip joints and the pubic symphysis, including narrowing of the joint spaces and sclerosis.

There are no abnormalities of the imaged thoracic and lumbar spine.

SOFT TISSUES
The psoas muscle outline is visible bilaterally.

There are cutaneous fat folds projecting over the region of the abdomen.

OTHER
There are no additional radiopaque foreign bodies.

There are no vascular lines, drains or surgical clips.

REVIEW AREAS
Gallstones / Renal calculi: No radiopaque calculi.
Lung bases: Normal.
Spine: Normal.
Femoral heads: Bilateral degenerative change, including narrowing of joint spaces and sclerosis.

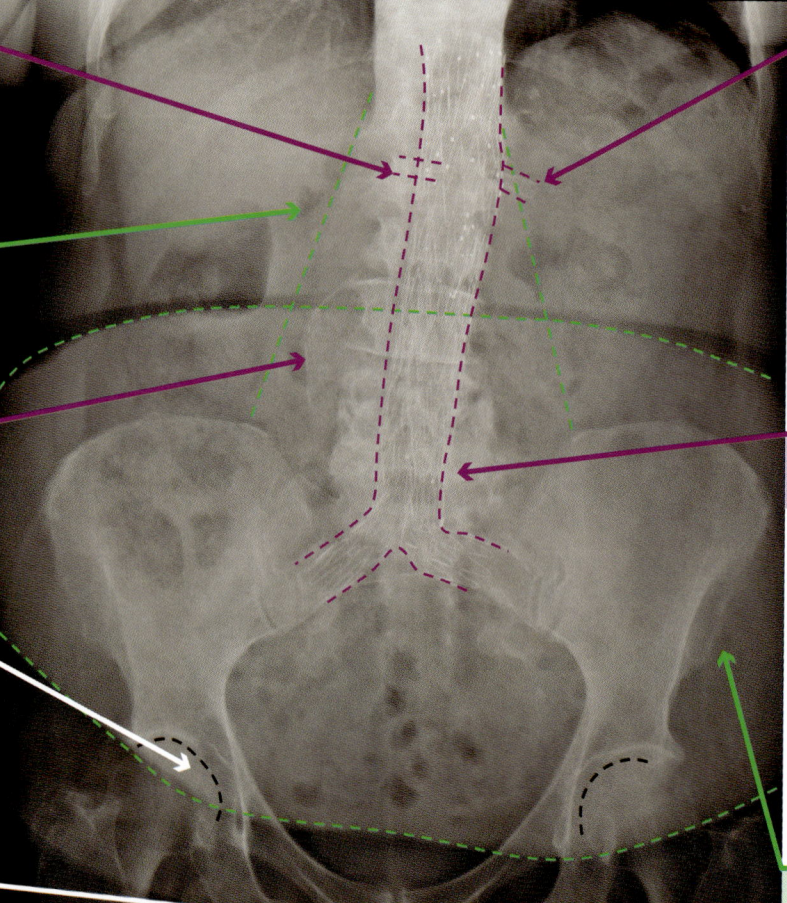

Right renal artery stent

Left renal artery stent

Psoas muscle outlines

Abdominal aorta aneurysm calcification

Endovascular iliac branch aortic stent

Joint space narrowing

Cutaneous fat folds

Sclerosis

SUMMARY
This X-ray demonstrates a multi-branched aortic stent within the abdominal aorta extending into the proximal left renal and bilateral common iliac arteries. The minor degenerative changes seen bilaterally within the hip joints and pubic symphysis are incidental findings.

INVESTIGATIONS AND MANAGEMENT
If the patient is otherwise well, no further investigations or imaging is required. The stents are adequately positioned. Degenerative changes should be correlated with clinical history, and lifestyle advice/analgesia should be considered in the first instance.

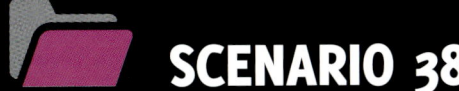

SCENARIO 38

A 55 year old male presents to the haematology outpatient clinic as a referral from his primary care physician due to abnormal haematology results with a markedly raised WBC. He has no significant past medical history and is a non-smoker. On examination, he has saturations of 99% in room air and a temperature of 36.6°C. His HR is 66 bpm, RR is 14 and blood pressure is 120/70 mmHg. The abdomen is soft and there is no tenderness, although massive splenomegaly is detected. Bowel sounds are normal and urine dipstick is unremarkable.

An abdominal X-ray is requested to assess for possible bone abnormalities and organomegaly.

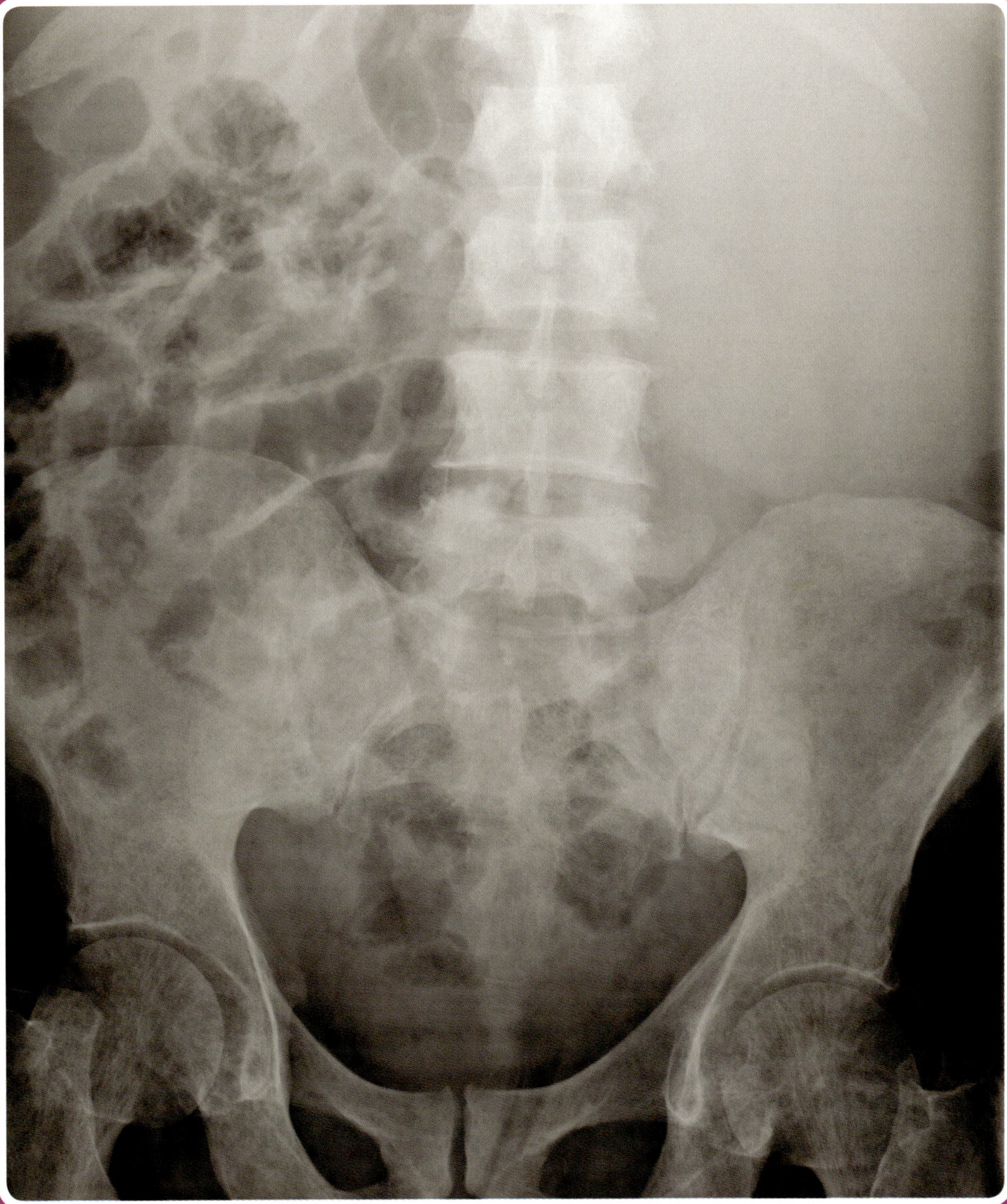

REPORT – SPLENOMEGALY AND BONE LESIONS

REPORT
Patient ID: Anonymous.
Projection: AP supine.
Rotation: Adequate.
Penetration: Adequate – the spinous processes are visible.
Coverage: Inadequate – the anterior ribs have not been included.

BOWEL GAS PATTERN
The bowel is displaced to the right by a homogeneous opacification in the left upper quadrant of the abdomen.

BOWEL WALL
There is no evidence of mural thickening or intramural gas within the large or small bowel.

PNEUMOPERITONEUM
There is no evidence of free intra-abdominal gas.

SOLID ORGANS
There is a large homogeneous opacification within the left upper quadrant of the abdomen, in keeping with an enlarged spleen.

VASCULAR
No abnormal vascular calcification.

BONES
There is a mottled appearance of the bones of the pelvis and the imaged femur.

There are no abnormalities of the imaged thoracic and lumbar spine.

SOFT TISSUES
The psoas muscle outline is visible bilaterally.

The extra-abdominal soft tissues are unremarkable.

OTHER
There are no radiopaque foreign bodies.

There are no vascular lines, drains or surgical clips.

REVIEW AREAS
Gallstones / Renal calculi: No radiopaque calculi.
Lung bases: Not fully included.
Spine: Normal.
Femoral heads: Mottled appearance of bones.

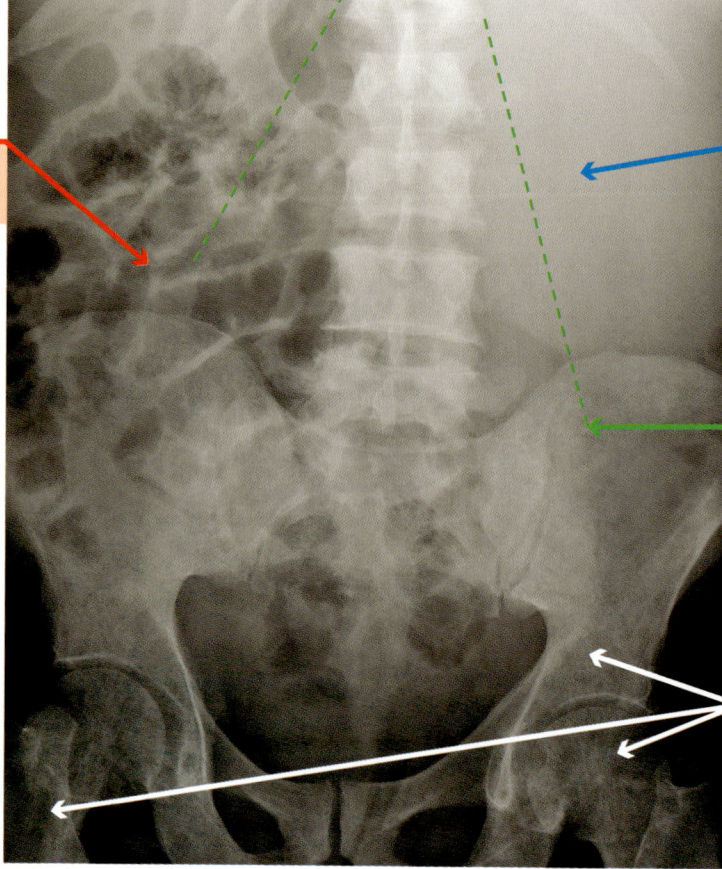

Lateral displacement of bowel to right of abdomen

Enlarged spleen

Psoas muscle outlines

Mottled appearance of bones

SUMMARY
This X-ray demonstrates splenomegaly with displacement of the bowel to the right. It also demonstrates an associated mottled appearance of the bones of the pelvis and femurs. Given the clinical history, these findings are suggestive of a myeloproliferative disorder.

INVESTIGATIONS AND MANAGEMENT
Bloods should be taken, including FBC, U&Es, LFTs, CRP, ESR, bone profile, LDH, coagulation, hepatitis screening, cytomegalovirus and Epstein-Barr virus screening, ESR, blood gas, and blood film. Additional tests such as flow cytometry, fluorescence in situ hybridisation (FISH) and polymerase chain reaction (PCR) testing for BCR-ABL/JAK2 should be considered, as well as a bone marrow biopsy. An abdominal USS should be performed to confirm splenomegaly, and further evaluate the abdominal solid organs.

The patient should be followed up by haematology. Diagnosis and treatment will depend on the results of the above tests and the patient's wishes. Treatment options potentially include observation, chemotherapy, radiation therapy, biological therapies, or stem cell transplantation.

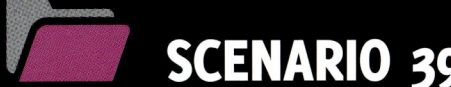

SCENARIO 39

A 35 year old female presents to ED with worsening back pain and pyrexia of unknown origin. She has no significant past medical history but has recently travelled to Thailand. She is a non-smoker. On examination, she has saturations of 98% in room air and a temperature of 38.6°C. Her HR is 96 bpm, RR is 20 and blood pressure is 105/62 mmHg. The abdomen is rigid and there is generalised tenderness with normal bowel sounds. Urine dipstick is unremarkable and a pregnancy test is negative.

An abdominal X-ray is requested to assess for possible bowel obstruction.

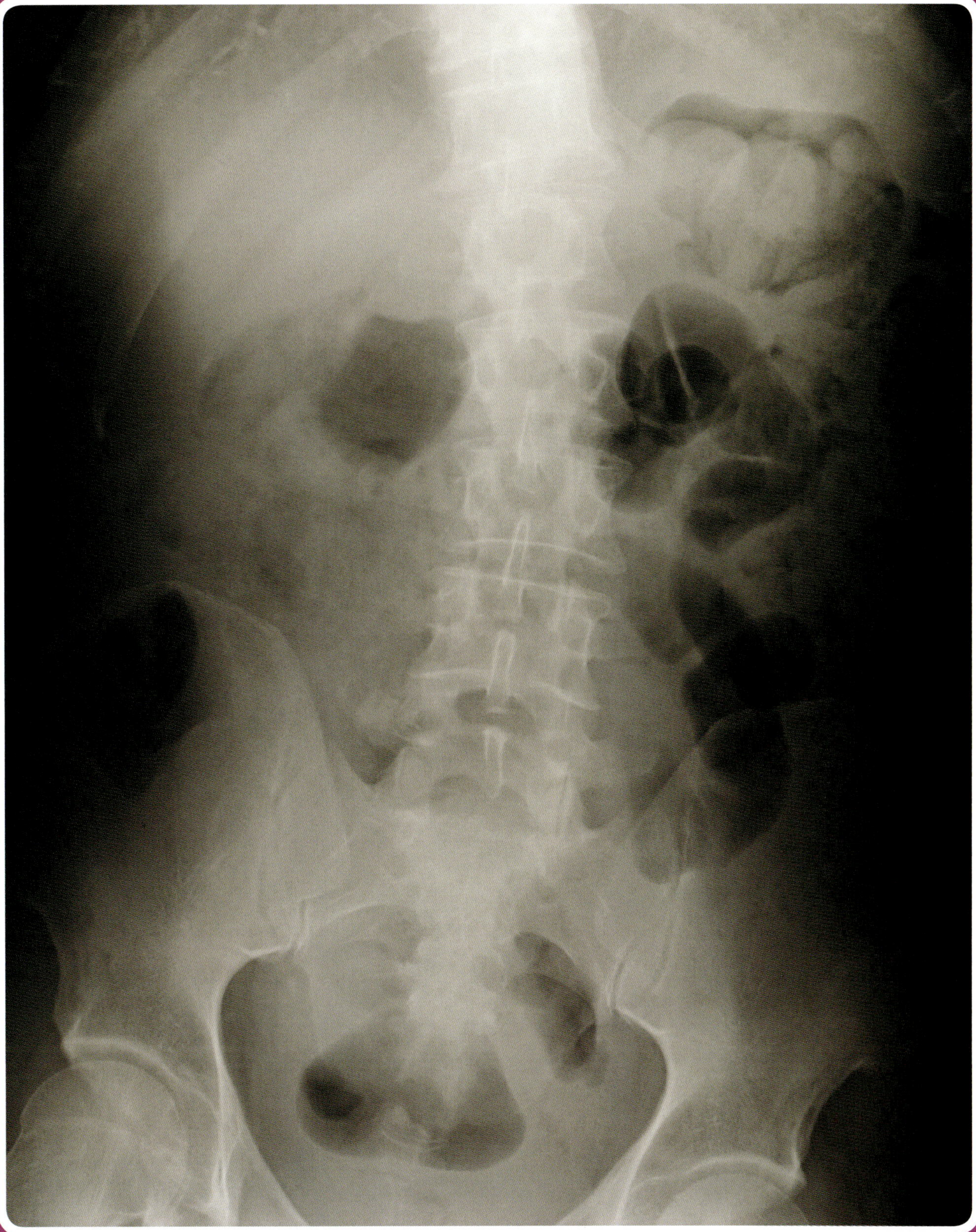

REPORT
Patient ID: Anonymous.
Projection: AP supine.
Rotation: Adequate.
Penetration: Adequate – the spinous processes are visible.
Coverage: Inadequate – the pubic symphysis, inferior pubic rami and hip joints have not been fully included.

BOWEL GAS PATTERN
The bowel gas pattern is normal.

There are hard faeces in the distal transverse colon and a small volume of faecal material present throughout the descending colon.

BOWEL WALL
There is no evidence of mural thickening or intramural gas within the large or small bowel.

PNEUMOPERITONEUM
There is no evidence of free intra-abdominal gas.

SOLID ORGANS
The solid organ contours are within normal limits with no solid organ calcification.

VASCULAR
No abnormal vascular calcification.

BONES
There is thoracolumbar scoliosis seen convex to the left, centred at the L1/L2 level. No fractures or destructive bone lesions are visible in the imaged skeleton.

SOFT TISSUES
There is a mottled appearance projecting over the right psoas muscle outline and the left psoas muscle outline is not visible.

The extra-abdominal soft tissues are unremarkable.

OTHER
There are no radiopaque foreign bodies.

There are no vascular lines, drains or surgical clips.

REVIEW AREAS
Gallstones / Renal calculi: No radiopaque calculi.
Lung bases: Not fully included.
Spine: Thoracolumbar scoliosis convex to the left, centred at the L1/L2 level.
Femoral heads: Not fully included.

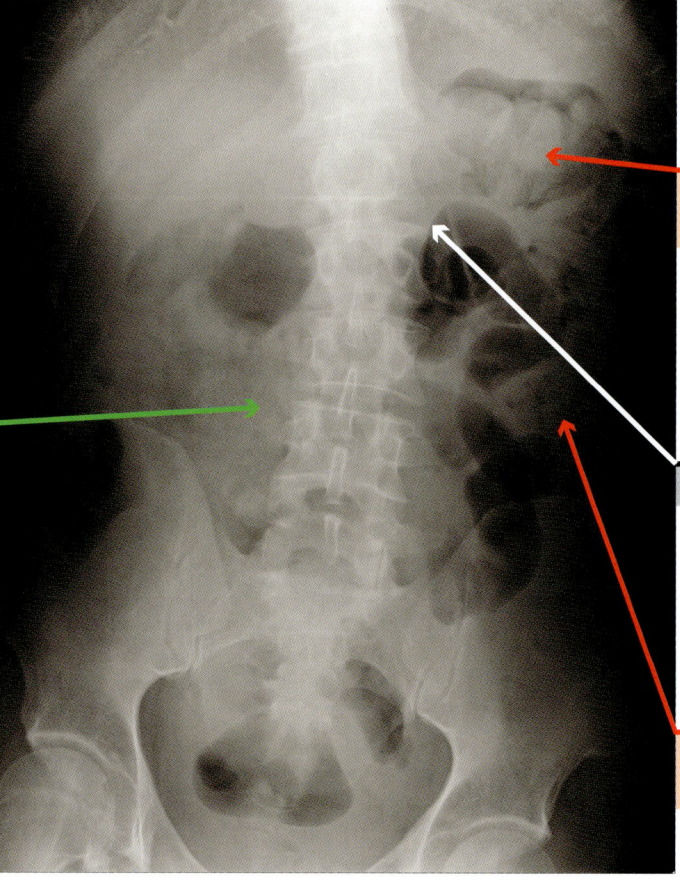

Hard faeces in distal transverse colon

Mottled appearance overlying right psoas muscle shadow

Scoliosis

Faecal material throughout descending colon

SUMMARY
This X-ray demonstrates a mottled appearance overlying the right psoas muscle outline. Given the clinical history, this is likely to represent a psoas abscess. The lumbar scoliosis is an incidental finding but may be secondary to the abscess.

INVESTIGATIONS AND MANAGEMENT
The patient should be resuscitated using an ABCDE approach.

Adequate analgesia and hydration should be provided.

Urgent bloods should be taken, including FBC, U&Es, CRP, bone profile, LFTs, clotting, blood cultures, a blood gas, and group and save.

Broad spectrum antibiotics should be prescribed. The patient should be made NBM and started on IV fluids.

The sepsis 6 pathway should be started immediately, including administration of oxygen, IV antibiotics and consideration of a fluid bolus as well as measurement of lactate and urinary output and taking blood cultures.

A CT scan of the abdomen/pelvis with IV contrast should be considered for further evaluation of the possible abscess and the general surgical team should be involved for consideration of possible percutaneous drainage or surgical management.

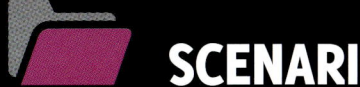

SCENARIO 40

A 63 year old female presents to ED with an increasing sensation of fullness of the abdomen and worsening bilateral pedal oedema. She has no significant past medical history and is a non-smoker. On examination, she has saturations of 97% in room air and a temperature of 36.6°C. Her HR is 72 bpm, RR is 14 and blood pressure is 122/76 mmHg. The abdomen is distended and soft with no tenderness and normal bowel sounds. Urine dipstick is unremarkable.

An abdominal X-ray is requested to assess for possible bowel obstruction.

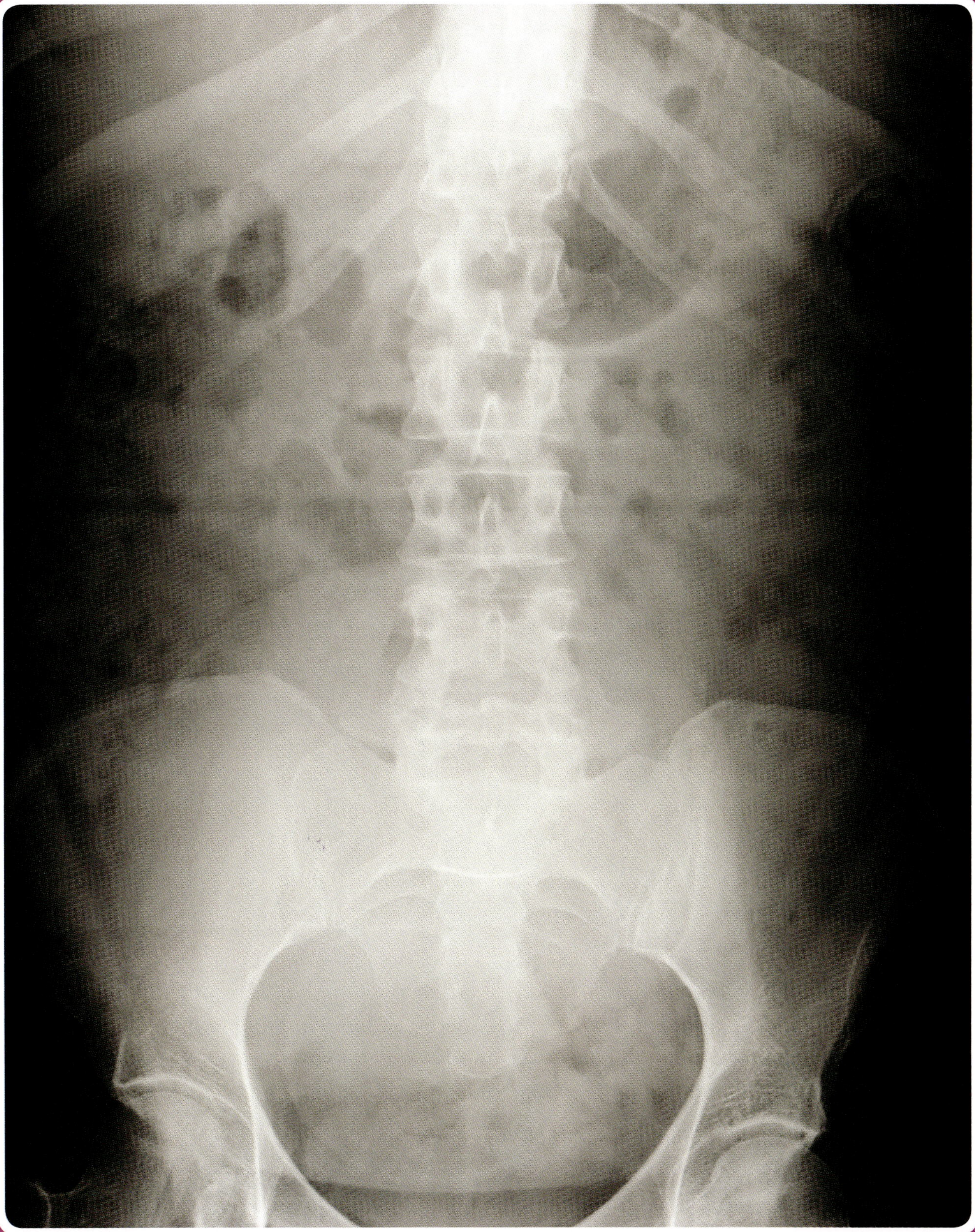

REPORT

Patient ID: Anonymous.
Projection: AP supine.
Rotation: Adequate.
Penetration: Adequate – the spinous processes are visible.
Coverage: Inadequate – the pubic symphysis, inferior pubic rami and hip joints have not been included.

BOWEL GAS PATTERN

The bowel gas pattern is normal.

BOWEL WALL

There is no evidence of mural thickening or intramural gas within the large or small bowel.

PNEUMOPERITONEUM

There is no evidence of free intra-abdominal gas.

SOLID ORGANS

The solid organ contours are within normal limits with no solid organ calcification.

VASCULAR

No abnormal vascular calcification.

BONES

There are no abnormalities of the imaged thoracic and lumbar spine, or within the pelvis.

SOFT TISSUES

The psoas muscle outline is not visible bilaterally, which is non-specific.

There is a large, rounded, well-circumscribed soft-tissue density mass centred around the right sacrum projecting over the lower abdomen and pelvis with a smaller well-circumscribed soft tissue density mass centred projecting over the right pelvis.

The urinary bladder is visualised separate to these two masses.

The extra-abdominal soft tissues are unremarkable.

OTHER

There are no radiopaque foreign bodies.

There are no vascular lines, drains or surgical clips.

REVIEW AREAS

Gallstones / Renal calculi: No radiopaque calculi.
Lung bases: Not fully included.
Spine: Normal.
Femoral heads: Not visible.

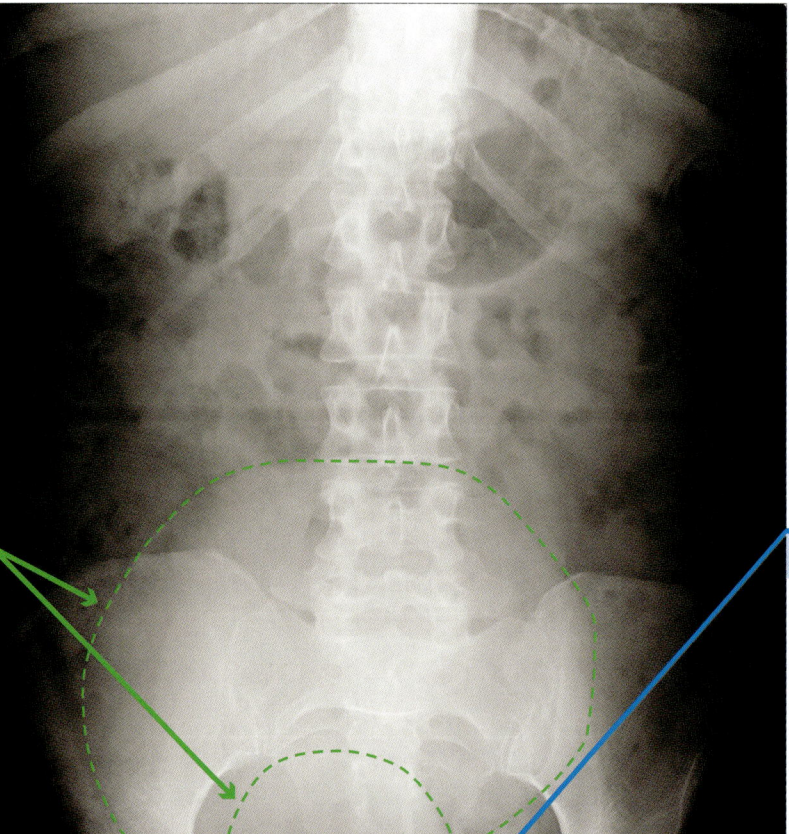

Pelvic masses

Urinary bladder

SUMMARY

This X-ray demonstrates two rounded, well-circumscribed masses of soft-tissue density projecting over the pelvis and lower abdomen, which appear separate from the urinary bladder. Differentials include fibroids and ovarian masses, both malignant and benign.

INVESTIGATIONS AND MANAGEMENT

Adequate analgesia and hydration should be provided.

Urgent bloods should be taken, including FBC, U&Es, CRP, LFTs, bone profile, blood gas, and tumour markers (including CA-125).

The patient should be referred to gynaecology. An ultrasound scan of the abdomen and pelvis may be helpful to better assess the masses with a view to a CT or MRI scan of the abdomen and pelvis for further assessment.

SCENARIO 41

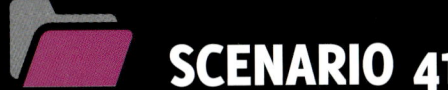

A 4 year old boy presents to ED with right iliac fossa pain, nausea, vomiting, and pyrexia. He has no significant past medical history. On examination, he has saturations of 99% in room air and a temperature of 38.6°C. His HR is 120 bpm, RR is 28 and blood pressure is 90/50 mmHg. The abdomen is soft and there is tenderness in the right iliac fossa with normal bowel sounds. Urine dipstick is unremarkable.

An abdominal X-ray is requested to assess for possible bowel obstruction.

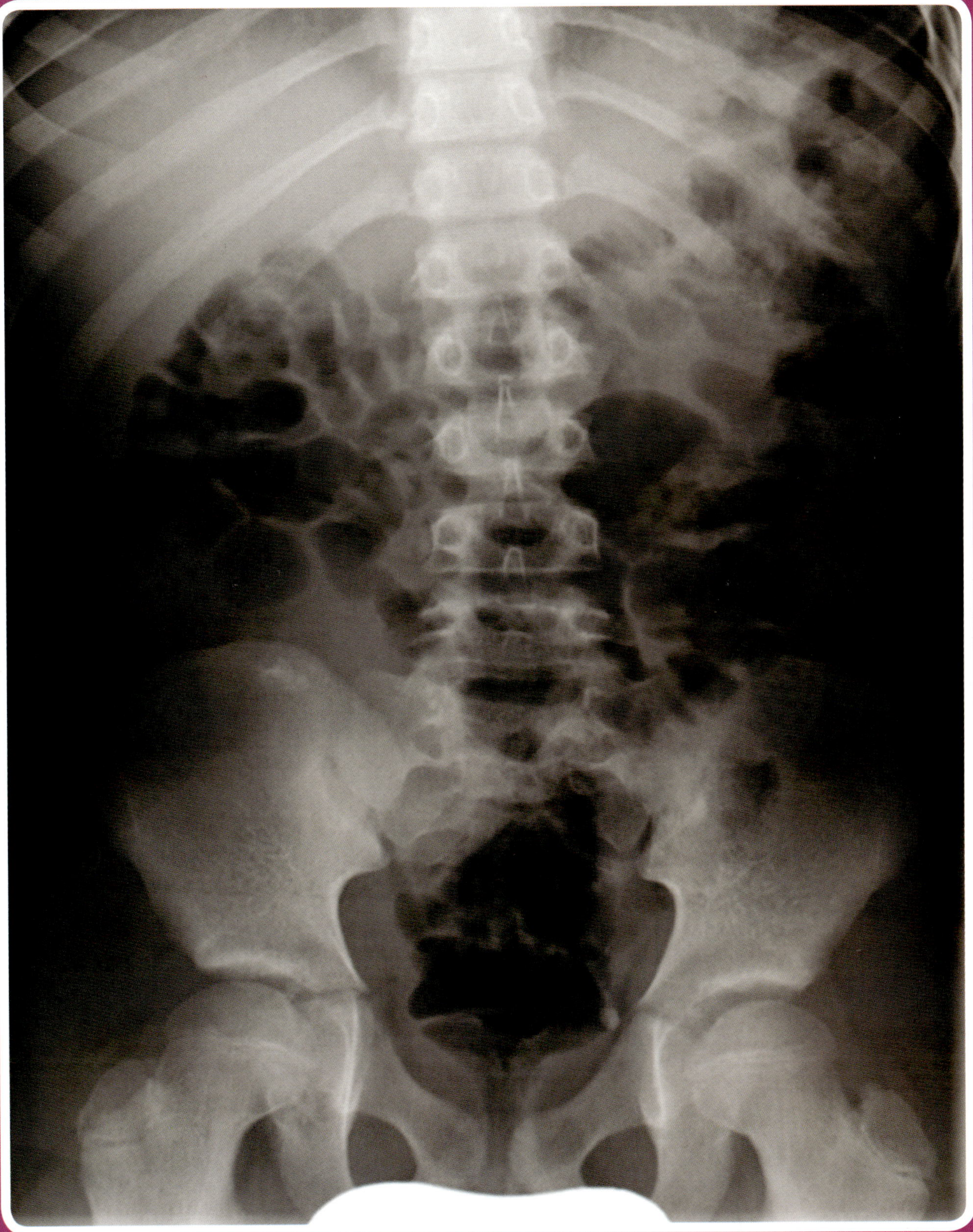

REPORT
Patient ID: Anonymous.
Projection: AP supine.
Rotation: Adequate.
Penetration: Adequate – the spinous processes are visible.
Coverage: Adequate – the anterior ribs are visible superiorly and the inferior pubic rami are visible.

BOWEL GAS PATTERN
The bowel gas pattern is normal.

BOWEL WALL
There is no evidence of mural thickening or intramural gas within the large or small bowel.

PNEUMOPERITONEUM
There is no evidence of free intra-abdominal gas.

SOLID ORGANS
The solid organ contours are within normal limits with no solid organ calcification.

VASCULAR
No abnormal vascular calcification.

BONES
There are no abnormalities of the imaged thoracic and lumbar spine, or within the pelvis.

There are growth plates at the femoral head, greater trochanter and acetabulum as the ossification centres have not yet fused, which is a normal finding in a child of this age.

SOFT TISSUES
The psoas muscle outline is visible bilaterally.

The extra-abdominal soft tissues are unremarkable.

OTHER
There is a radiopaque density projected over the region of the right iliac fossa.

There is a gonadal shield in situ.

There are no vascular lines, drains or surgical clips.

REVIEW AREAS
Gallstones / Renal calculi: No radiopaque calculi.
Lung bases: Normal.
Spine: Normal.
Femoral heads: Normal – growth plates present.

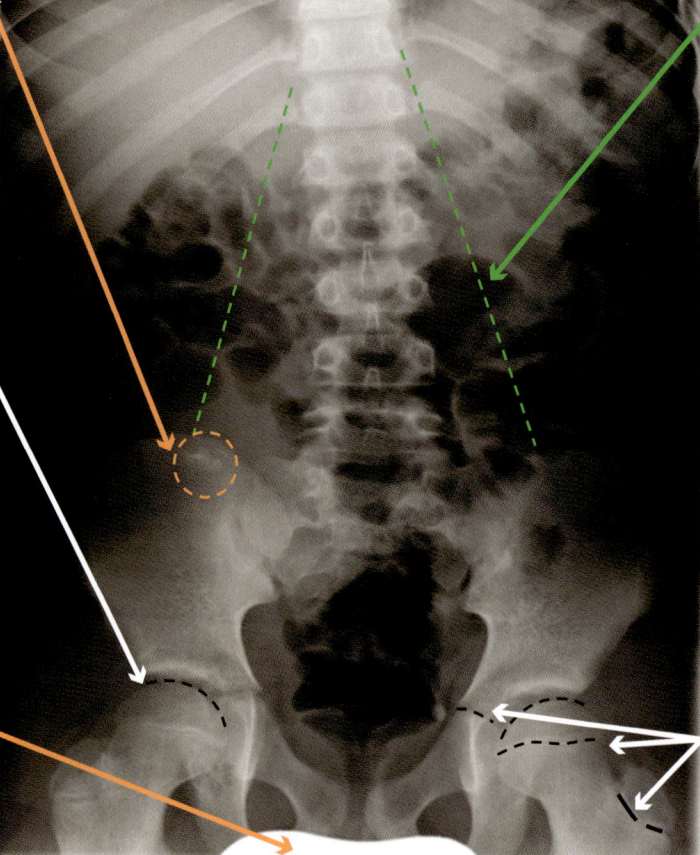

Appendicolith

Psoas muscle outlines

Femoral heads normal

Gonadal shield

Growth plates

SUMMARY
This X-ray demonstrates a radiopaque density projected over the region of the right iliac fossa, in keeping with an appendicolith within the appendix. There is no evidence of bowel obstruction or pneumoperitoneum.

INVESTIGATIONS AND MANAGEMENT
The patient should be resuscitated using an ABCDE approach.

Adequate analgesia and hydration should be provided.

The patient should be made NBM and started on IV fluids.

Urgent bloods should be taken including FBC, U&Es, blood culture, blood gas, coagulation, group and save, and CRP.

The patient should be commenced on broad spectrum antibiotics.

The patient should be referred urgently to the paediatric surgeons for consideration of an appendicectomy.

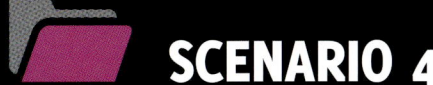

SCENARIO 42

A 3 day old baby boy, currently admitted on SCBU, is acutely unwell and deteriorating rapidly. He was born prematurely at 32 weeks but has been progressing well up until this point. On examination, he has saturations of 96% in room air and a temperature of 38.5°C. His HR is 245 bpm and RR is 68. The abdomen is rigid with tinkling bowel sounds.

An abdominal X-ray is requested to assess for possible necrotising enterocolitis.

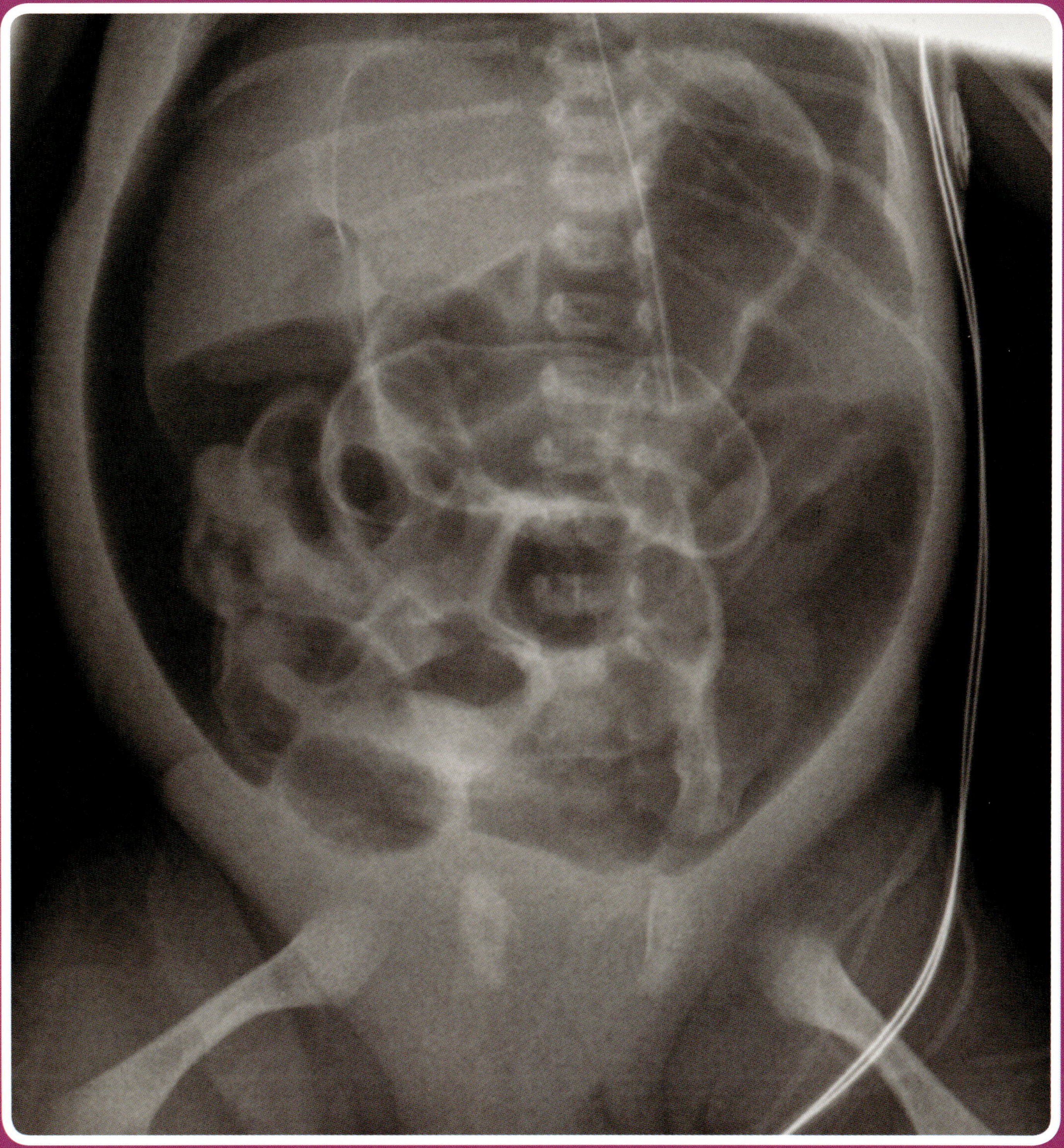

REPORT

Patient ID: Anonymous.
Projection: AP supine.
Rotation: Asymmetrical appearances of the pelvis with deviation of the spine to the left in keeping with patient rotation to the right.
Penetration: Adequate – the spine is visible.
Coverage: Inadequate –the hemidiaphragms have not been included.

BOWEL GAS PATTERN

There are multiple loops of dilated bowel seen centrally within the abdomen. There is no gas within the rectum.

BOWEL WALL

There is no evidence of mural thickening or intramural gas within the large or small bowel.

PNEUMOPERITONEUM

There is evidence of free intra-abdominal gas, in keeping with pneumoperitoneum.

Rigler's sign (double wall sign) can be seen, in keeping with air present on both the luminal and peritoneal sides of the bowel wall.

The falciform ligament sign can be seen, in keeping with a large amount of air present within the abdomen outlining the falciform ligament.

The football sign can be seen, in keeping with a large amount of air present within the abdomen outlining the entire abdominal cavity.

SOLID ORGANS

The liver and falciform ligament are well-outlined by free gas in the abdomen.

VASCULAR

No abnormal vascular calcification.

BONES

There are no abnormalities of the imaged thoracic and lumbar spine, or within the pelvis.

There is cartilage present between the pelvic bones and femurs as they have not yet fused, which is a normal finding in a child of this age.

There is cartilage seen between the vertebrae, which is a normal finding in a child of this age.

SOFT TISSUES

The psoas muscle outline is not seen bilaterally, which is non-specific, particularly in a child of this age.

The extra-abdominal soft tissues are unremarkable.

OTHER

There is an NG tube in situ, although given how straight it is, there is a possibility it has perforated the oesophagus.

There is an electrode and lead external to the patient on the left, in keeping with cardiopulmonary monitoring.

There are no vascular lines, drains or surgical clips.

REVIEW AREAS

Gallstones / Renal calculi: No radiopaque calculi.
Lung bases: Not fully included.
Spine: Normal – cartilage between vertebrae.
Femoral heads: Normal – growth plates present.

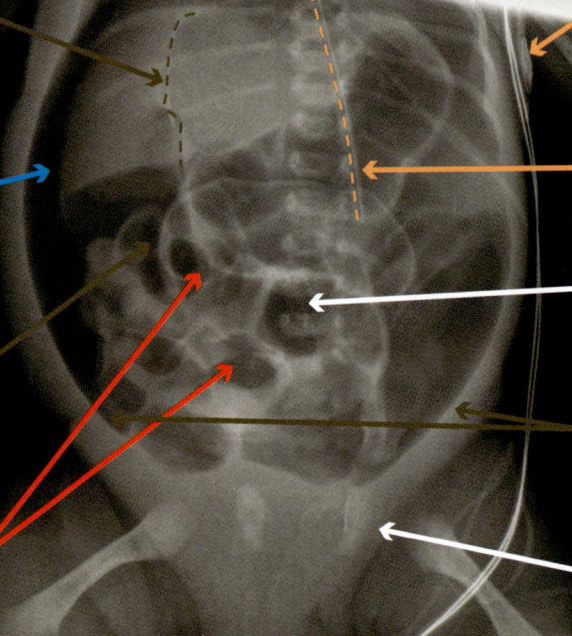

Falciform ligament sign of pneumoperitoneum

Liver outlined by free intra-abdominal gas

Rigler's sign of pneumoperitoneum

Dilated loops of bowel

Electrode for cardiopulmonary monitoring

NG tube

Cartilage between unfused vertebrae

Football sign of pneumoperitoneum

Cartilage between unfused bones

SUMMARY

This X-ray demonstrates multiple loops of dilated bowel throughout the abdomen with evidence of pneumoperitoneum. There is no gas within the rectum. Given the clinical history, the most likely diagnosis is bowel perforation, which may be due to necrotising enterocolitis. The NG tube should be checked to ensure there is a gastric aspirate.

INVESTIGATIONS AND MANAGEMENT

The baby should be resuscitated using an ABCDE approach.

The baby should be started on broad spectrum antibiotics, made NBM and started on IV fluids.

The baby needs to be intubated given the perforation.

Urgent bloods should be taken, including FBC, U&Es, CRP, bone profile, LFTs, coagulation, blood cultures, blood gas, and group and save. A lateral shoot-through AXR would be helpful to confirm perforation, and NG position.

The patient should be referred urgently to the neonatal surgeons for ongoing management.

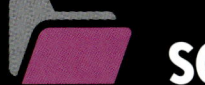

SCENARIO 43

A 14 year old male attends the spinal outpatient clinic for a routine follow up appointment, but is noted to be vomiting. His past medical history is significant for spina bifida occulta. On examination, he has saturations of 99% in room air and a temperature of 37.0°C. His HR is 80 bpm, RR is 15 and blood pressure is 120/72 mmHg. The abdomen is soft but mildly tender with normal bowel sounds.

An abdominal X-ray is requested to assess for possible bowel obstruction.

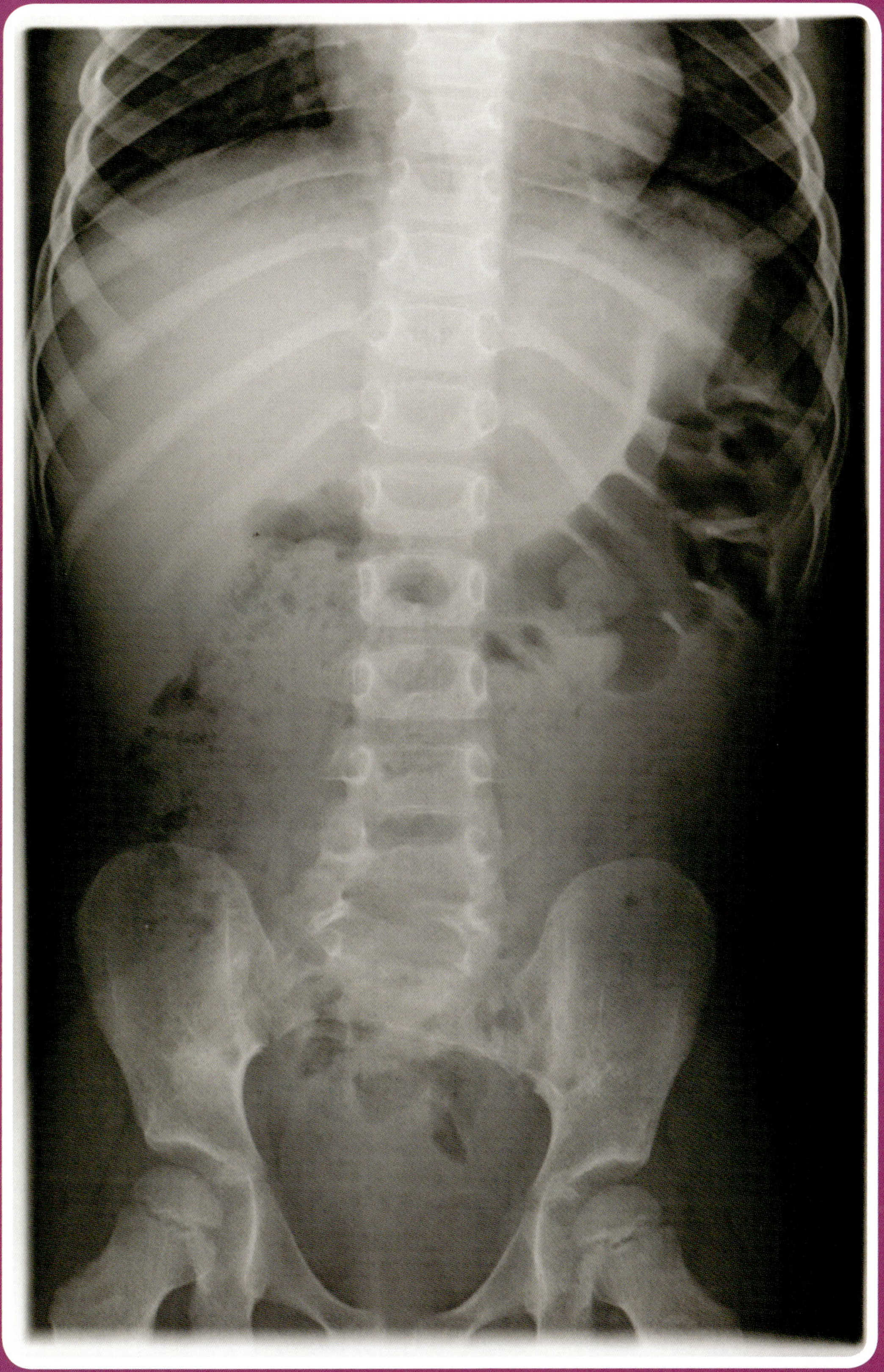

REPORT
Patient ID: Anonymous.
Projection: AP supine.
Rotation: Adequate.
Penetration: Adequate – the spine is visible.
Coverage: Inadequate - the pubic symphysis and inferior pubic rami are not fully included.

BOWEL GAS PATTERN
There is a mild to moderate volume of faecal residue present in the ascending and proximal transverse colon.

BOWEL WALL
There is no evidence of mural thickening or intramural gas within the large or small bowel.

PNEUMOPERITONEUM
There is no evidence of free intra-abdominal gas.

SOLID ORGANS
The solid organ contours are within normal limits with no solid organ calcification.

VASCULAR
No abnormal vascular calcification.

BONES
There is a lateral hemivertebra segmentation anomaly present at the level of L5, however no associated scoliosis.

There is lumbarisation of S1.

There are growth plates at the femoral head and acetabulum (triradiate cartilage) as the ossification centres have not yet fused, which is a normal finding in a child of this age.

SOFT TISSUES
The psoas muscle outline is visible bilaterally.

The extra-abdominal soft tissues are unremarkable.

OTHER
There are no radiopaque foreign bodies.

There are no vascular lines, drains or surgical clips.

REVIEW AREAS
Gallstones / Renal calculi: No radiopaque calculi.
Lung bases: Normal.
Spine: Normal.
Femoral heads: Normal – growth plates present.

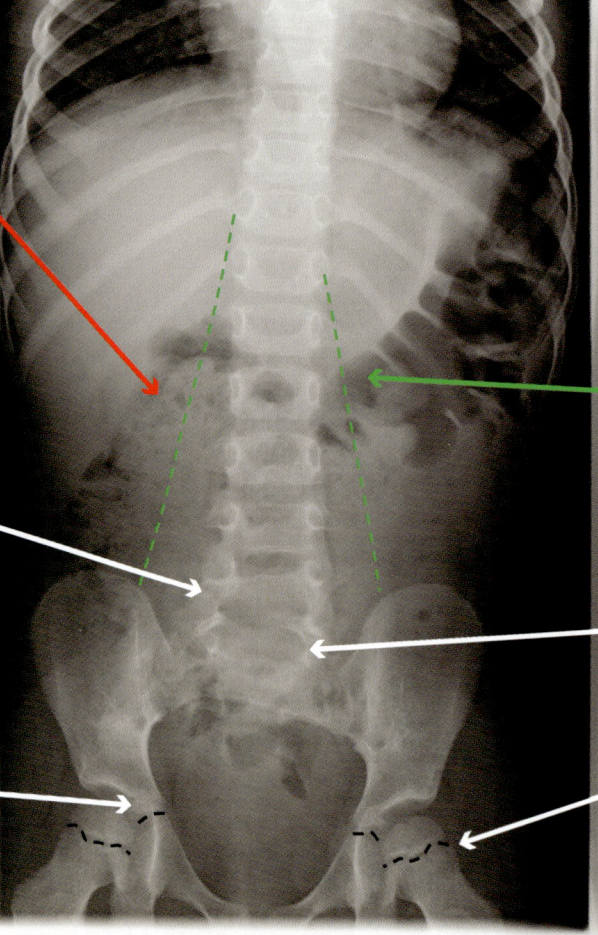

Faecal residue in the ascending and proximal transverse colon

Psoas muscle outlines

L5 hemivertebra

Lumbarisation of S1

Triradiate cartilage

Growth plates

SUMMARY
This X-ray demonstrates mild to moderate volume of faecal residue in the ascending and proximal transverse colon. There is an L5 hemivertebra, in keeping with the patient's background history of spina bifida occulta, and lumbarisation of S1.

INVESTIGATIONS AND MANAGEMENT
If the patient is otherwise well, no further investigation or imaging is required at present. If the patient is clinically constipated, current medications should be reviewed and laxatives considered. Advice should be given regarding lifestyle adjustments, including adequate fluid intake, sufficient dietary fibre and exercise if clinically appropriate.

SCENARIO 44

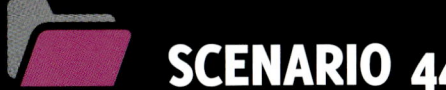

A 70 year old male has recently had an abdominal aortic aneurysm repaired, but is otherwise well and is a non smoker. On examination, he has saturations of 99% in room air and a temperature of 37.0°C. His HR is 70 bpm, RR is 18 and blood pressure is 120/72 mmHg. The abdomen is soft but mildly tender with normal bowel sounds.

You are given his post operative X-ray to review.

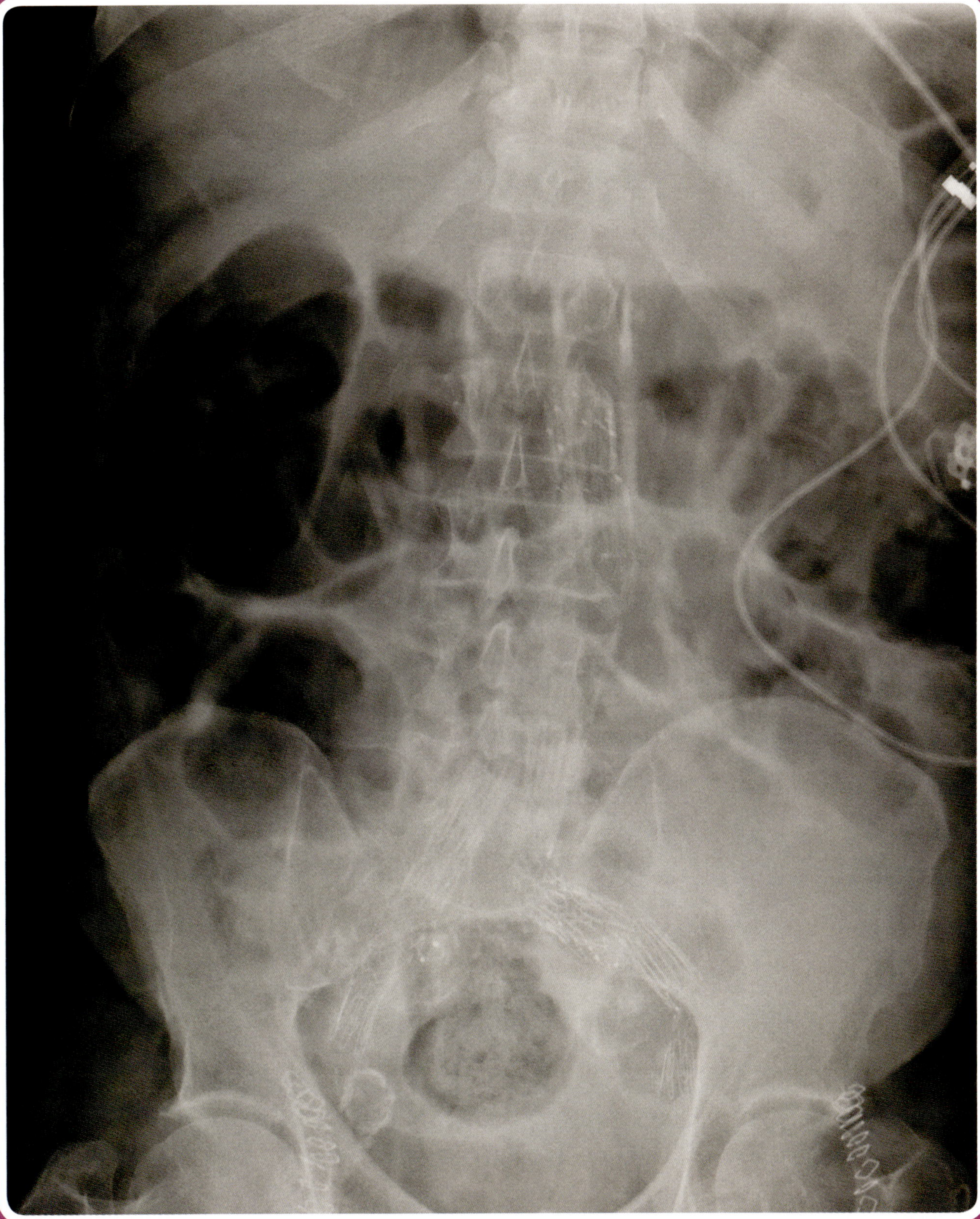

REPORT – ENDOVASCULAR ILIAC BRANCH AORTIC STENT

REPORT
Patient ID: Anonymous.
Projection: AP supine.
Rotation: Asymmetrical appearances of the pelvis in keeping with mild patient rotation.
Penetration: Adequate.
Coverage: Inadequate – inferior pubic rami not included.

BOWEL GAS PATTERN
There is a prominent transverse colon loop however no significant dilatation.

BOWEL WALL
There is no evidence of mural thickening or intramural gas within the large or small bowel.

PNEUMOPERITONEUM
There is no evidence of free intra-abdominal gas.

SOLID ORGANS
The solid organ contours are within normal limits with no solid organ calcification.

VASCULAR
There is a fenestrated endovascular iliac branch aortic stent seen within the abdominal aorta, extending into the common iliac arteries bilaterally.

BONES
There are osteophytes in the spine in keeping with mild degenerative changes.

SOFT TISSUES
The psoas muscle outline is visible bilaterally.

Extra-abdominal soft tissues are unremarkable.

OTHER
There is a radiopaque ECG lead seen external to the patient on the left side.

There are surgical clips projecting over the femoral regions bilaterally.

There are no vascular lines or drains.

REVIEW AREAS
Gallstones / Renal calculi: No radiopaque calculi.
Lung bases: Not fully included.
Spine: Mild degenerative changes.
Femoral heads: Normal.

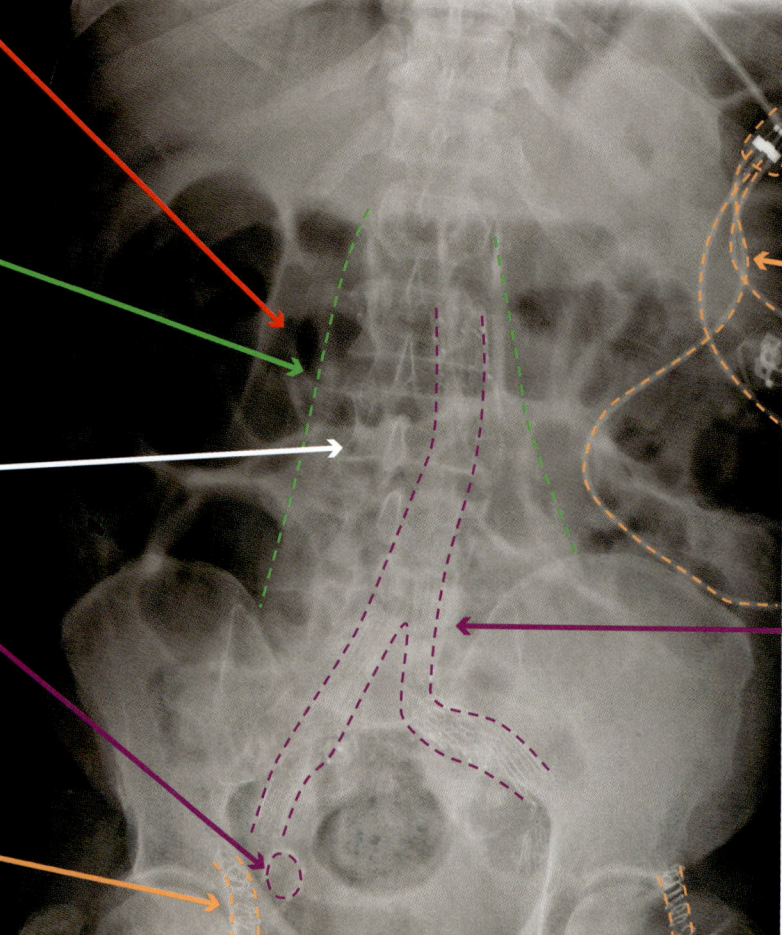

Prominent transverse colon

Psoas muscle outlines

Degenerative changes

Vascular calcification

Surgical clips

External line

Endovascular aortic stent

SUMMARY
There is a fenestrated endovascular iliac branch aortic stent seen within the abdominal aorta, extending into the common iliac arteries bilaterally. The surgical clips projecting over the femoral regions bilaterally are in keeping with the recent endovascular aneurysm repair (EVAR).

INVESTIGATIONS AND MANAGEMENT
The iliac branch aortic stent is appropriately sited, and there are no other abnormalities to report on the AXR.

Ruptured AAA patients should initially be cared for in ICU / HDU, but elective patients may be suitable for ward-level care. It is important to ensure that adequate maintenance fluids are prescribed to limit renal damage following CT contrast. Long term follow up includes monitoring for signs of AAA increasing in size, and ensuring of compliance with medications and optimal lifestyle strategies to minimise cardiovascular risk.

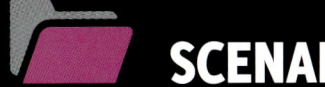

SCENARIO 45

A 64 year old male presents to ED with right iliac fossa pain and lethargy. His past medical history is significant for type II diabetes mellitus and he is a non-smoker. On examination, he has saturations of 95% in air and a temperature of 38.6°C. His HR is 80 bpm, RR is 18 and blood pressure is 120/85 mmHg. The abdomen is soft and there is tenderness in the right iliac fossa with tinkling bowel sounds. Urine dipstick is unremarkable.

An abdominal X-ray is requested to assess for possible bowel obstruction.

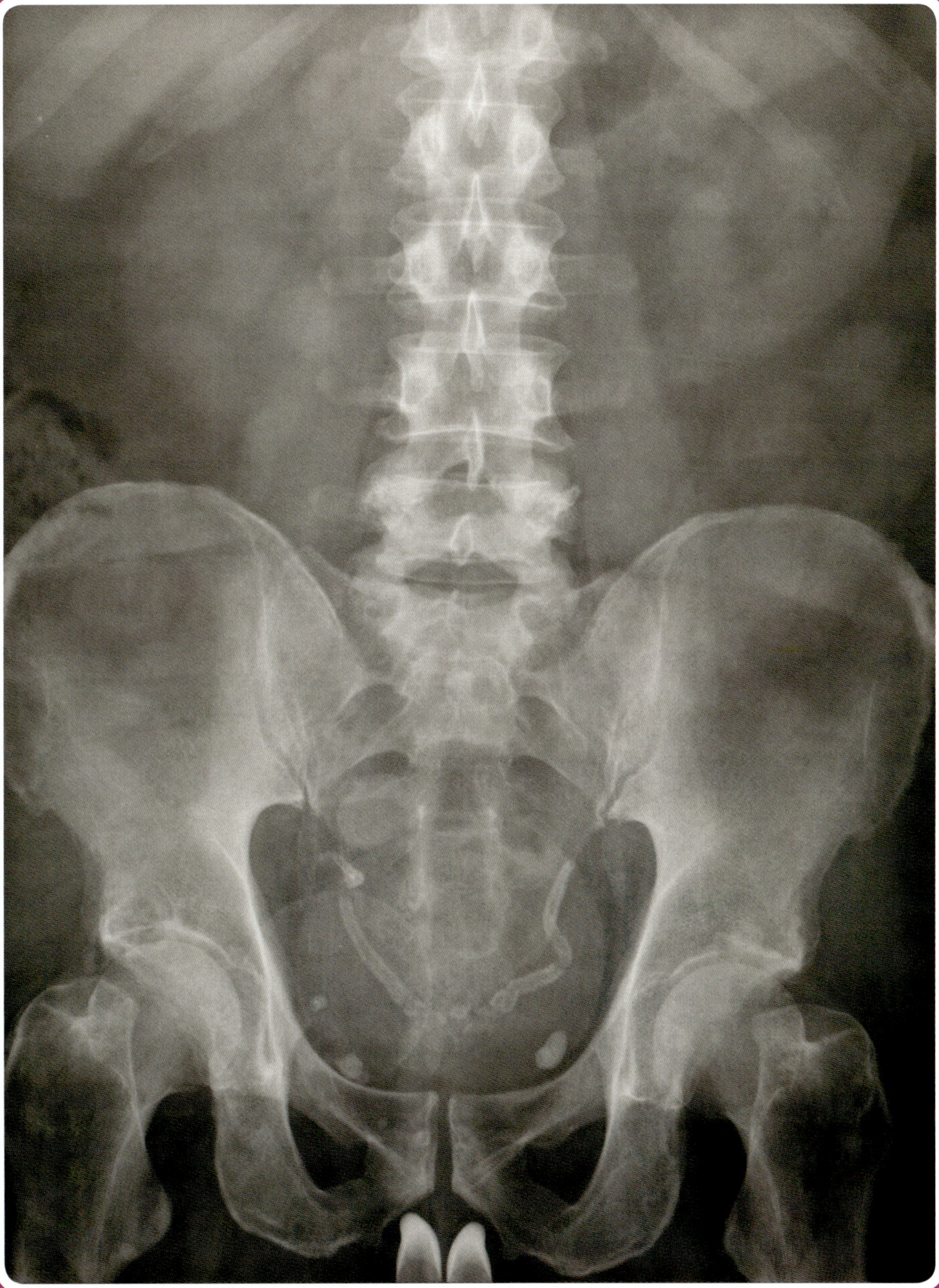

REPORT – DIABETIC PATIENT WITH PENILE IMPLANT

REPORT
Patient ID: Anonymous.
Projection: AP supine.
Rotation: Adequate.
Penetration: Adequate – the spinous processes are visible.
Coverage: Adequate – the anterior ribs are visible superiorly and the inferior pubic rami are visible.

BOWEL GAS PATTERN
The bowel gas pattern is normal.

There is a small volume of faecal residue present in the ascending colon.

BOWEL WALL
There is no evidence of mural thickening or intramural gas within the large or small bowel.

PNEUMOPERITONEUM
There is no evidence of free intra-abdominal gas.

SOLID ORGANS
The solid organ contours are within normal limits with no solid organ calcification.

VASCULAR
No abnormal vascular calcification.

BONES
There are no abnormalities of the imaged lumbar spine, or within the pelvis.

SOFT TISSUES
The psoas muscle outline is visible bilaterally.

The extra-abdominal soft tissues are unremarkable.

OTHER
There are bilateral serpiginous radiopacities projected over the region of the pelvis, which most likely represents vas deferens calcification.

There are several rounded radiopaque densities projected over the region of the pelvis, which most likely represent phleboliths.

There is a penile implant in situ and a penile implant reservoir projecting over the right hemipelvis.

There are no vascular lines, drains or surgical clips.

REVIEW AREAS
Gallstones / Renal calculi: No radiopaque calculi.
Lung bases: Not fully included.
Spine: Normal.
Femoral heads: Normal.

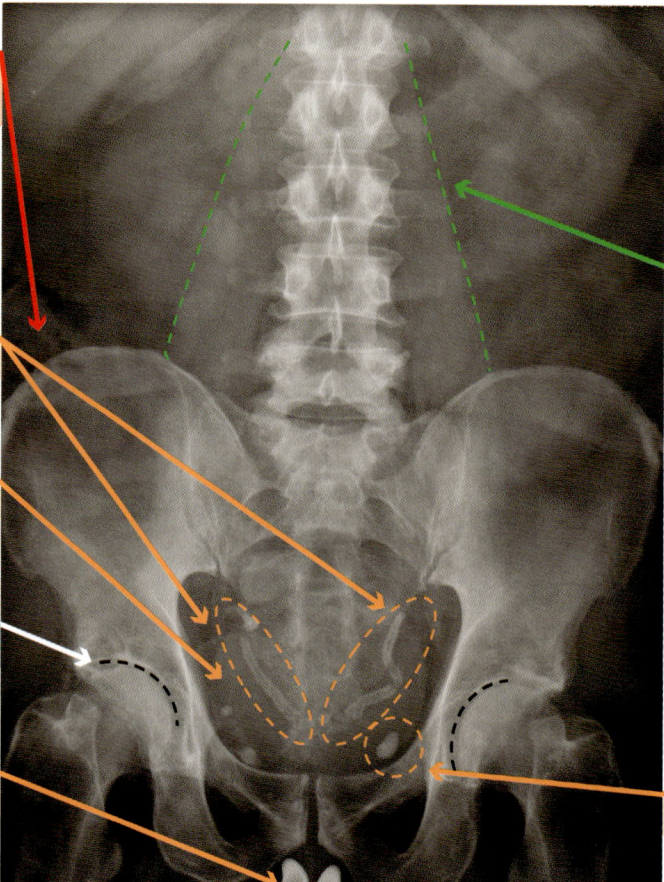

Faecal residue in ascending colon

Calcification of vas deferens

Penile implant reservoir

Femoral heads normal

Penile implant

Psoas muscle outlines

Phleboliths

SUMMARY
This X-ray demonstrates serpiginous calcification bilaterally within the pelvis, in keeping with calcification of the vas deferens. It also demonstrates several rounded calcific densities projected over the region of the pelvis, in keeping with phleboliths (areas of calcification within a vein). The penile implant is an incidental finding, likely related to the patient's diabetes resulting in impotence. There is no evidence of bowel obstruction or pneumoperitoneum.

INVESTIGATIONS AND MANAGEMENT
The patient should be resuscitated using an ABCDE approach.

Adequate analgesia and hydration should be provided.

Bloods should be taken including FBC, U&Es, LFTs, amylase, bone profile, CRP, coagulation, blood gas, blood cultures, and group and save.

A CT scan of the abdomen/pelvis with IV contrast may be considered for further evaluation of the abdomen and surgical input should be sought.

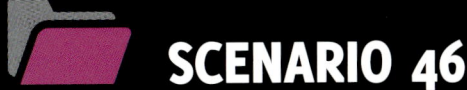
A 21 year old female presents to ED with worsening, repeated episodes of bloody diarrhoea for the past 48 hours. She has no significant past medical history and is a non-smoker. On examination, she has saturations of 98% in room air and a temperature of 37.9°C. Her HR is 104 bpm, RR is 21 and blood pressure is 128/72 mmHg. The abdomen is soft with generalised tenderness and normal bowel sounds. Urine dipstick is unremarkable and a pregnancy test is negative.

An abdominal X-ray is requested to assess for possible colitis.

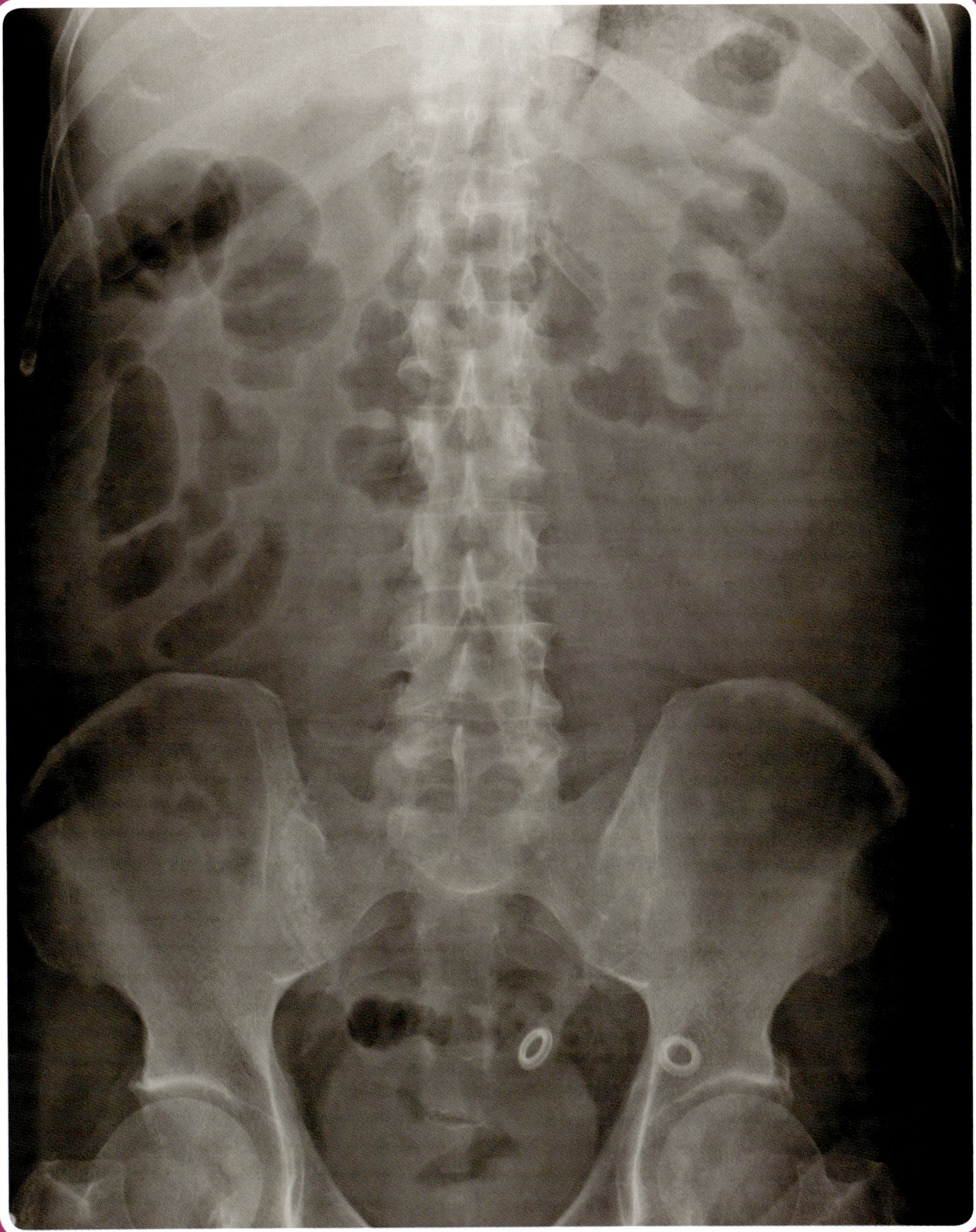

REPORT – COLITIS

REPORT
Patient ID: Anonymous.
Projection: AP supine.
Rotation: Adequate.
Penetration: Adequate – the spinous processes are visible.
Coverage: Inadequate – the pubic symphysis and inferior pubic rami have not been included.

BOWEL GAS PATTERN
The bowel gas pattern is normal.

BOWEL WALL
There is mural thickening of the transverse colon in the left upper quadrant, with loss of the normal colonic haustral folds and evidence of 'thumbprinting', in keeping with mural oedema.

There is no evidence of intramural gas within the large or small bowel.

PNEUMOPERITONEUM
There is no evidence of free intra-abdominal gas.

SOLID ORGANS
The solid organ contours are within normal limits with no solid organ calcification.

VASCULAR
No abnormal vascular calcification.

BONES
There are no abnormalities of the imaged thoracic and lumbar spine, or within the pelvis.

SOFT TISSUES
The psoas muscle outline is visible bilaterally.

The extra-abdominal soft tissues are unremarkable.

OTHER
There are two rounded radiopaque bodies seen projected over the left hemi-pelvis in keeping with clothing artefact.

There are no vascular lines, drains or surgical clips.

REVIEW AREAS
Gallstones / Renal calculi: No radiopaque calculi.
Lung bases: Not fully included.
Spine: Normal.
Femoral heads: Normal.

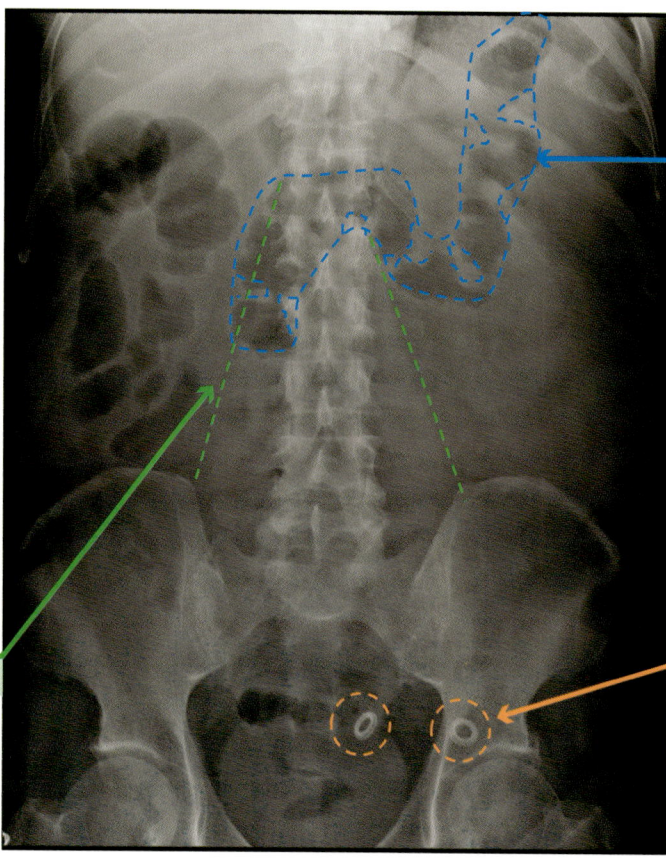

Mural oedema of transverse colon with loss of haustral folds and thumbprinting

Psoas muscle outlines

External foreign bodies

SUMMARY
This X-ray demonstrates mural oedema of the transverse colon, with loss of the normal colonic haustral folds and evidence of thumbprinting, suggestive of colitis. Given the clinical history, this is likely infective or inflammatory in nature.

INVESTIGATIONS AND MANAGEMENT
This patient should be resuscitated using an ABCDE approach.

Adequate analgesia and hydration should be provided.

Urgent bloods should be taken, including FBC, U&Es, LFTs, ESR, CRP, iron studies, folate, blood gas, and group and save. A stool sample should be sent.

Urgent referral to the gastroenterology team should be considered.

A CT scan of the abdomen/pelvis with IV contrast should be considered for better visualisation of the anatomy and to assess for complications such as pneumoperitoneum and abscess formation.

Treatment will depend on the results of further investigations, as well as the clinical state of the patient.

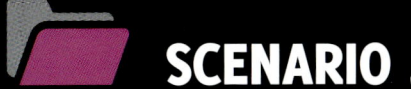

A 20 year old female presents to ED with repeated episodes of bloody diarrhoea that have been getting worse over the past 24 hours. She has no significant past medical history and is a non-smoker. On examination, she has saturations of 98% in room air and a temperature of 39.2°C. Her HR is 88 bpm, RR is 20 and blood pressure is 120/68 mmHg. The abdomen is rigid and there is generalised tenderness with normal bowel sounds. Urine dipstick is unremarkable and a pregnancy test is negative.

An abdominal X-ray is requested as assess for possible bowel obstruction.

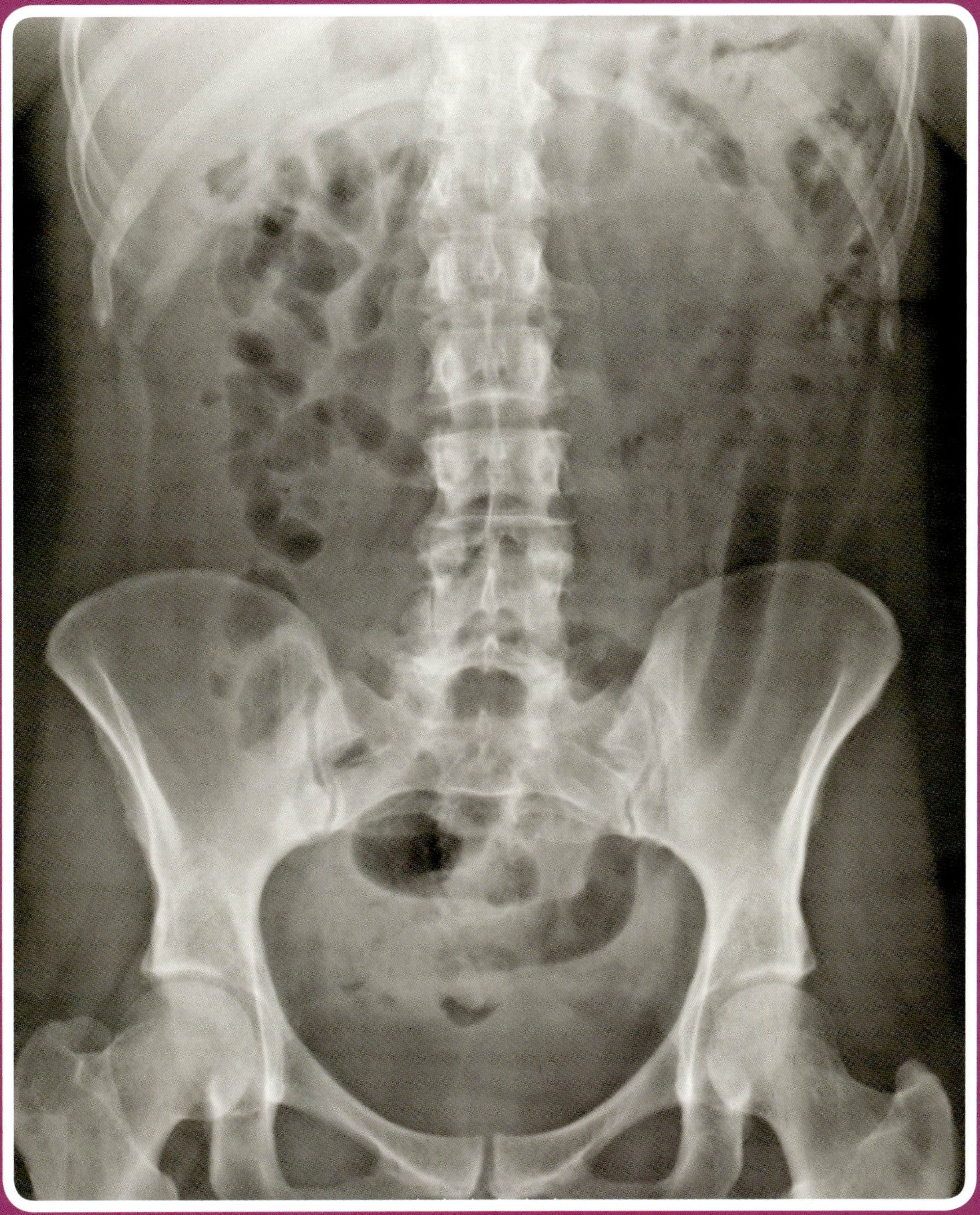

REPORT
Patient ID: Anonymous.
Projection: AP supine.
Rotation: Adequate.
Penetration: Adequate – the spinous processes are visible.
Coverage: Adequate – the anterior ribs are visible superiorly and the pubic rami are visible inferiorly.

BOWEL GAS PATTERN
The bowel gas pattern is normal.

BOWEL WALL
There is evidence of mural thickening within the distal descending and sigmoid colon in the left lower quadrant, with loss of the normal colonic haustral folds,

in keeping with mural oedema. This is termed 'lead pipe colon'.

There is no evidence of intramural gas within the large or small bowel.

PNEUMOPERITONEUM
There is no evidence of free intra-abdominal gas.

SOLID ORGANS
The solid organ contours are within normal limits with no solid organ calcification.

VASCULAR
No abnormal vascular calcification.

BONES
There is lumbarisation of S1, which is a normal anatomical variant. There are no

other abnormalities of the imaged thoracic and lumbar spine, or within the pelvis.

SOFT TISSUES
The psoas muscle outline is visible bilaterally.

The extra-abdominal soft tissues are unremarkable.

OTHER
There are no radiopaque foreign bodies.

There are no vascular lines, drains or surgical clips.

REVIEW AREAS
Gallstones / Renal calculi: No radiopaque calculi.
Lung bases: Not fully included.
Spine: Normal.
Femoral heads: Normal.

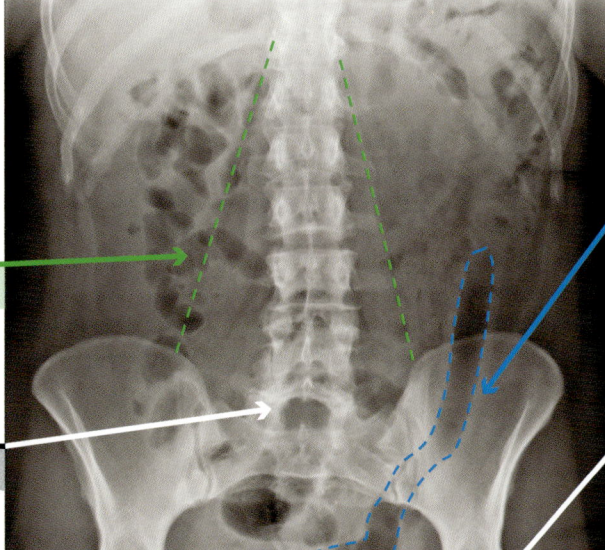

Psoas muscle outlines

Mural oedema of descending and sigmoid colon with loss of haustral folds

Lumbarisation of S1

Femoral heads normal

SUMMARY
This X-ray demonstrates mural oedema of the distal descending and sigmoid colon, with loss of the normal colonic haustral folds. Given the clinical history, these findings are likely secondary to acute colitis which is infective or inflammatory in nature.

INVESTIGATIONS AND MANAGEMENT
This patient should be resuscitated using an ABCDE approach.

Adequate analgesia and hydration should be provided.

Urgent bloods should be taken, including FBC, U&Es, LFTs, ESR, CRP, iron studies, folate, blood gas, and group and save. A stool sample should be sent.

Urgent referral to the gastroenterology team should be considered.

A CT scan of the abdomen/pelvis with IV contrast should be considered for better visualisation of the anatomy and to assess for complications such as pneumoperitoneum and abscess formation.

Treatment will depend on the results of further investigations as well as the clinical state of the patient.

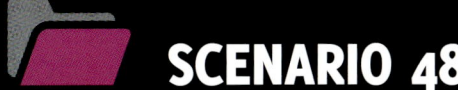

SCENARIO 48

A 17 year old male presents to ED with abdominal pain, vomiting and an inability to bear weight on his left leg. His past medical history is significant for congenital spinal problems and he is a non-smoker. He has a VP shunt in situ and is awaiting a PEG-J tube due to severe reflux. On examination, he has saturations of 99% in room air and a temperature of 36.4°C. His HR is 95 bpm, RR is 23 and blood pressure is 126/69 mmHg. The abdomen is soft with generalised mild tenderness and normal bowel sounds. He is unable to perform any voluntary movements of the back or left hip due to pain.

An abdominal X-ray is requested to assess for the position of the VP shunt, and for possible bowel obstruction.

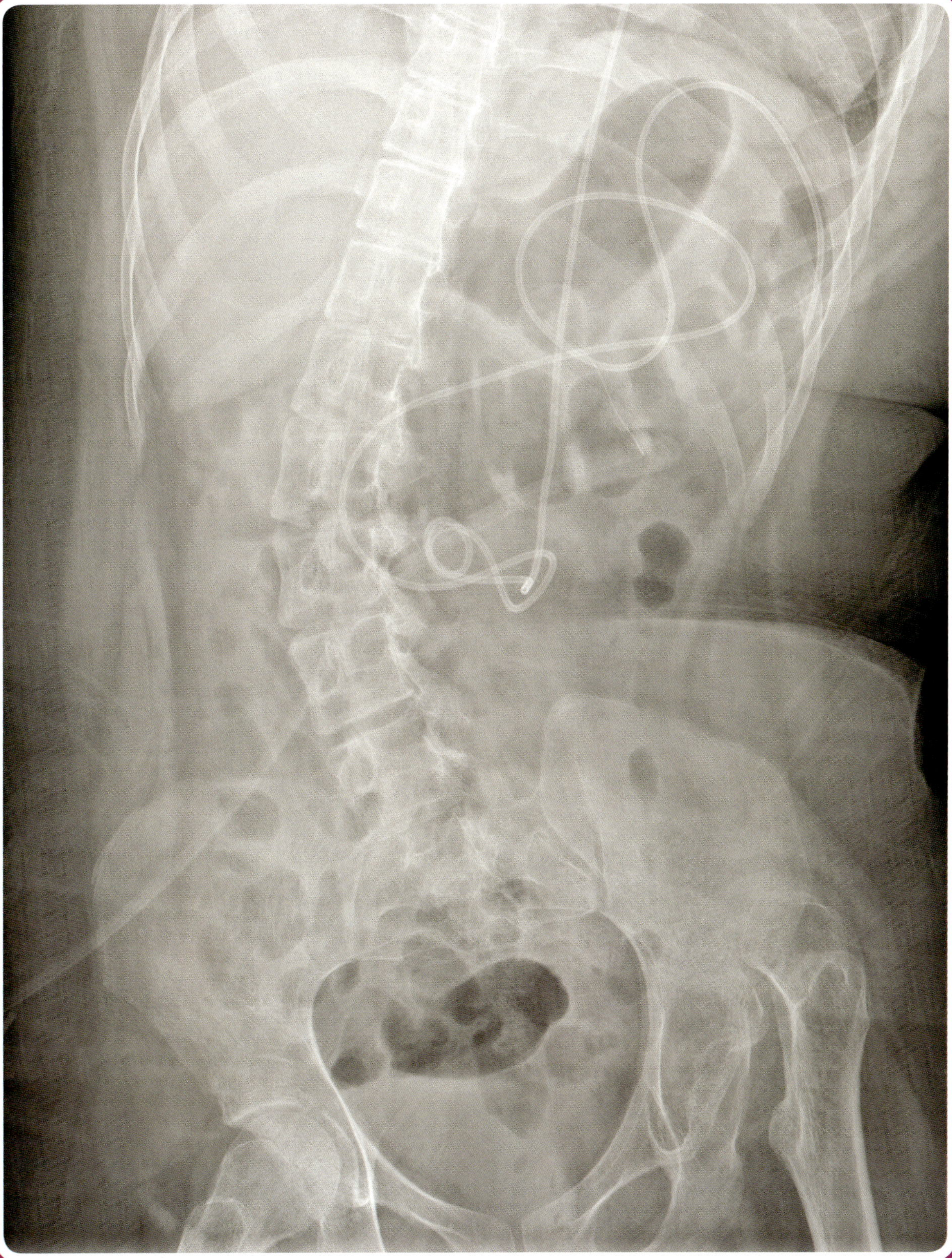

REPORT – SCOLIOSIS AND DISLOCATED LEFT HIP

REPORT
Patient ID: Anonymous.
Projection: AP supine.
Rotation: Adequate.
Penetration: Adequate – the spinous processes are visible.
Coverage: Inadequate – the pubic symphysis and inferior pubic rami have not been fully included.

BOWEL GAS PATTERN
The bowel gas pattern is normal.

BOWEL WALL
There is no evidence of mural thickening or intramural gas within the large or small bowel.

PNEUMOPERITONEUM
There is no evidence of free intra-abdominal gas.

SOLID ORGANS
The solid organ contours are within normal limits with no solid organ calcification.

VASCULAR
No abnormal vascular calcification.

BONES
There is a moderate thoracolumbar scoliosis seen convex to the right, centred on the L2 vertebral body.

There are osteophytes in the lower thoracic and upper lumbar spine with left-sided bridging osteophyte formation.

The left femoral head is abnormally positioned superolaterally to the acetabulum in keeping with a posterior hip dislocation. There is no associated fracture.

SOFT TISSUES
The psoas muscle outline is visible bilaterally.

The extra-abdominal soft tissues are unremarkable.

OTHER
There is a VP shunt in situ, which appears intact with its tip projecting over the left upper quadrant.

There is a radiopaque line seen, which is likely external to the patient, projected across the abdomen of indeterminate significance.

There are no vascular lines, drains or surgical clips.

REVIEW AREAS
Gallstones / Renal calculi: No radiopaque calculi.
Lung bases: Right lung base not fully included.
Spine: Thoracolumbar scoliosis convex to the right, centred on the L2 vertebral body with osteophyte formation and bridging osteophytes on the left.
Femoral heads: The contours of the left hip are abnormal. The acetabulum is shallow and there is superolateral displacement of the left femoral head consistent with a posterior hip dislocation. The femoral head is also dysplastic.

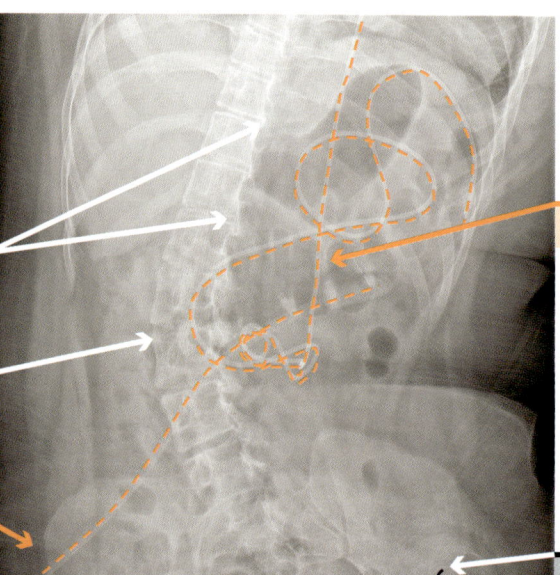

Osteophytes

Scoliosis

External line

VP shunt

Acetabular dysplasia

Deformed left hip dislocation

SUMMARY
This X-ray demonstrates a moderate thoracolumbar scoliosis convex to the right, centred on the L2 vertebral body, bridging osteophyte formation in the lower thoracic and upper lumbar spine, and an associated left hip posterior dislocation, which is likely to be chronic given the dysplasia of the acetabulum and femoral head. There is no evidence of any other significant abnormalities. Note is made of the VP shunt with its tip projecting over the left upper quadrant.

INVESTIGATIONS AND MANAGEMENT
This patient should be resuscitated using an ABCDE approach.

Adequate analgesia should be provided.

Bloods should be taken, including FBC, U&Es, bone profile, LFTs, CRP, coagulation and group and save.

Previous imaging should be reviewed to confirm the age of the hip dislocation, which appears chronic, as well as the scoliosis, and should be discussed with the orthopaedic team.

The patient should be referred to the paediatric team with input from neurosurgery to exclude VP shunt dysfunction.

SCENARIO 49

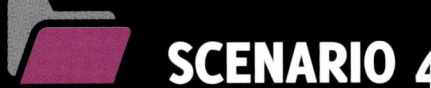

A 2 year old male presents to ED with worsening abdominal pain. His past medical history is significant for faltering growth, for which he is requiring PEG feeding. On examination, he has saturations of 97% in room air and a temperature of 37.2°C. His HR is 152 bpm and RR is 40. The abdomen is soft and there is generalised tenderness with normal bowel sounds. Urine dipstick is unremarkable.

An abdominal X-ray is requested to assess for possible bowel obstruction.

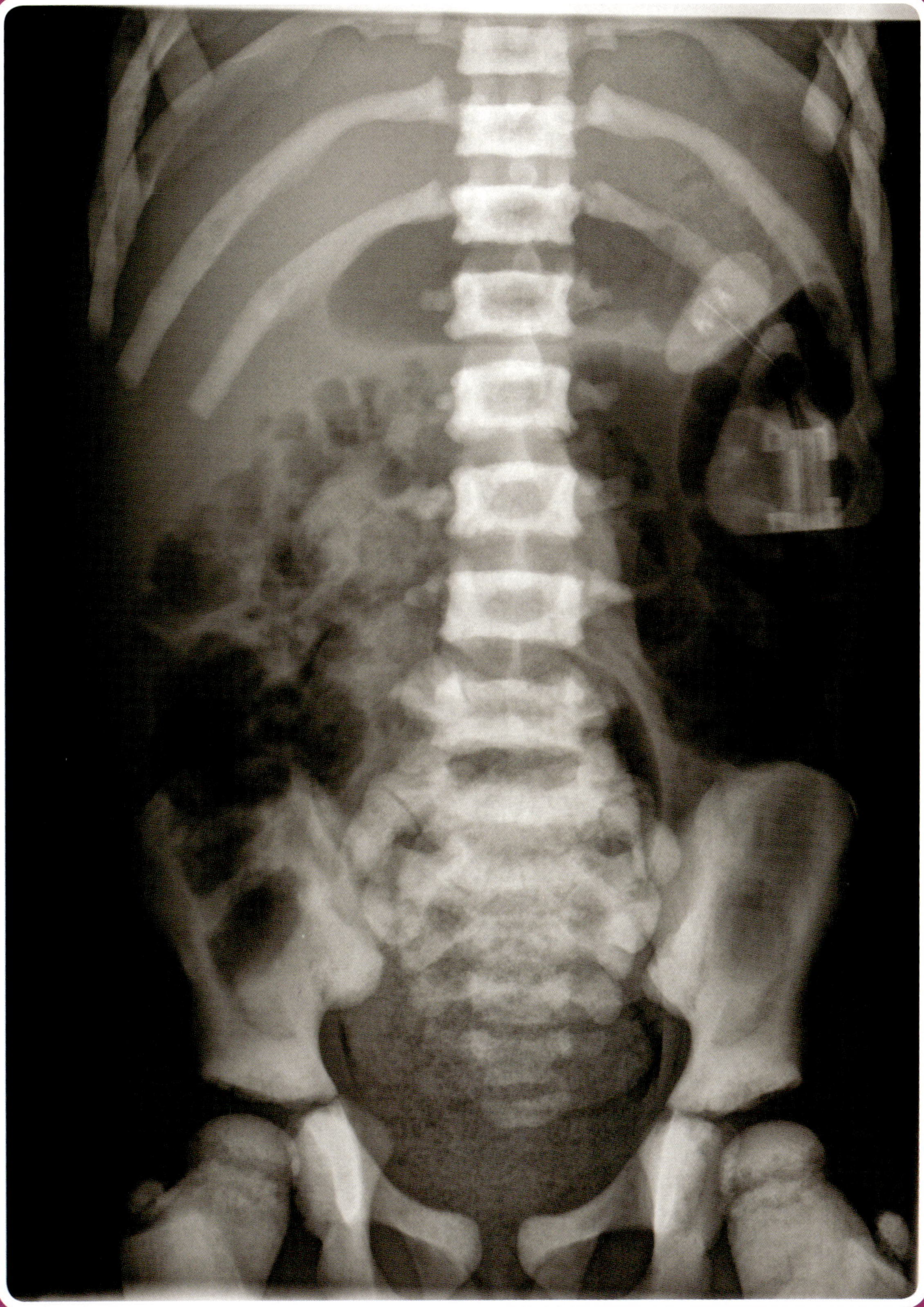

REPORT
Patient ID: Anonymous.
Projection: AP supine.
Rotation: Adequate.
Penetration: Adequate – the spinous processes are visible.
Coverage: Inadequate – the inferior pubic rami have not been fully included.

BOWEL GAS PATTERN
There is a significant volume of faecal residue in the rectum. There is no bowel dilatation.

BOWEL WALL
There is no evidence of mural thickening or intramural gas within the large or small bowel.

PNEUMOPERITONEUM
There is no evidence of free intra-abdominal gas.

SOLID ORGANS
The solid organ contours are within normal limits with no solid organ calcification.

VASCULAR
No abnormal vascular calcification.

BONES
There is homogeneous sclerosis and increased density of the bones diffusely.

The vertebrae demonstrate multi-level subendplate densities with relative central vertebral lucencies in keeping with 'rugger-jersey spine' appearance.

There is metaphyseal splaying of the femoral necks bilaterally.

There are growth plates at the femoral head, greater trochanter and acetabulum as the ossification centres have not yet fused, which is a normal finding in a child of this age.

SOFT TISSUES
The psoas muscle outline is not visible bilaterally, which is non-specific, particularly in a child of this age.

The extra-abdominal soft tissues are unremarkable.

OTHER
There is a port and radiopaque tube projecting over the left upper quadrant, in keeping with a PEG.

There are no vascular lines, drains or surgical clips.

REVIEW AREAS
Gallstones / Renal calculi: No radiopaque calculi.
Lung bases: Not fully included.
Spine: Rugger-jersey appearance.
Femoral heads: Metaphyseal splaying of femoral necks bilaterally and growth plates present.

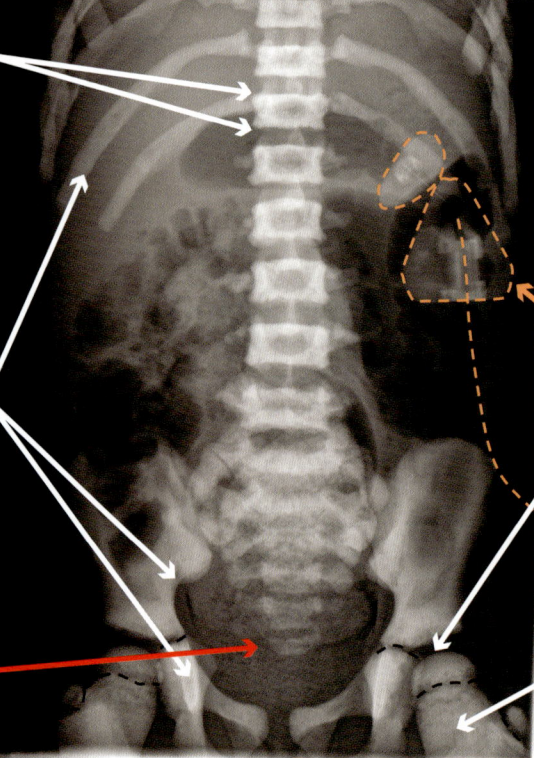

Subendplate sclerosis with relative central lucency – 'rugger-jersey spine'

Sclerosis

Faecal residue in the rectum

PEG

Growth plates

Metaphyseal splaying of femoral necks

SUMMARY
This X-ray demonstrates diffuse increased bone density, a 'rugger-jersey' spine appearance and metaphyseal splaying of the femoral necks bilaterally. Given the clinical history, the most likely diagnosis is osteopetrosis. Note is made of the PEG gastrostomy in the left upper quadrant. There is a significant volume of faecal residue in the rectum, however no evidence of bowel obstruction.

INVESTIGATIONS AND MANAGEMENT
Adequate analgesia and hydration should be provided.

Bloods should be taken, including FBC, U&Es, bone profile, LFTs, CRP, blood gas and group and save.

There are no clear findings on the abdominal X-ray to explain the patient's abdominal pain. Surgical input should be sought.

The patient should be referred on to a specialist for further assessment and management of possible osteopetrosis.

Given the complex needs including faltering growth and PEG feeding, the patient is likely to require multidisciplinary team input.

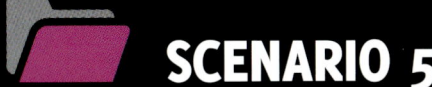

SCENARIO 50

An 80 year old female presents to ED with worsening abdominal distension, nausea and bilious vomiting. Her past medical history is significant for hypertension, osteoarthritis and type II diabetes mellitus. She is a smoker. On examination, she has saturations of 100% in room air and a temperature of 37.2°C. Her HR is 100 bpm, RR is 22 and blood pressure is 145/90 mmHg. The abdomen is rigid with generalised tenderness and tinkling bowel sounds. Urine dipstick is unremarkable.

An abdominal X-ray is requested to assess for possible bowel obstruction.

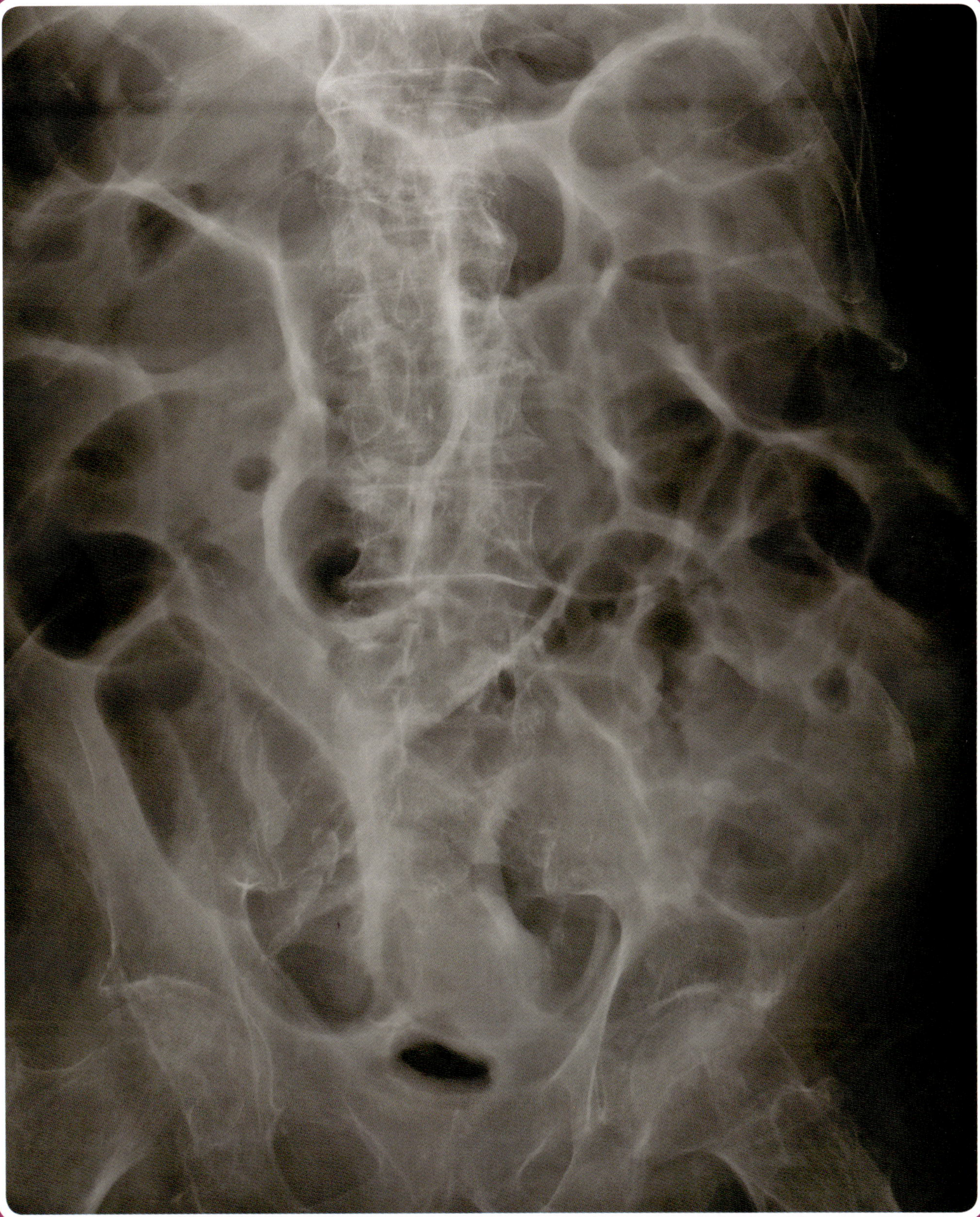

REPORT – MIXED SMALL AND LARGE BOWEL OBSTRUCTION

REPORT
Patient ID: Anonymous.
Projection: AP supine.
Rotation: Adequate.
Penetration: Adequate – the spinous processes are visible.
Coverage: Adequate – the anterior ribs are visible superiorly and the inferior pubic rami are visible.

BOWEL GAS PATTERN
There are multiple loops of dilated small and large bowel seen centrally and peripherally within the abdomen, in keeping with bowel obstruction.

BOWEL WALL
There is no evidence of mural thickening or intramural gas within the large or small bowel.

PNEUMOPERITONEUM
There is no evidence of free intra-abdominal gas.

SOLID ORGANS
The solid organ contours are within normal limits with no solid organ calcification.

VASCULAR
There is calcification of the right femoral artery and iliac arteries bilaterally.

BONES
There is moderate to severe degenerative change with osteophyte formation and intervertebral disc space narrowing seen throughout the spine.

There is moderate osteoarthritic change seen within both hip joints, including subchondral sclerosis and narrowing of the joint spaces.

There is diffuse osteopenia of the bones.

SOFT TISSUES
The psoas muscle outline is not visible bilaterally, which is non-specific.

The extra-abdominal soft tissues are unremarkable.

OTHER
There are no radiopaque foreign bodies.

There are no vascular lines, drains or surgical clips.

REVIEW AREAS
Gallstones / Renal calculi: No radiopaque calculi.
Lung bases: Not fully included.
Spine: Moderate to severe degenerative change.
Femoral heads: Moderate degenerative change.

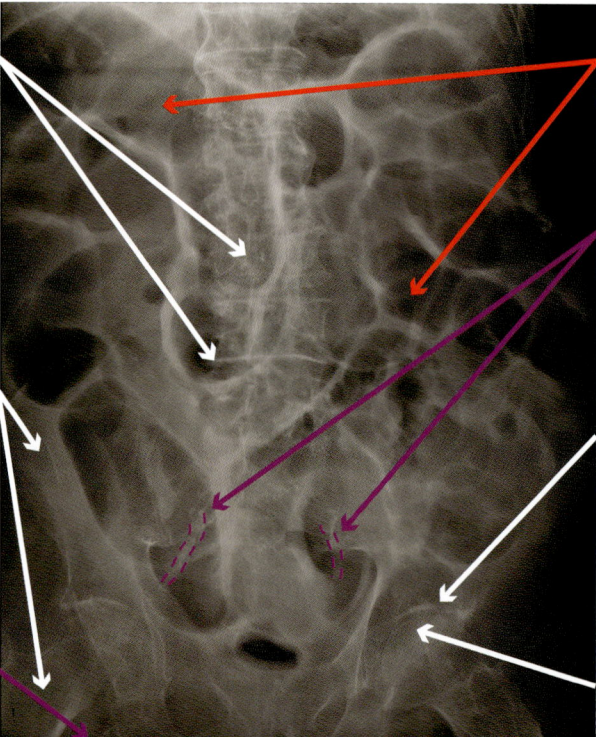

Degenerative change in the spine

Bowel dilatation

Calcified iliac arteries

Diffuse osteopenia

Subchondral sclerosis

Calcified femoral artery

Joint space narrowing

SUMMARY
This X-ray demonstrates multiple loops of dilated small and large bowel seen centrally and peripherally within the abdomen, in keeping with bowel obstruction. This is an open-loop obstruction. No cause for this is visible on the X-ray. The moderate to severe degenerative spinal changes, bilateral moderate hip joint degenerative changes and diffuse osteopaenia are incidental findings.

INVESTIGATIONS AND MANAGEMENT
The patient should be resuscitated using an ABCDE approach.

Adequate analgesia and hydration should be provided.

The patient should be kept NBM and an NG tube inserted on free drainage to relieve the pressure in the small bowel. IV fluids should be commenced.

Urgent bloods should be taken, including FBC, U&Es, CRP, bone profile, LFTs, coagulation, blood gas, and group and save.

The general surgical team should be contacted urgently and a CT scan of the abdomen/pelvis with IV contrast should be considered for better visualisation of the anatomy and further assessment.

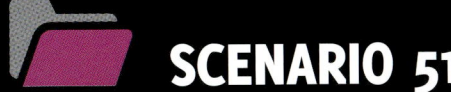
A 75 year old female presents to ED with worsening bone pain and abdominal pain, having not opened her bowels for 5 days. Her past medical history is significant for renal cell carcinoma (awaiting surgery) and she is a non-smoker. On examination, she has saturations of 95% in room air and a temperature of 37.1°C. Her HR is 88 bpm, RR is 19 and blood pressure is 130/75 mmHg. The abdomen is soft and non-tender with normal bowel sounds. Urine dipstick is unremarkable.

An abdominal X-ray is requested to assess for possible bowel obstruction.

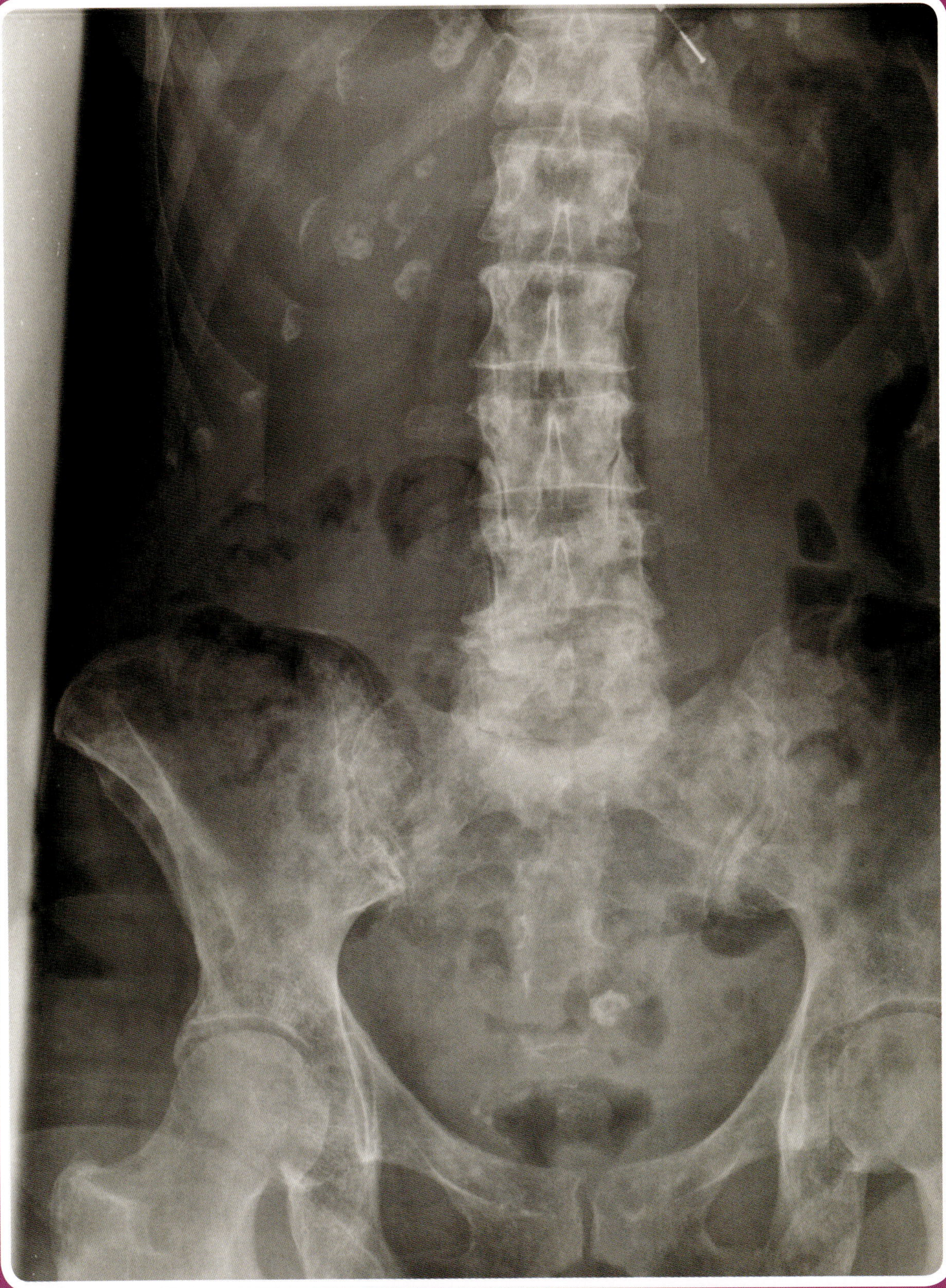

REPORT
Patient ID: Anonymous.
Projection: AP supine.
Rotation: Adequate.
Penetration: Adequate – the spinous processes are visible.
Coverage: Inadequate – the lateral aspect of the left ilium and inferior pubic rami have not been included.

BOWEL GAS PATTERN
There is mild volume of faecal residue predominantly in the ascending colon.

BOWEL WALL
There is no evidence of mural thickening or intramural gas within the large or small bowel.

PNEUMOPERITONEUM
There is no evidence of free intra-abdominal gas.

SOLID ORGANS
The solid organ contours are within normal limits with no solid organ calcification.

VASCULAR
No abnormal vascular calcification.

BONES
There are multiple mixed lytic/sclerotic bone lesions throughout the axial skeleton, including in the spine and the pelvis bilaterally.

There are moderate degenerative changes in the distal lumbar spine.

There is bilateral costochondral calcification.

SOFT TISSUES
The psoas muscle outline is visible bilaterally.

The extra-abdominal soft tissues are unremarkable.

OTHER
There is a cardiac pacing lead projecting to the left of the T12 vertebral body likely within the right ventricle.

There is an area of calcification projecting within the pelvis likely to represent mesenteric lymph node calcification.

There are no vascular lines, drains or surgical clips.

REVIEW AREAS
Gallstones / Renal calculi: No radiopaque calculi.
Lung bases: Not fully included.
Spine: Mixed lytic/sclerotic spinal lesions with moderate degenerative changes in the distal lumbar spine.
Femoral heads: Multiple lytic bone lesions.

Costochondral calcification

Degenerative changes

Faecal residue in ascending colon

Pacemaker lead

Mixed lytic/sclerotic bone lesions

Calcification in pelvis

SUMMARY
This X-ray demonstrates multiple mixed lytic/sclerotic bone lesions throughout the degenerative axial skeleton likely to represent metastases secondary to the renal cell carcinoma. There is no evidence of bowel obstruction or pneumoperitoneum. Incidental note is made of the cardiac pacing wire.

INVESTIGATIONS AND MANAGEMENT
The patient should be resuscitated using an ABCDE approach.

Adequate analgesia and hydration should be provided.

Urgent bloods should be taken, including FBC, U&Es, CRP, LFTs, bone profile, blood gas, and tumour markers.

If no recent imaging has been performed, a staging CT scan of the chest, abdomen and pelvis with IV contrast should be considered to assess the known renal cell carcinoma and for disease progression.

The patient should be referred to oncology for further management, which may include biopsy and MDT discussion. Treatment, which may include surgery, radiotherapy, chemotherapy, or palliative treatment, will depend on the outcome of the MDT investigations and the patients' wishes.

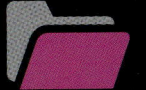

SCENARIO 52

A 25 year old female presents to ED with diarrhoea. Her past medical history is significant for Crohn's disease and she is a non-smoker. On examination, she has saturations of 98% in room air and a temperature of 37.4°C. Her HR is 82 bpm, RR is 14 and blood pressure is 110/60 mmHg. The abdomen is soft and there is generalised tenderness with normal bowel sounds. Urine dipstick is unremarkable and a pregnancy test is negative.

An abdominal X-ray is requested to assess for possible colitis.

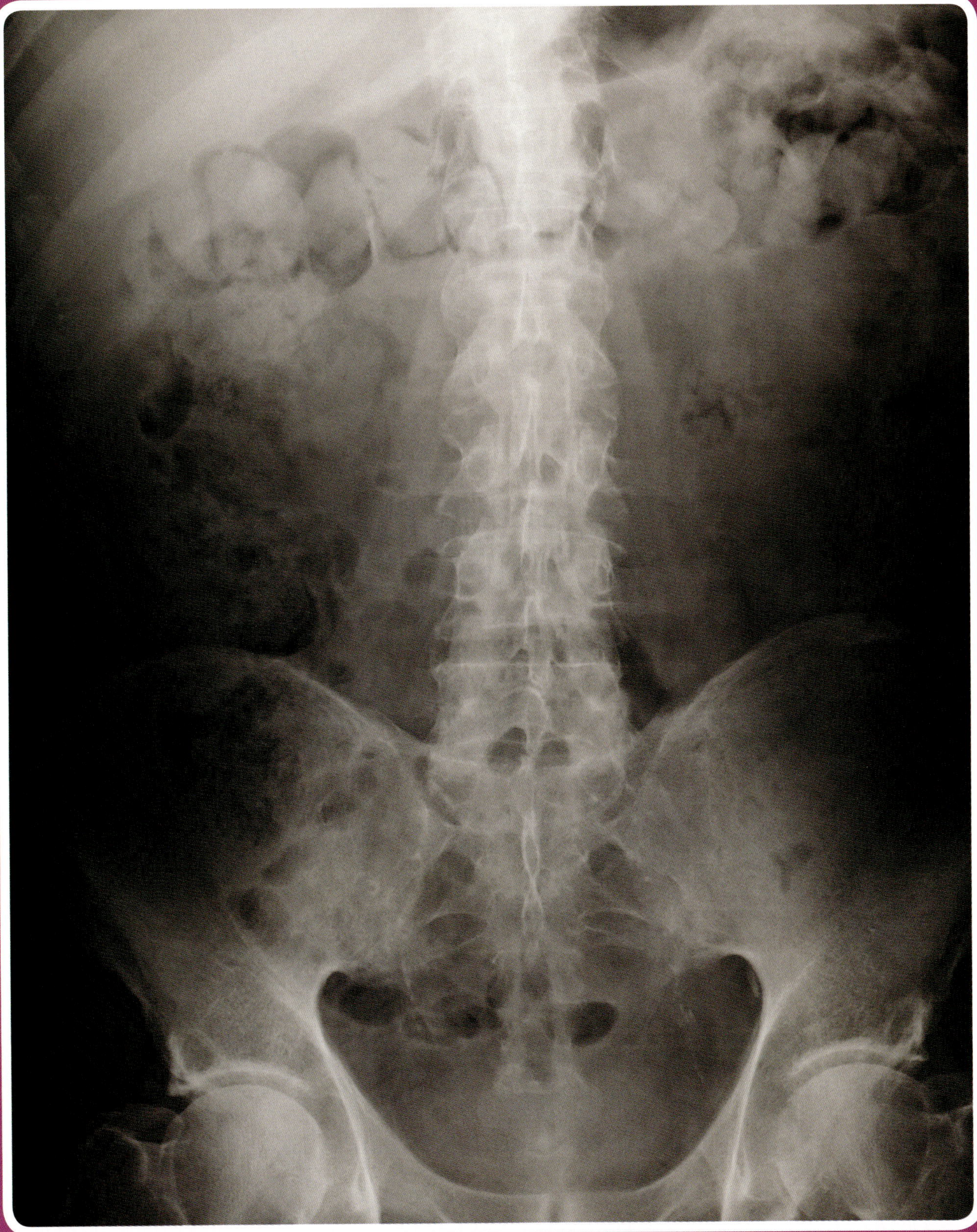

REPORT
Patient ID: Anonymous.
Projection: AP supine.
Rotation: Adequate.
Penetration: Adequate – the spinous processes are visible.
Coverage: Inadequate – the pubic symphysis and inferior pubic rami have not been fully included.

BOWEL GAS PATTERN
The bowel gas pattern is normal.

There is a moderate volume of faecal residue present throughout the ascending colon and hard faeces within the transverse colon.

BOWEL WALL
There is no evidence of mural thickening or intramural gas within the large or small bowel.

PNEUMOPERITONEUM
There is no evidence of free intra-abdominal gas.

SOLID ORGANS
The solid organ contours are within normal limits with no solid organ calcification.

VASCULAR
No abnormal vascular calcification.

BONES
There is fusion of the sacroiliac joints bilaterally.

There are no abnormalities of the imaged thoracic and lumbar spine.

SOFT TISSUES
The psoas muscle outline is visible bilaterally.

The extra-abdominal soft tissues are unremarkable.

OTHER
There are no radiopaque foreign bodies.

There are no vascular lines, drains or surgical clips.

REVIEW AREAS
Gallstones / Renal calculi: No radiopaque calculi.
Lung bases: Not fully included.
Spine: Normal.
Femoral heads: Normal.

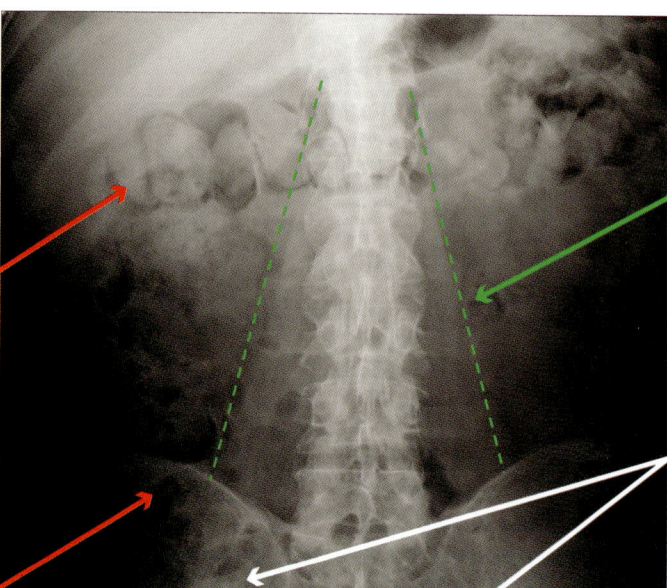

Hard faeces throughout transverse colon

Faecal residue throughout ascending colon

Psoas muscle outlines

Fusion of sacroiliac joints

Femoral heads normal

SUMMARY
This X-ray demonstrates a moderate volume of faecal residue in the ascending colon with hard faeces in the transverse colon, however no evidence of mural oedema or active colitis. Findings may suggest overflow diarrhoea given the clinical history. The bilateral fusion of the sacroiliac joints is an incidental finding and likely related to enteropathic arthritis.

INVESTIGATIONS AND MANAGEMENT
The patient should be resuscitated using an ABCDE approach.

Adequate analgesia and hydration should be provided.

Treatment should aim to disimpact the patient's bowel with either oral laxatives or an enema, and then advice should be given regarding lifestyle adjustments, including adequate fluid intake, sufficient dietary fibre and exercise.

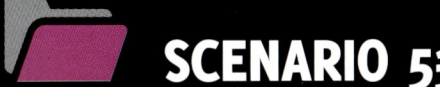

A 42 year old male presents to ED with abdominal distension, night sweats, lymphadenopathy, and weight loss. He is currently undergoing investigations for this. He is a non-smoker. On examination, he has saturations of 99% in room air and a temperature of 36.2°C. His HR is 80 bpm, RR is 19 and blood pressure is 120/72 mmHg. His abdomen is soft and grossly distended and there is no tenderness. Massive hepatosplenomegaly is detected. Bowel sounds are normal. Urine dipstick is unremarkable.

An abdominal X-ray is requested to assess for possible bowel obstruction.

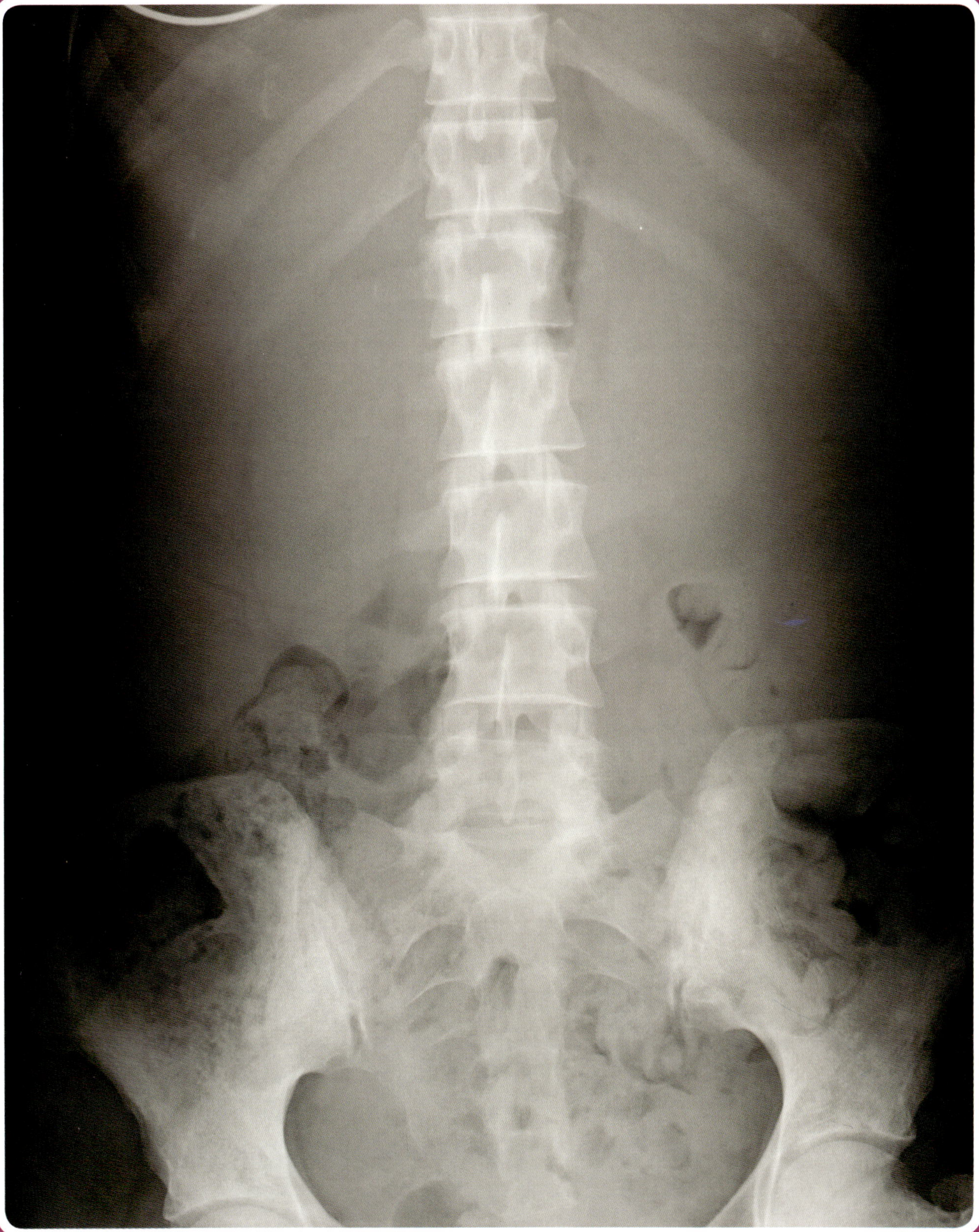

REPORT – HEPATOSPLENOMEGALY

REPORT
Patient ID: Anonymous.
Projection: AP supine.
Rotation: Adequate.
Penetration: Adequate – the spinous processes are visible.
Coverage: Inadequate – the pubic symphysis, inferior pubic rami and hip joints have not been fully included.

BOWEL GAS PATTERN
The bowel is displaced inferiorly into the lower abdomen and pelvis by a homogeneous opacification in the upper abdomen.

There is faecal residue present throughout the large bowel.

BOWEL WALL
There is no evidence of mural thickening or intramural gas within the large or small bowel.

PNEUMOPERITONEUM
There is no evidence of free intra-abdominal gas.

SOLID ORGANS
There is a large homogeneous opacification projecting across the upper abdomen bilaterally, in keeping with massive hepatosplenomegaly.

VASCULAR
No abnormal vascular calcification.

BONES
There are no abnormalities of the imaged thoracic and lumbar spine.

SOFT TISSUES
The psoas muscle outline is visible bilaterally.

The extra-abdominal soft tissues are unremarkable.

OTHER
There is a radiopaque line projected over the region of the right upper quadrant, likely representing an external line.

There are no vascular lines, drains or surgical clips.

REVIEW AREAS
Gallstones / Renal calculi: No radiopaque calculi.
Lung bases: Not fully included.
Spine: Normal.
Femoral heads: Not visible.

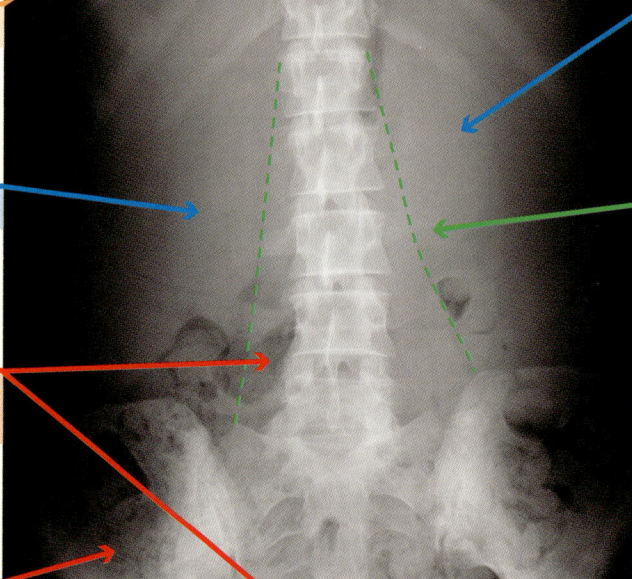

External line

Enlarged spleen

Enlarged liver

Psoas muscle outlines

Inferior displacement of large bowel towards the pelvis

Faecal residue throughout large bowel

SUMMARY
This X-ray demonstrates a large homogeneous opacification in the upper abdomen causing inferior displacement of the bowel into the lower abdomen and pelvis, in keeping with massive hepatosplenomegaly.

INVESTIGATIONS AND MANAGEMENT
The patient should be resuscitated using an ABCDE approach.

Adequate analgesia and hydration should be provided.

Urgent bloods should be taken, including FBC, U&Es, CRP, ESR, LFTs, bone profile, LDH, Hepatitis screening, cytomegalovirus (CMV) and Epstein-Barr virus (EBV) screening, clotting, tumour markers, blood gas, and blood film.

An USS of the abdomen should be considered in the first instance to image the liver and spleen more clearly, and to assess for any associated portal hypertension.

A CT scan of the chest, abdomen and pelvis with IV contrast should be considered for further evaluation and to assess for nodal enlargement elsewhere.

Depending on the above results, a referral to haematology and/or oncology services should be considered for further management, which may include biopsy and MDT discussion. Treatment, which may include surgery, radiotherapy, chemotherapy, or palliative treatment, will depend on the outcome of the MDT, investigations and the patient's wishes.

SCENARIO 54

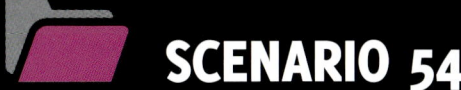

A 12 day old baby boy born at 34 weeks presents to ED with abdominal distension and vomiting. He has not opened his bowels for over 24 hours. He has no significant past medical history. On examination, he has saturations of 97% in room air and a temperature of 37.0°C. His HR is 220 bpm and RR is 62. The abdomen is soft and a hernia is noted in the left groin. Urine dipstick is unremarkable.

An abdominal X-ray is requested to assess for possible bowel obstruction.

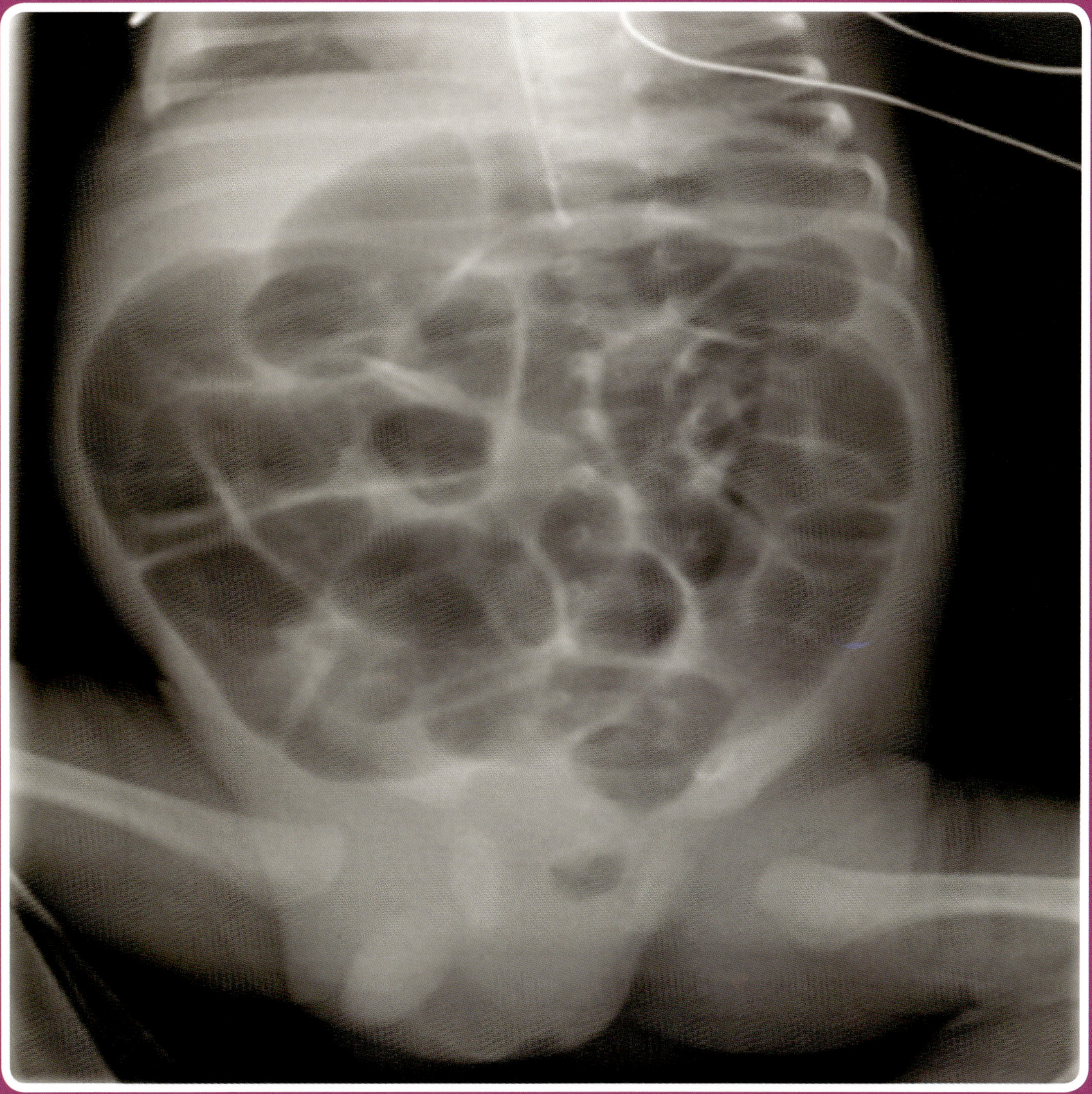

REPORT – LEFT INGUINAL HERNIA WITH BOWEL OBSTRUCTION

REPORT
Patient ID: Anonymous.
Projection: AP supine – frog leg lateral view.
Rotation: Asymmetrical appearances of the pelvis with deviation of the spine to the left due to patient rotation to the right.
Penetration: Adequate – the spine is visible.
Coverage: Adequate – the anterior ribs are visible superiorly and the inferior pubic rami are visible.

BOWEL GAS PATTERN
There are multiple loops of dilated bowel seen centrally in the abdomen.

There is an air-filled loop of bowel seen within the pelvis in the inguinal region, most likely to represent an incarcerated inguinal hernia.

BOWEL WALL
There is no evidence of mural thickening or intramural gas within the large or small bowel.

PNEUMOPERITONEUM
There is no evidence of free intra-abdominal gas.

SOLID ORGANS
The solid organ contours are within normal limits with no solid organ calcification.

VASCULAR
No abnormal vascular calcification.

BONES
The spine appears to be deviated to the left which is due to the rotation of the patient to the right.

There is cartilage present between the pelvic bones and femurs as they have not yet fused, which is a normal finding in a child of this age.

SOFT TISSUES
The psoas muscle outline is not visible bilaterally, which is non-specific, particularly in a child of this age.

The extra-abdominal soft tissues are unremarkable.

OTHER
There is an NG tube in situ, with its tip seen in the left upper quadrant.

There are radiopaque lines projected over the upper abdomen and chest on the left which likely represent external lines.

There are no vascular lines, drains or surgical clips.

REVIEW AREAS
Gallstones / Renal calculi: No radiopaque calculi.
Lung bases: Normal.
Spine: Deviated to the left, due to the rotation of the patient to the right.
Femoral heads: Normal – growth plates present.

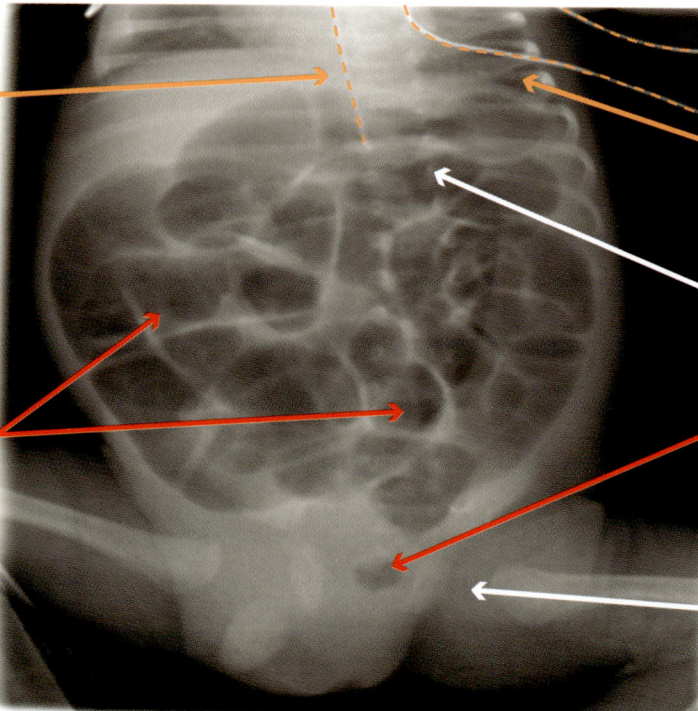

NG tube

External line

Deviated spinal column

Dilated loops of bowel

Incarcerated inguinal hernia

Cartilage between unfused bones

SUMMARY
This X-ray demonstrates multiple loops of dilated bowel seen centrally within the abdomen and an air-filled loop of bowel within the left inguinal region. This is likely to represent bowel obstruction secondary to an incarcerated left inguinal hernia. There is an NG tube in situ but it may be worth advancing to ensure it is in the body of the stomach.

INVESTIGATIONS AND MANAGEMENT
The baby should be resuscitated using an ABCDE approach.

Adequate analgesia and hydration should be provided.

The baby should be started on broad spectrum antibiotics, made NBM and commenced on IV fluids.

Urgent bloods should be taken including FBC, U&Es, blood culture, blood gas, coagulation, group and save, and CRP.

The baby should be referred urgently to the neonatal surgeons for hernia assessment and repair.

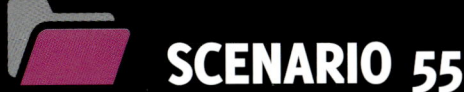

SCENARIO 55

A 48 year old male presents to ED with generalised abdominal pain and abdominal distension. He is unable to pass flatus or open his bowels. He has no significant past medical history and is a smoker. On examination he has saturations of 94% in air and a temperature of 35.9°C. His HR is 104 bpm, RR is 26 and blood pressure is 140/90 mmHg. The abdomen is peritonitic and there are tinkling bowel sounds. Urine dipstick is unremarkable.

An abdominal X-ray is requested to assess for possible bowel obstruction.

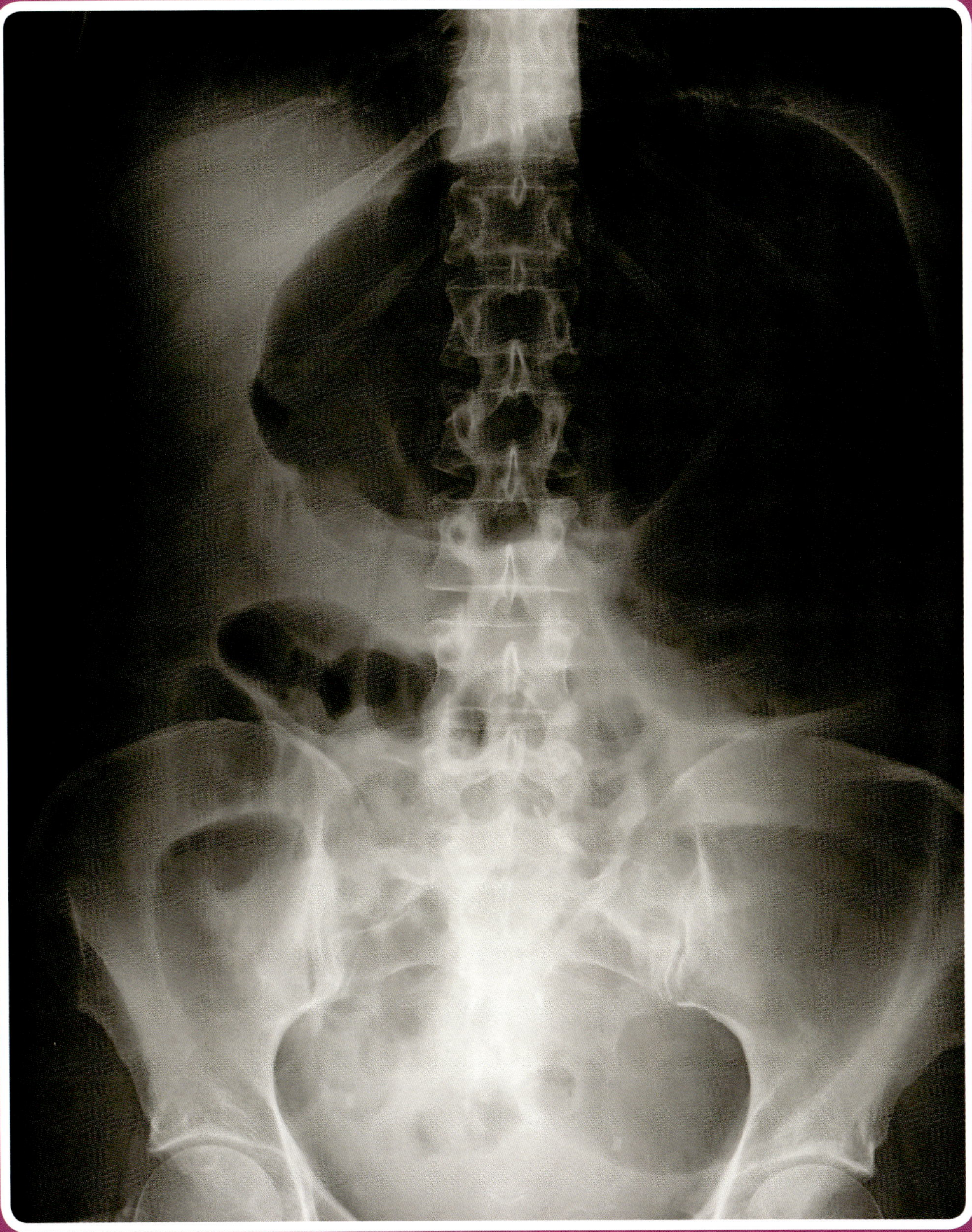

REPORT – CAECAL VOLVULUS

REPORT
Patient ID: Anonymous.
Projection: AP supine.
Rotation: Adequate.
Penetration: Adequate – the spinous processes are visible.
Coverage: Inadequate – the pubic symphysis, inferior pubic rami and hip joints have not been included.

BOWEL GAS PATTERN
The caecum is very distended and in an abnormal position. There are no dilated small bowel loops.

BOWEL WALL
There is no evidence of mural thickening or intramural gas within the large or small bowel.

PNEUMOPERITONEUM
There is no evidence of free intra-abdominal gas.

SOLID ORGANS
The solid organ contours are within normal limits with no solid organ calcification.

VASCULAR
No abnormal vascular calcification.

BONES
There are no abnormalities of the imaged thoracic and lumbar spine, or within the pelvis.

SOFT TISSUES
The psoas muscle outline is not visible on the left side, which is non-specific.

The extra-abdominal soft tissues are unremarkable.

OTHER
There are no radiopaque foreign bodies.

There are no vascular lines, drains or surgical clips.

REVIEW AREAS
Gallstones / Renal calculi: No radiopaque calculi.
Lung bases: Not fully included.
Spine: Normal.
Femoral heads: Normal.

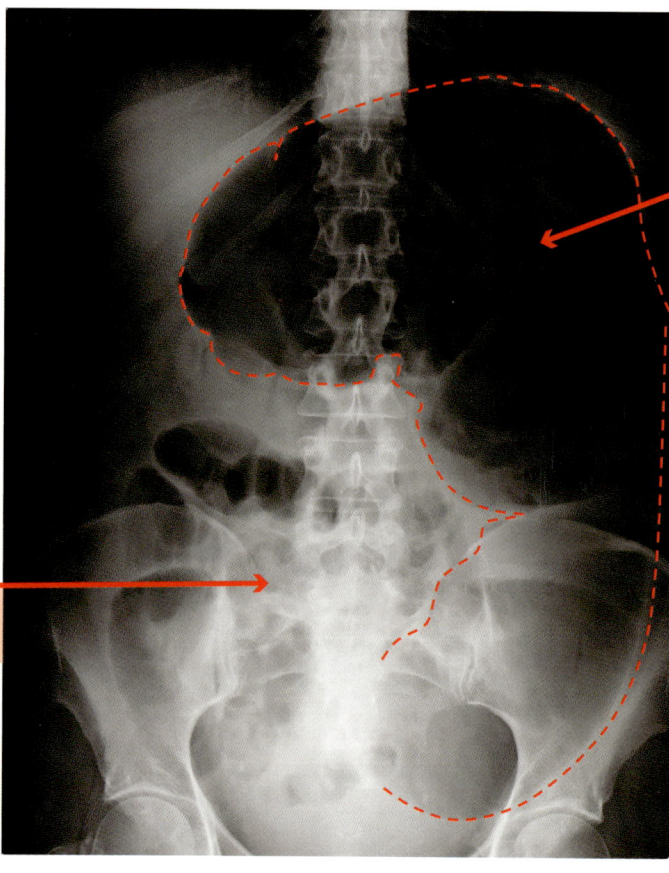

Caecal volvulus

Lateral and inferior displacement of small bowel

SUMMARY
This X-ray demonstrates a large gas filled loop of large bowel in keeping with caecal volvulus.

INVESTIGATIONS AND MANAGEMENT
The patient should be resuscitated using an ABCDE approach.

Adequate analgesia and hydration should be provided.

The patient should be kept NBM and an NG tube inserted on free drainage. IV fluids should be commenced.

Urgent bloods should be taken, including FBC, U&Es, CRP, LFTs, coagulation, blood gas, and group and save.

The general surgical team should be contacted urgently. Management will be with either endoscopic decompression or surgical intervention via detorsion and caecotomy.

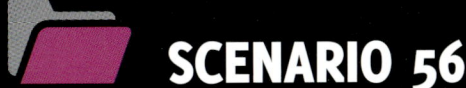
An 18 year old female presents to ED with severe lower abdominal pain. She has no significant past medical history and is a non-smoker. On examination, she has saturations of 97% in air and a temperature of 37.2°C. Her HR is 80 bpm, RR is 18 and blood pressure is 120/85 mmHg. The abdomen is rigid and there is generalised tenderness, particularly in the left iliac fossa, with normal bowel sounds. Urine dipstick is unremarkable and a pregnancy test is negative.

An abdominal X-ray is requested to assess for possible bowel obstruction.

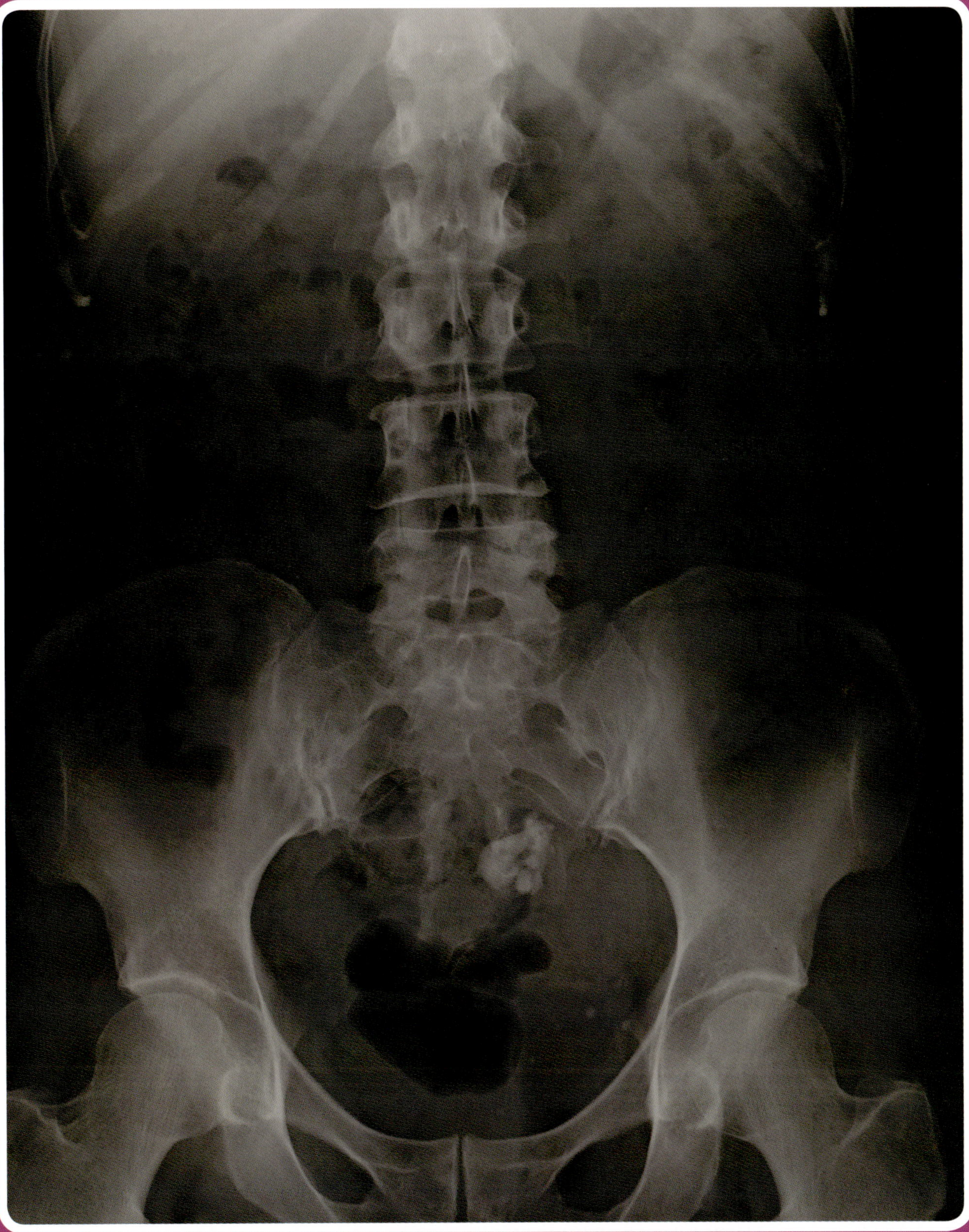

REPORT – DERMOID CYST

REPORT
Patient ID: Anonymous.
Projection: AP supine.
Rotation: Adequate.
Penetration: Adequate – the spinous processes are visible.
Coverage: Adequate – the anterior ribs are visible superiorly and the inferior pubic rami are visible.

BOWEL GAS PATTERN
The bowel gas pattern is normal.

BOWEL WALL
There is no evidence of mural thickening or intramural gas within the large or small bowel.

PNEUMOPERITONEUM
There is no evidence of free intra-abdominal gas.

SOLID ORGANS
The solid organ contours are within normal limits with no solid organ calcification.

VASCULAR
No abnormal vascular calcification.

BONES
There are no abnormalities of the imaged thoracic and lumbar spine, or within the pelvis.

SOFT TISSUES
The psoas muscle outline is visible bilaterally.

The extra-abdominal soft tissues are unremarkable.

OTHER
There is a rounded radiopaque density projected over the region of the left hemi-pelvis, which demonstrates tooth-like calcifications and may represent an ovarian dermoid cyst.

There are several rounded radiopaque densities projected over the lower pelvis that most likely represent phleboliths.

There are no vascular lines, drains or surgical clips.

REVIEW AREAS
Gallstones / Renal calculi: No radiopaque calculi.
Lung bases: Not fully included.
Spine: Normal.
Femoral heads: Normal.

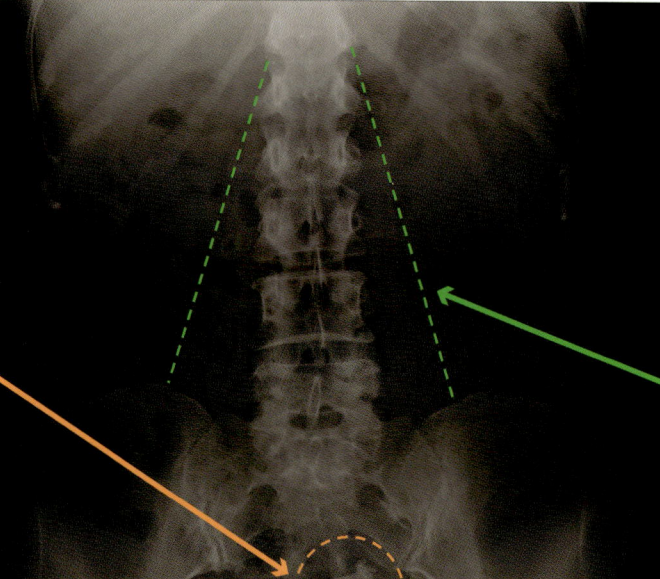

Calcified pelvic cyst

Psoas muscle outlines

Phleboliths

SUMMARY
This X-ray demonstrates a circular radiopaque density projected over the region of the left hemi-pelvis with tooth-like calcification, which may represent a potentially torted ovarian dermoid cyst (teratoma) or a fibroid. There is no evidence of bowel obstruction.

INVESTIGATIONS AND MANAGEMENT
The patient should be resuscitated using an ABCDE approach.

Adequate analgesia and hydration should be provided.

Urgent bloods should be taken including FBC, U&Es, CRP, bone profile, LFTs, tumour markers, coagulation, blood gas, and group and save.

An ultrasound scan of the pelvis should be considered to better assess the pelvic lesion and the patient should be referred urgently to gynaecology. Whilst the most likely diagnosis is an ovarian dermoid cyst (teratoma), other differential diagnoses should be considered depending on the blood test results and clinical findings.

An MRI scan of the pelvis may be required depending on the ultrasound results to further assess the pelvic lesion.

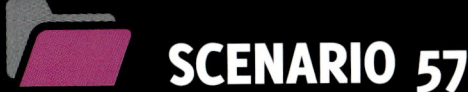
A 79 year old female presents to ED with severe central abdominal pain, nausea, vomiting and diarrhoea. Her past medical history is significant for hypertension, atrial fibrillation and osteoporosis. She is a non-smoker. On examination, she has saturations of 94% on 4L of oxygen and a temperature of 39.0°C. Her HR is 100 bpm, RR is 22 and blood pressure is 96/52 mmHg. The abdomen is rigid and there is generalised tenderness with normal bowel sounds. Rectal examination reveals liquid faeces with a small amount of fresh blood. Urine dipstick is unremarkable.

An abdominal X-ray is requested to assess for possible colitis.

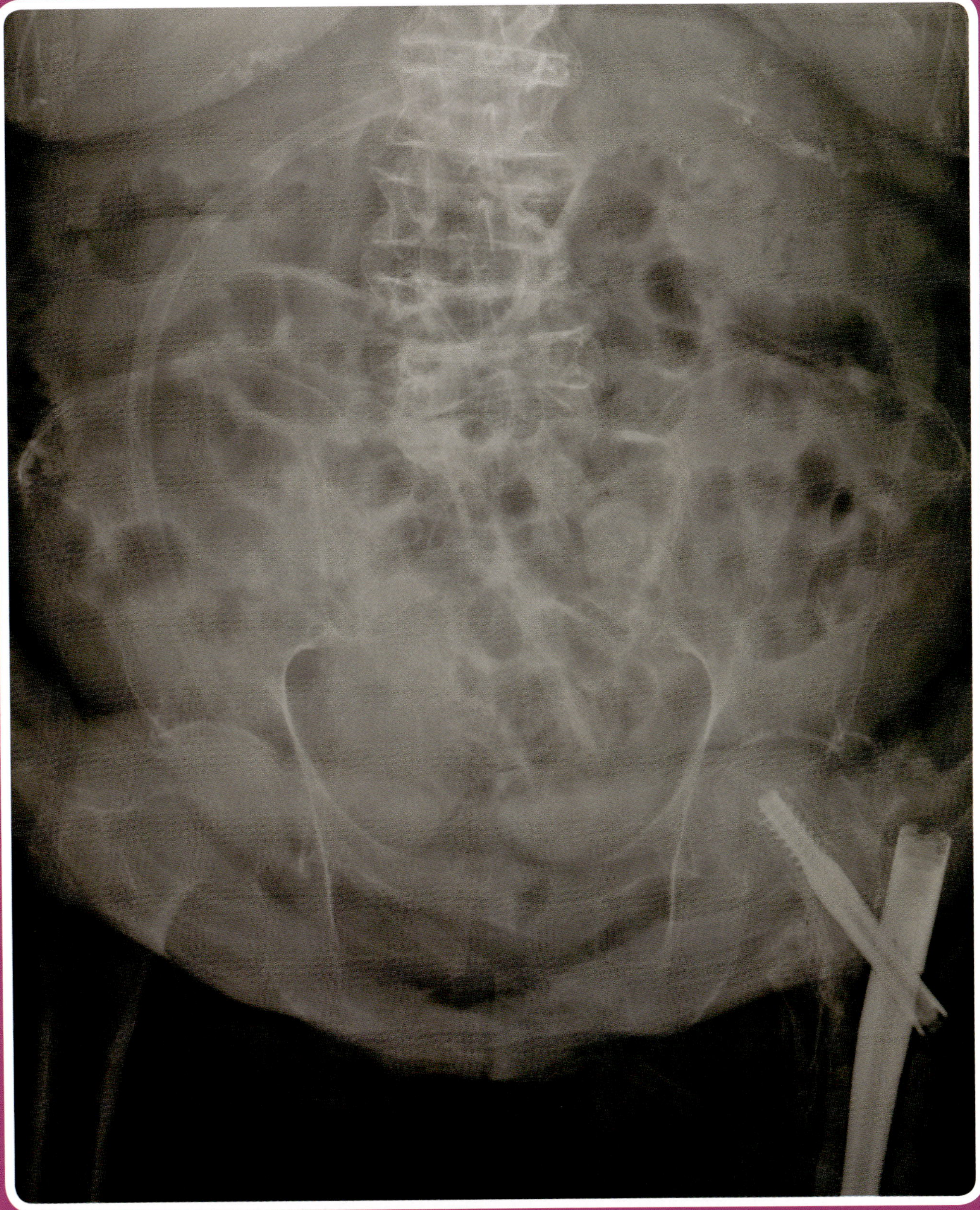

REPORT
Patient ID: Anonymous.
Projection: AP supine.
Rotation: Adequate.
Penetration: Adequate – the spinous processes are visible.
Coverage: Inadequate – the upper abdomen and diaphragm have not been included.

BOWEL GAS PATTERN
Bowel gas pattern is normal.

BOWEL WALL
There is no evidence of mural thickening or intramural gas within the large or small bowel.

PNEUMOPERITONEUM
There is no evidence of free intra-abdominal gas.

SOLID ORGANS
The solid organ contours are within normal limits with no solid organ calcification.

VASCULAR
No abnormal vascular calcification.

BONES
There is diffuse osteopenia of the skeleton, particularly of the vertebrae.

There are significant degenerative changes throughout the spine and in the sacroiliac and hip joints.

There are vertebral body compression (likely insufficiency) fractures at L3, L4 and L5.

There is an old left subtrochanteric femoral fracture, which has been repaired by internal fixation using a proximal femoral nail. Bony remodelling and heterotopic ossification is seen adjacent to this.

SOFT TISSUES
The psoas muscle outline is not visible bilaterally, which is non-specific.

The extra-abdominal soft tissues are unremarkable.

OTHER
There is a left-sided proximal femoral nail in situ but there are no other radiopaque foreign bodies.

There is an external line projected over the right side of the abdomen and the pelvis, which most likely represents oxygen tubing. The patient's hands are visible across the pelvis.

There are no vascular lines, drains or surgical clips.

REVIEW AREAS
Gallstones / Renal calculi: No radiopaque calculi.
Lung bases: Not visible.
Spine: Vertebral body compression fractures at L3, L4 and L5.
Femoral heads: Old left subtrochanteric fracture with left-sided proximal femoral nail in situ.

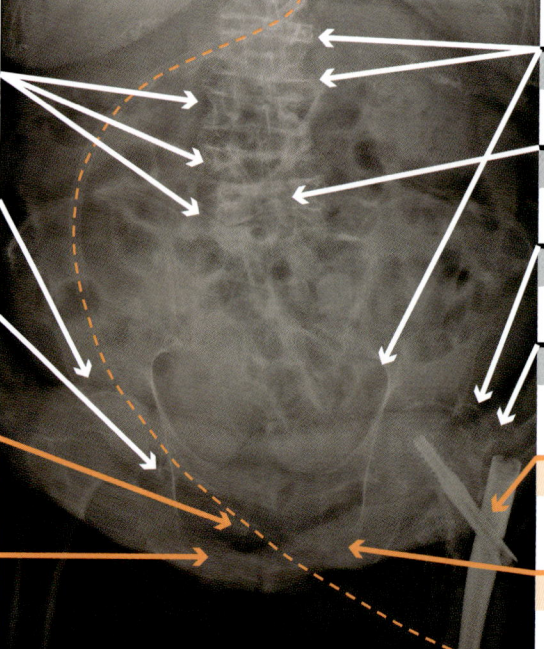

Vertebral body compression fractures

Joint space narrowing

Osteophytes

External line – likely oxygen tubing

Patient's hand

Degenerative change

Diffuse osteopenia

Heterotopic ossification

Bony remodelling

Proximal femoral nail

Patient's hand

SUMMARY
This X-ray demonstrates a normal bowel appearance with no evidence of colitis, intramural gas or pneumoperitoneum. It also demonstrates age-indeterminate vertebral body compression (insufficiency) fractures at L3, L4 and L5, on a background of diffuse osteopenia and significant degenerative changes throughout the spine, sacroiliac and hip joints. The left-sided proximal femoral nail is an incidental finding in keeping with a previous subtrochanteric femur fracture with associated bony remodelling and heterotopic ossification.

INVESTIGATIONS AND MANAGEMENT
The patient should be resuscitated using an ABCDE approach.

Adequate analgesia and hydration should be provided.

Urgent bloods should be taken, including FBC, U&Es, LFTs, amylase, CRP, blood gas, coagulation, blood gas, and group and save. Broad spectrum antibiotics should be prescribed.

There are no clear findings on the abdominal X-ray to explain the patient's clinical presentation.

A CT scan of the abdomen and pelvis with IV contrast should be considered for further assessment and the patient should be referred to general surgery.

Chronic management of vertebral crush fractures may involve lifestyle modification, physiotherapy, and pain medication, but further history/examination should be sought, and previous images reviewed.

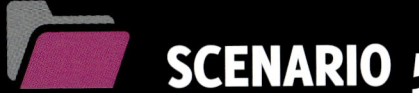

A 42 year old male presents to ED following a collapse and abdominal pain at home. She is diagnosed with septic shock secondary to pneumonia. He has no significant past medical history and is a non-smoker. On examination, he has saturations of 80% in room air and a temperature of 38.4°C. His HR is 95 bpm, RR is 30 and blood pressure is 90/50 mmHg. The abdomen is firm and there is some tenderness centrally with normal bowel sounds. Urine dipstick is unremarkable. He is intubated and vascular access is established as part of his ABCDE resuscitation.

An abdominal X-ray is requested to assess the position of his femoral line and assess for possible bowel obstruction.

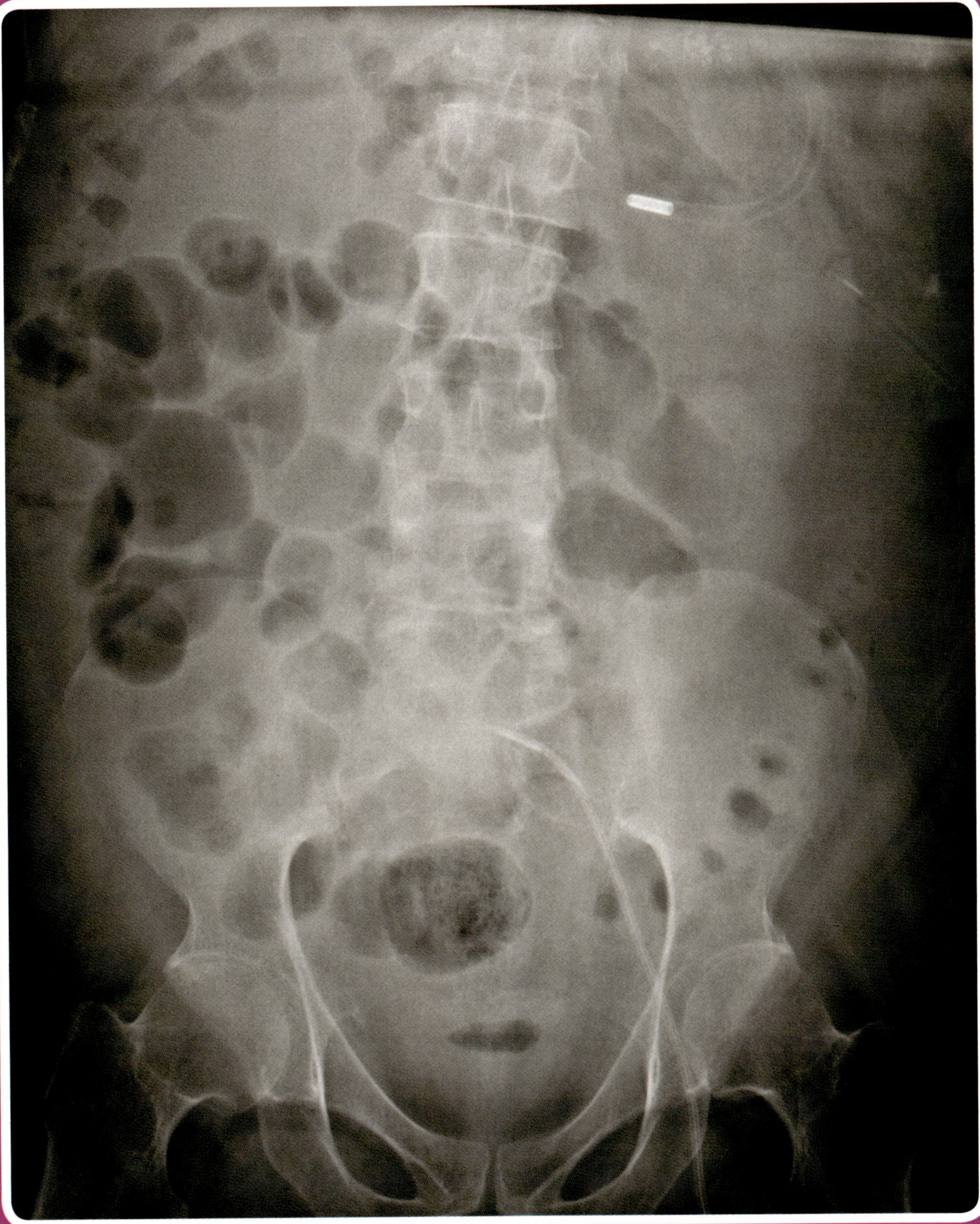

REPORT
Patient ID: Anonymous.
Projection: AP supine.
Rotation: Adequate.
Penetration: Adequate – the spinous processes are visible.
Coverage: Adequate – the anterior ribs are visible superiorly and the inferior pubic rami are visible.

BOWEL GAS PATTERN
The bowel gas pattern is normal.

BOWEL WALL
There is no evidence of mural thickening or intramural gas within the large or small bowel.

PNEUMOPERITONEUM
There is no evidence of free intra-abdominal gas.

SOLID ORGANS
The solid organ contours are within normal limits with no solid organ calcification.

VASCULAR
There is a left sided femoral venous catheter with its tip projecting over the inferior endplate of L5, likely at the site of the inferior vena cava bifurcation.

The abdominal aorta appears normal.

BONES
There are no abnormalities of the imaged thoracic and lumbar spine, or within the pelvis.

SOFT TISSUES
The psoas muscle outline is visible bilaterally.

The extra-abdominal soft tissues are unremarkable.

OTHER
There is an NG tube in situ, with its tip seen in the left upper quadrant within the stomach.

There are no drains or surgical clips.

REVIEW AREAS
Gallstones / Renal calculi: No radiopaque calculi.
Lung bases: Not fully included.
Spine: Normal.
Femoral heads: Normal.

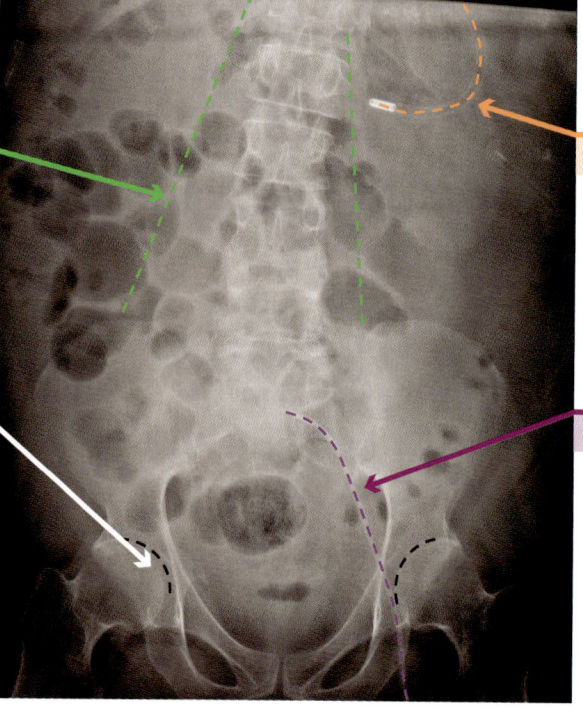

Psoas muscle outlines

NG tube

Femoral heads normal

Left sided femoral venous catheter

SUMMARY
This X-ray demonstrates an NG tube in situ, with its tip situated within the gastric fundus. It also demonstrates a left sided femoral venous catheter with its tip projecting over the proximal left common iliac vein. There is no evidence of any other significant abnormality.

INVESTIGATIONS AND MANAGEMENT
The patient should be resuscitated using an ABCDE approach.

Adequate analgesia and hydration should be provided.

Urgent bloods should be taken including FBC, U&Es, CRP, bone profile, LFTs, coagulation, blood culture, blood gas, and group and save.

The sepsis 6 pathway should be started immediately, including administration of oxygen, IV broad spectrum antibiotics and consideration of a fluid bolus as well as measurement of lactate and urinary output and blood cultures.

The patient should be made NBM and started on IV fluids.

There are no clear findings on the abdominal X-ray to explain the patient's abdominal pain. A CT scan of the abdomen/pelvis with IV contrast may be considered for further evaluation of the abdomen and the general surgical team should be involved.

Intensive care should be informed about the patient as their input may be required.

SCENARIO 59

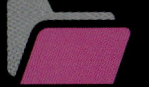

A 1 day old baby boy is currently admitted on NICU after a premature birth at 34 weeks. On examination, he has saturations of 99%, is intubated in 40% oxygen and has a temperature of 36.5°C. His HR is 190 bpm and RR is 40. The abdomen is soft and bowel sounds are normal.

An abdominal X-ray is requested to assess the position of the ET tube and umbilical lines that have just been inserted.

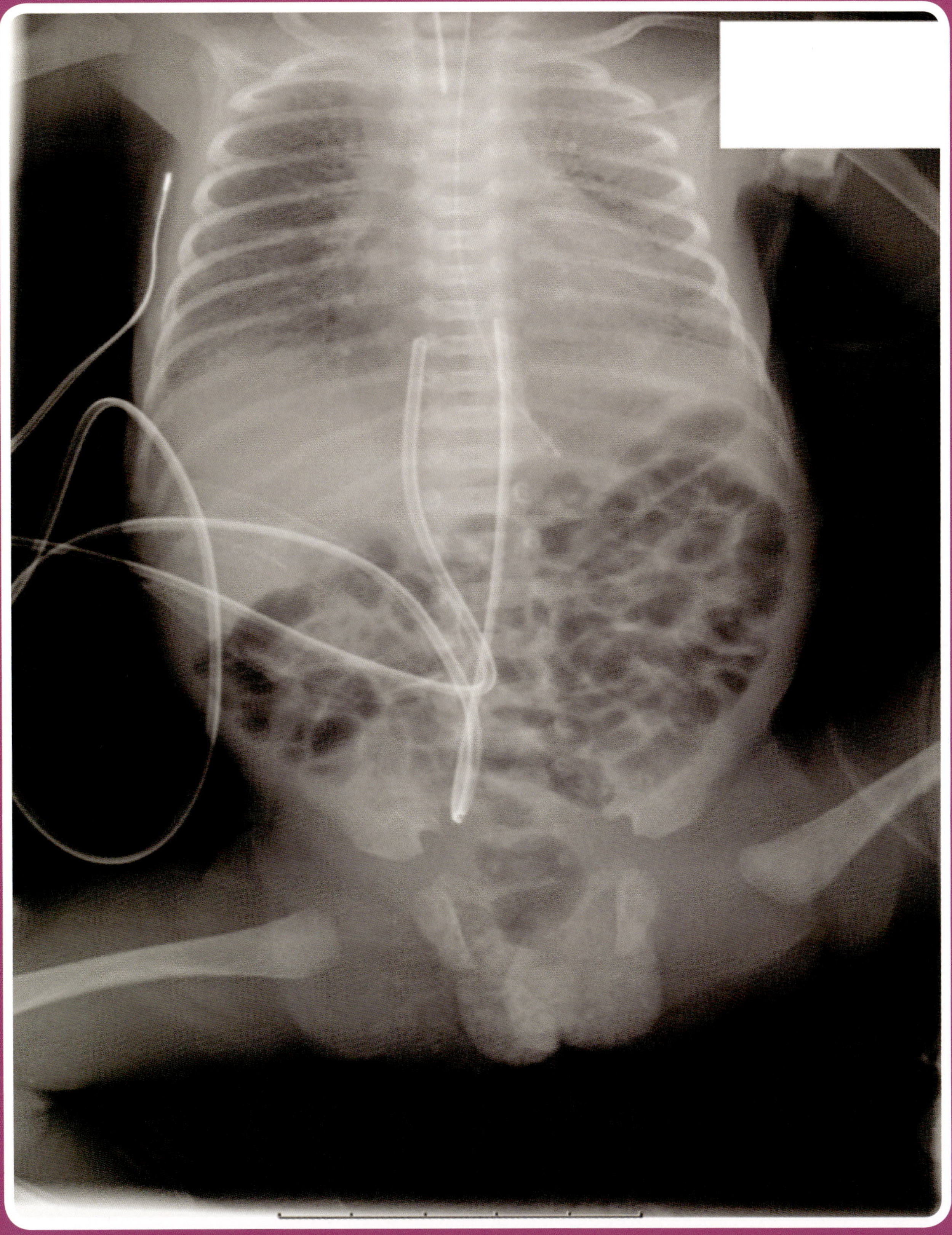

REPORT

Patient ID: Anonymous.
Projection: AP supine.
Rotation: Adequate.
Penetration: Adequate – the spine is visible.
Coverage: Adequate – the anterior ribs are visible superiorly and the inferior pubic rami are visible.

BOWEL GAS PATTERN

The bowel gas pattern is normal. There is faeces projecting over the pelvis and external to the patient with a nappy.

BOWEL WALL

There is no evidence of mural thickening or intramural gas within the large or small bowel.

PNEUMOPERITONEUM

There is no evidence of free intra-abdominal gas.

SOLID ORGANS

The solid organ contours are within normal limits with no solid organ calcification.

There is bilateral ground glass shadowing in the lung fields.

VASCULAR

No abnormal vascular calcification.

There is an umbilical artery catheter. Its tip is seen appropriately sited at the level of T9.

There is an umbilical venous catheter with its tip seen appropriately sited projecting over the diaphragm at the level of T9/10 in the inferior vena cava.

BONES

There are no abnormalities of the imaged thoracic and lumbar spine, or within the pelvis.

There is cartilage present between the pelvic bones and femurs as they have not yet fused, which is a normal finding in a child of this age.

There is cartilage seen between vertebrae which is a normal finding in a child of this age.

SOFT TISSUES

The psoas muscle outline is not visible bilaterally, which is non-specific, particularly in a child of this age.

The extra-abdominal soft tissues are unremarkable.

OTHER

There is an NG tube in situ, with its tip seen in the left upper quadrant of the abdomen, within the stomach.

There is an ET tube in situ, with its tip seen in the midline between the medial border of the clavicles and above the carina in a satisfactory position.

There is an electrode and lead external to the patient, in keeping with a skin temperature probe.

There are no drains or surgical clips.

REVIEW AREAS

Gallstones / Renal calculi: No radiopaque calculi.
Lung bases: Bilateral ground glass shadowing.
Spine: Normal – cartilage between vertebrae.
Femoral heads: Normal – growth plates present.

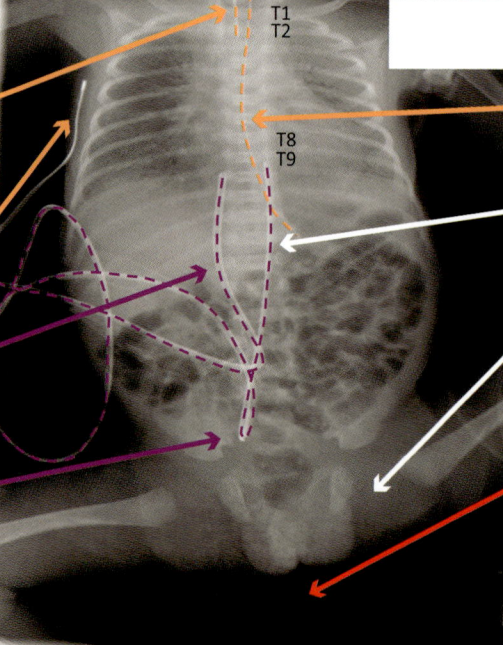

ET tube

Temperature probe

Umbilical venous catheter

Umbilical artery catheter

T1
T2

T8
T9

NG tube

Cartilage between unfused vertebrae

Cartilage between unfused bones

Faeces in nappy

SUMMARY

This X-ray demonstrates an NG tube, ET tube, skin temperature probe, umbilical artery catheter and umbilical venous catheter, all appropriately sited. There is bilateral ground glass shadowing in the lung fields, in keeping with respiratory distress syndrome.

INVESTIGATIONS AND MANAGEMENT

The ET tube and vascular lines are in satisfactory positions.

If not already done, surfactant should be given. The baby should be started on broad spectrum antibiotics, and kept NBM on IV fluids.

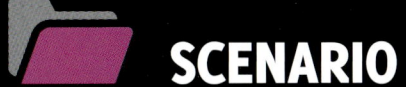

SCENARIO 60

A 39 year old female presents to ED with abdominal distension and increasing frequency of diarrhoea and passing mucus. Her past medical history is significant for ulcerative colitis and she is a smoker. On examination, she has saturations of 99% in room air and a temperature of 38.1°C. Her HR is 88 bpm, RR is 19 and blood pressure is 125/65 mmHg. The abdomen is soft and there is generalised tenderness with normal bowel sounds. Urine dipstick is unremarkable and a pregnancy test is negative.

An abdominal X-ray is requested to assess for active colitis.

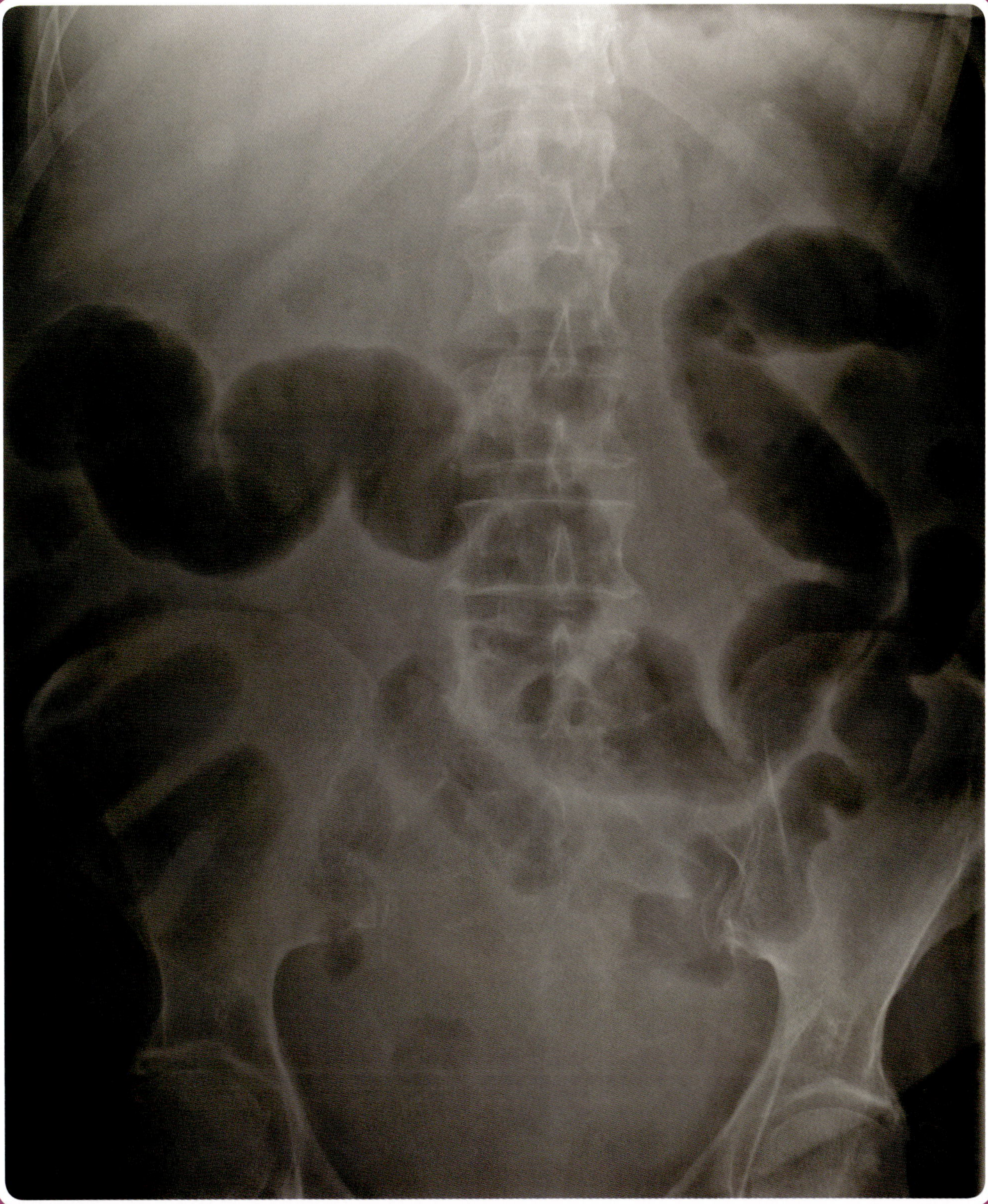

REPORT
Patient ID: Anonymous.
Projection: AP supine.
Rotation: Adequate.
Penetration: Adequate – the spinous processes are visible.
Coverage: Inadequate – the pubic symphysis and inferior pubic rami have not been included.

BOWEL GAS PATTERN
There is dilatation of the large bowel, in particular the ascending and transverse colon.

BOWEL WALL
There is mural thickening of the entire transverse colon in the right and left upper quadrants, and of the sigmoid colon, with loss of the normal colonic haustral folds, in keeping with mural oedema. This is termed 'lead pipe colon'.

There is no evidence of intramural gas within the large or small bowel.

PNEUMOPERITONEUM
There is no evidence of free intra-abdominal gas.

SOLID ORGANS
The solid organ contours are within normal limits with no solid organ calcification.

VASCULAR
No abnormal vascular calcification.

BONES
There are no abnormalities of the imaged thoracic and lumbar spine, or within the pelvis.

SOFT TISSUES
The psoas muscle outline is visible bilaterally.

The extra-abdominal soft tissues are unremarkable.

OTHER
There are no radiopaque foreign bodies.

There are no vascular lines, drains or surgical clips.

REVIEW AREAS
Gallstones / Renal calculi: No radiopaque calculi.
Lung bases: Not fully included.
Spine: Normal.
Femoral heads: Normal.

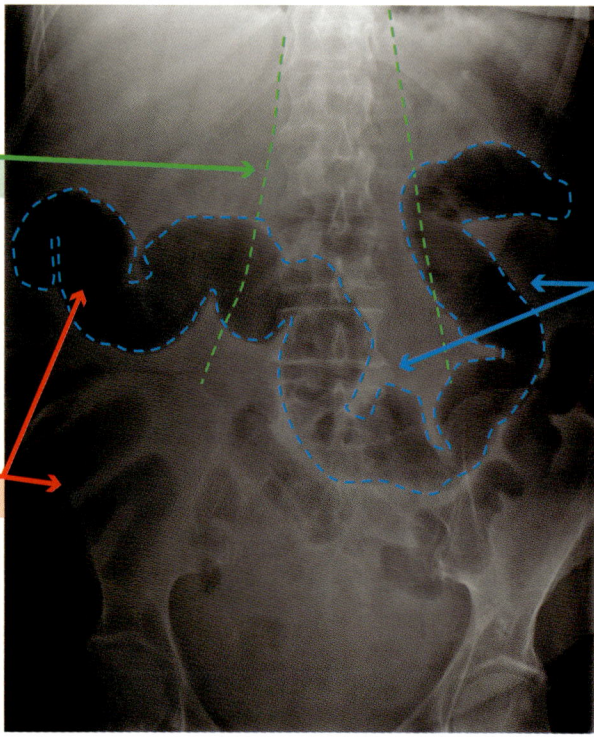

Psoas muscle outlines

Dilated large bowel

Mural oedema of transverse colon with loss of haustral folds

SUMMARY
This X-ray demonstrates mural oedema of the transverse and sigmoid colon with loss of the normal colonic haustral folds. There is also dilatation of the ascending and transverse colon. Given the clinical history, findings are in keeping with an acute exacerbation of ulcerative colitis.

INVESTIGATIONS AND MANAGEMENT
The patient should be resuscitated using an ABCDE approach.

Adequate analgesia and hydration should be provided.

Urgent bloods should be taken, including FBC, U&Es, LFTs, ESR, CRP, iron studies, folate, blood gas, and group and save. A stool sample should be sent.

Urgent referral to the gastroenterology team should be considered.

A CT scan of the abdomen/pelvis with IV contrast should be considered for better visualisation of the anatomy and to assess the extent of the disease.

Treatment will depend on the results of further investigations, as well as the clinical state of the patient.

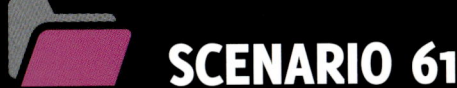

SCENARIO 61

A 70 year old male presents to ED with a 2 day history of nausea, vomiting and not passing flatus or opening his bowels. He has no significant past medical history and is a non-smoker. On examination, he has saturations of 98% in room air and a temperature of 36.5°C. His HR is 95 bpm, RR is 26 and blood pressure is 135/75 mmHg. The abdomen is rigid and there is generalised tenderness with tinkling bowel sounds. Urine dipstick is unremarkable.

An abdominal X-ray is requested to assess for possible bowel obstruction.

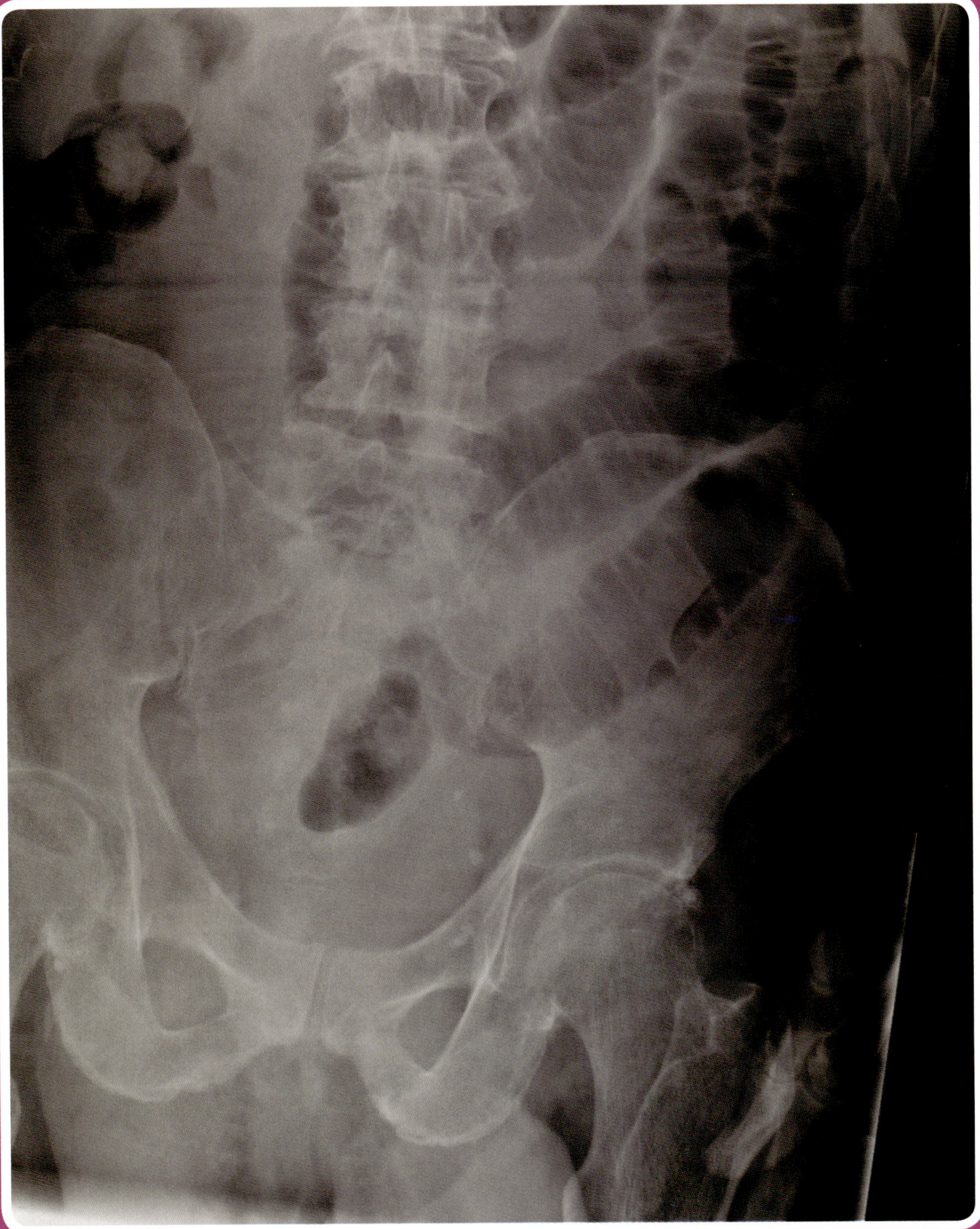

REPORT – INCARCERATED INGUINAL HERNIA WITH SMALL BOWEL OBSTRUCTION

REPORT
Patient ID: Anonymous.
Projection: AP supine.
Rotation: Adequate.
Penetration: Adequate – the spinous processes are visible.
Coverage: Inadequate – the anterior ribs, right hip joint and right ilium have not been fully included.

BOWEL GAS PATTERN
There are multiple loops of dilated bowel seen centrally within the abdomen, which demonstrate valvulae conniventes in keeping with small bowel obstruction.

There is abnormal bowel gas projecting over the groin below the inguinal ligament towards the scrotum, suggestive of an incarcerated indirect inguinal hernia.

BOWEL WALL
There is no evidence of mural thickening or intramural gas within the large or small bowel.

PNEUMOPERITONEUM
There is no evidence of free intra-abdominal gas.

SOLID ORGANS
The solid organ contours are within normal limits with no solid organ calcification.

VASCULAR
There is calcification of the iliac arteries bilaterally.

BONES
There is moderate degenerative change in the spine with osteophyte formation and mild degenerative change in the hip joints with osteophyte formation and subchondral sclerosis.

SOFT TISSUES
The psoas muscle outline is not visible.

The extra-abdominal soft tissues are unremarkable.

OTHER
There are multiple rounded radiopaque densities projected over the region of the pelvis, most likely phleboliths.

A hand has been exposed in the lower left hand side of the radiograph.

There are no vascular lines, drains or surgical clips.

REVIEW AREAS
Gallstones / Renal calculi: No radiopaque calculi.
Lung bases: Not included.
Spine: Moderate degenerative change.
Femoral heads: Mild degenerative change.

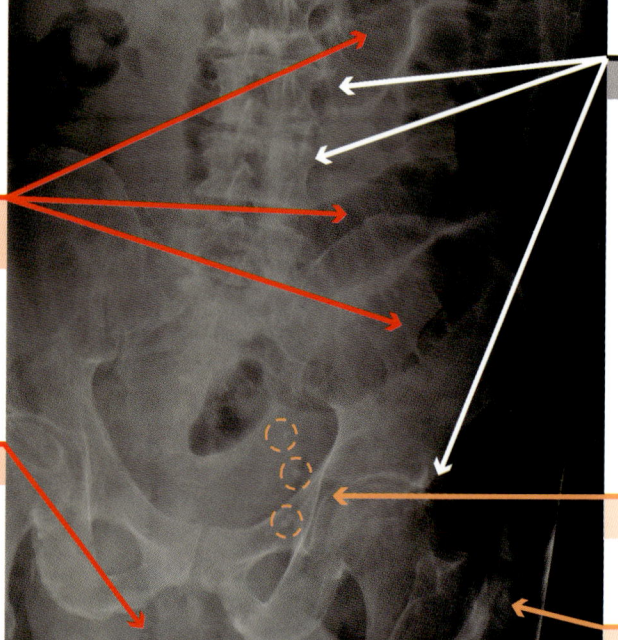

Small bowel dilatation with valvulae conniventes

Incarcerated inguinal hernia

Degenerative changes

Phleboliths

Hand

SUMMARY
This X-ray demonstrates multiple loops of dilated bowel seen centrally within the abdomen demonstrating valvulae conniventes, in keeping with small bowel obstruction. There is bowel gas seen projecting over the groin towards the scrotum, which most likely represents an incarcerated indirect inguinal hernia. The moderate degenerative changes in the spine, mild left hip degenerative changes and pelvic phleboliths are incidental findings.

INVESTIGATIONS AND MANAGEMENT
The patient should be resuscitated using an ABCDE approach.

Adequate analgesia and hydration should be provided.

The patient should be kept NBM and an NG tube inserted on free drainage to relieve the pressure in the small bowel. IV fluids should be commenced.

Urgent bloods should be taken, including FBC, U&Es, CRP, LFTs, coagulation, blood gas, and group and save.

The general surgical team should be contacted urgently for consideration of hernia repair.

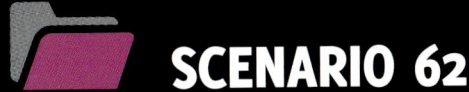

SCENARIO 62

A 50 year old male presents to ED with abdominal distension and generalised abdominal pain. He has not passed flatus or opened his bowels for 24 hours. He has chronic constipation and is a smoker. On examination, he has saturations of 99% in room air and a temperature of 36.5°C. His HR is 101 bpm, RR is 24 and blood pressure is 135/80 mmHg. The abdomen is rigid and there is generalised tenderness with tinkling bowel sounds. Urine dipstick is unremarkable.

An abdominal X-ray is requested to assess for possible bowel obstruction.

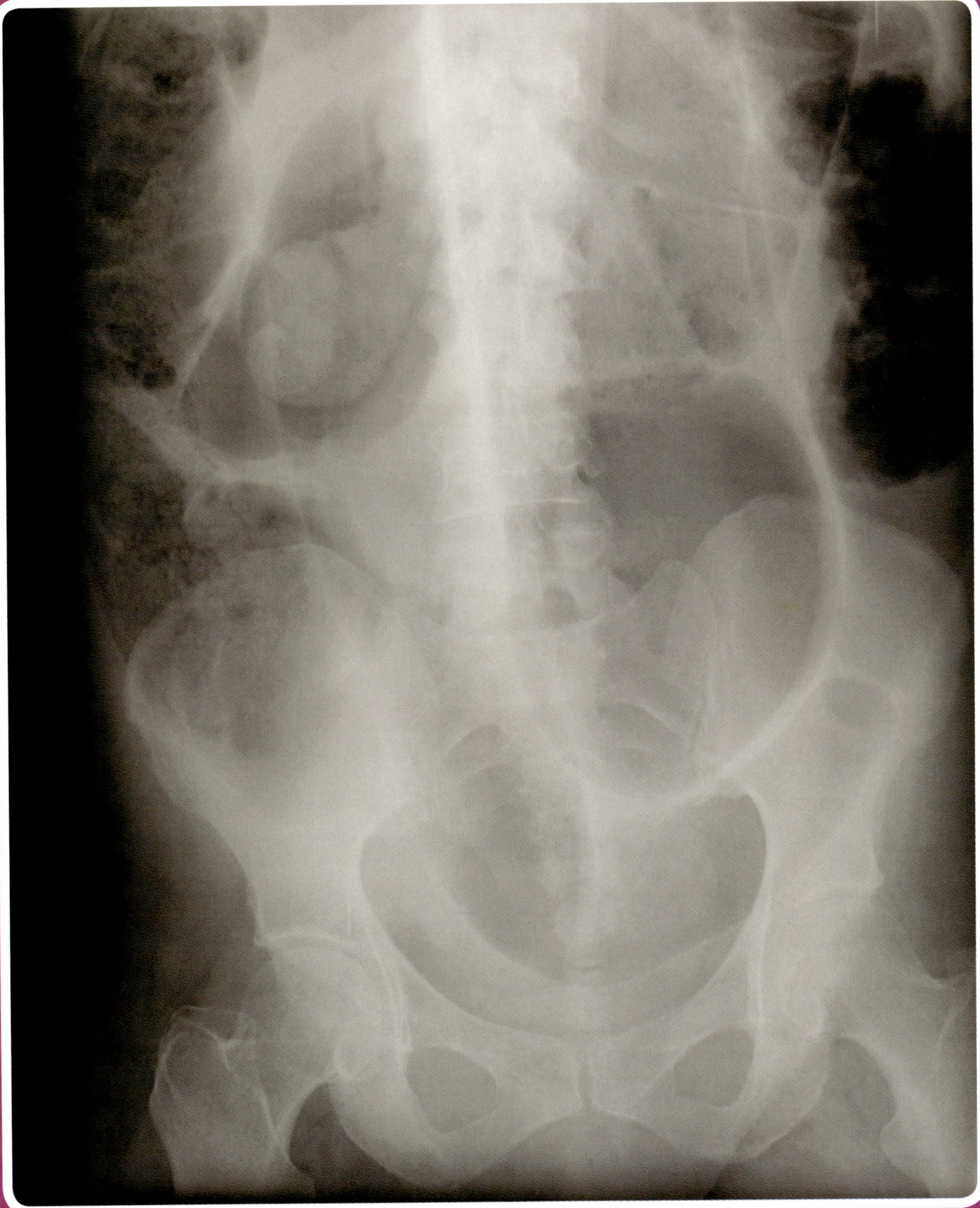

REPORT

Patient ID: Anonymous.
Projection: AP supine.
Rotation: Adequate.
Penetration: Adequate – the spinous processes are visible.
Coverage: Adequate – the anterior ribs are visible superiorly and the inferior pubic rami are visible.

BOWEL GAS PATTERN

There is a large gas filled loop of large bowel in the centre of the abdomen, with loss of the normal haustral markings, extending from the pelvis to the upper abdomen.

There are multiple loops of dilatated bowel seen within the abdomen demonstrating haustra, in keeping with large bowel dilatation.

Bowel gas is not seen in the rectum.

There is a moderate volume of faecal residue present within the ascending colon.

BOWEL WALL

There is no evidence of mural thickening or intramural gas within the large or small bowel.

PNEUMOPERITONEUM

There is no evidence of free intra-abdominal gas.

SOLID ORGANS

The solid organ contours are within normal limits with no solid organ calcification.

VASCULAR

No abnormal vascular calcification.

BONES

There is mild degenerative change in the spine.

There is mild osteoarthritic change seen within both hip joints, including subchondral sclerosis and narrowing of the joint spaces.

SOFT TISSUES

The psoas muscle outline is not visible bilaterally, which is non-specific.

The extra-abdominal soft tissues are unremarkable.

OTHER

There are no radiopaque foreign bodies.

There are no vascular lines, drains or surgical clips.

REVIEW AREAS

Gallstones / Renal calculi: No radiopaque calculi.
Lung bases: Normal.
Spine: Mild degenerative change.
Femoral heads: Moderate degenerative change.

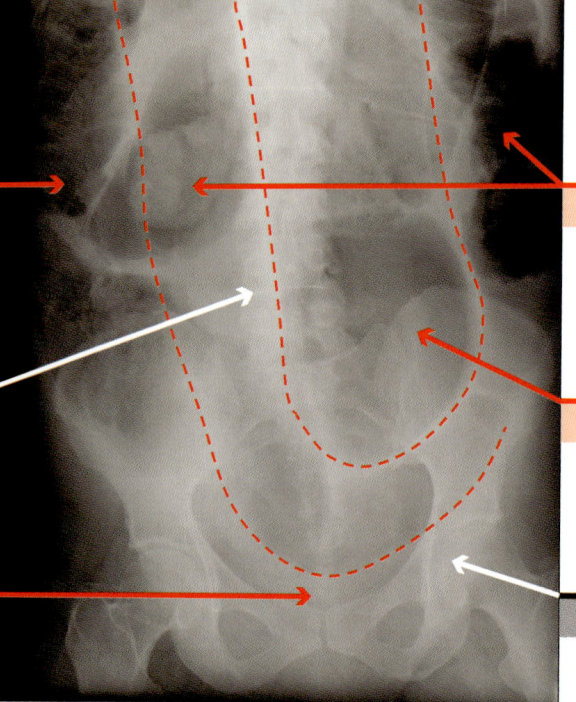

Faecal residue within ascending colon

Large bowel dilatation

Degenerative change throughout axial skeleton

Sigmoid volvulus

Empty rectum

Osteoarthritis of hip joints

SUMMARY

This X-ray demonstrates a large gas filled loop of large bowel, with loss of normal haustral markings. There is dilatation of the large bowel proximal to this, and an absence of bowel gas seen within the rectum distally. Findings are in keeping with sigmoid volvulus. The mild degenerative change in the spine and hip joints are incidental findings.

INVESTIGATIONS AND MANAGEMENT

The patient should be resuscitated using an ABCDE approach.

Adequate analgesia and hydration should be provided.

Urgent bloods should be taken, including FBC, U&Es, CRP, blood gas, coagulation and group and save.

The general surgical team should be contacted urgently.

Urgent decompression with sigmoidoscopy is required to relieve the obstruction, with a flatus tube left in situ.

Elective sigmoidectomy with primary anastomosis may then be undertaken to prevent reoccurrence.

Arthritic changes in the first instance should be managed with lifestyle changes and analgesia, depending on symptoms.

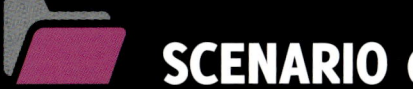

A 55 year old female presents to ED with a 4 day history of generalised abdominal pain. She has not opened her bowels in that time and feels nauseated but has not vomited. Her past medical history is significant for chronic back pain, for which she takes regular cocodamol and ibuprofen. She has no other significant past medical history and is a smoker. On examination, she has saturations of 95% in room air and a temperature of 36.5°C. Her HR is 77 bpm, RR is 18 and blood pressure is 118/64 mmHg. The abdomen is mildly distended with voluntary guarding and there is tenderness in the left iliac fossa with sluggish bowel sounds. Urine dipstick is unremarkable.

An abdominal X-ray is requested to assess for possible bowel obstruction.

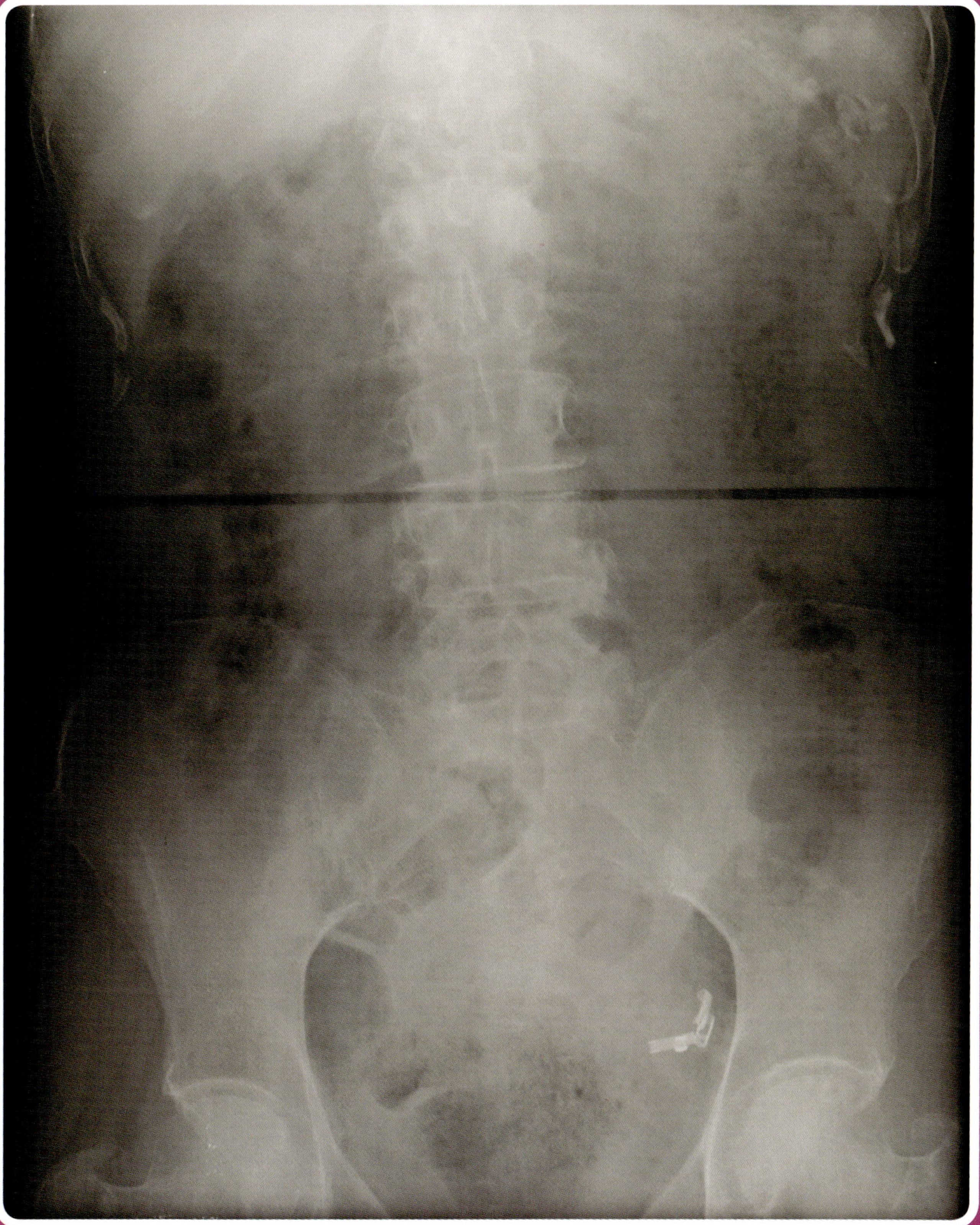

REPORT
Patient ID: Anonymous.
Projection: AP supine.
Rotation: Adequate.
Penetration: Adequate – the spinous processes are visible.
Coverage: Inadequate – the pubic symphysis and inferior pubic rami have not been fully included.

BOWEL GAS PATTERN
There is a paucity of bowel gas but no bowel dilatation is visible.

There is a moderate amount of faecal material present throughout the large bowel, extending from caecum to rectum.

BOWEL WALL
There is no evidence of mural thickening or intramural gas within the large or small bowel.

PNEUMOPERITONEUM
There is no evidence of free intra-abdominal gas.

SOLID ORGANS
The solid organ contours are within normal limits with no solid organ calcification.

VASCULAR
No abnormal vascular calcification.

BONES
There is degenerative change visible in the imaged thoracic and lumbar spine.

No fractures or destructive bone lesions are visible in the imaged skeleton.

SOFT TISSUES
The psoas muscle outline is visible bilaterally.

The extra-abdominal soft tissues are unremarkable.

OTHER
There are two sterilisation clips projecting over the left pelvis, indicating that one may have become loose.

There are no vascular lines or drains.

REVIEW AREAS
Gallstones / Renal calculi: No radiopaque calculi.
Lung bases: Not fully included.
Spine: Degenerative change.
Femoral heads: Normal.

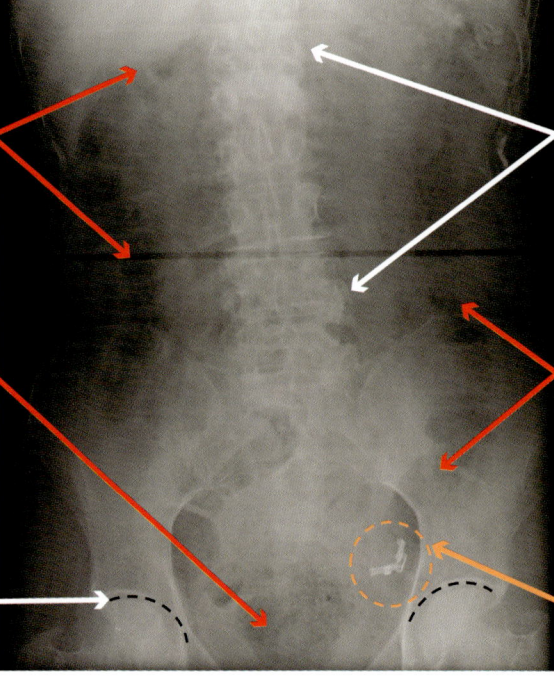

Faecal residue in ascending and transverse colon

Rectal faecal residue

Femoral heads normal

Degenerative change in thoracic and lumbar spine

Faecal residue in descending and sigmoid colon

Sterilisation clips

SUMMARY
This X-ray demonstrates a moderate volume of faecal residue throughout the large bowel. There are two sterilisation clips projecting over the left pelvis, indicating that one may have become loose. There is no evidence of bowel obstruction or pneumoperitoneum. There are moderate degenerative changes in the spine.

INVESTIGATIONS AND MANAGEMENT
If the patient is otherwise well, no further investigation or imaging is required.

If the patient is clinically constipated, current medications should be reviewed and laxatives considered. Advice should be given regarding lifestyle adjustments, including adequate fluid intake, sufficient dietary fibre and exercise if clinically appropriate.

In a premenopausal woman, the loose sterilisation clip would be of clinical importance as the patient may not be protected from conception and additional contraception may be required.

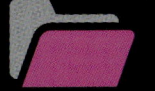

SCENARIO 64

A 25 year old female presents to ED with right sided abdominal pain. Her past medical history is significant for congenital hydrocephalus, for which she has a VP shunt, and she is a non-smoker. On examination, she has saturations of 98% in room air and a temperature of 36.5°C. Her HR is 88 bpm, RR is 23 and blood pressure is 130/82 mmHg. The abdomen is soft and there is widespread tenderness over the right side of the abdomen with normal bowel sounds. Urine dipstick is unremarkable and a pregnancy test is negative.

An abdominal X-ray is requested to assess for a possible bowel obstruction.

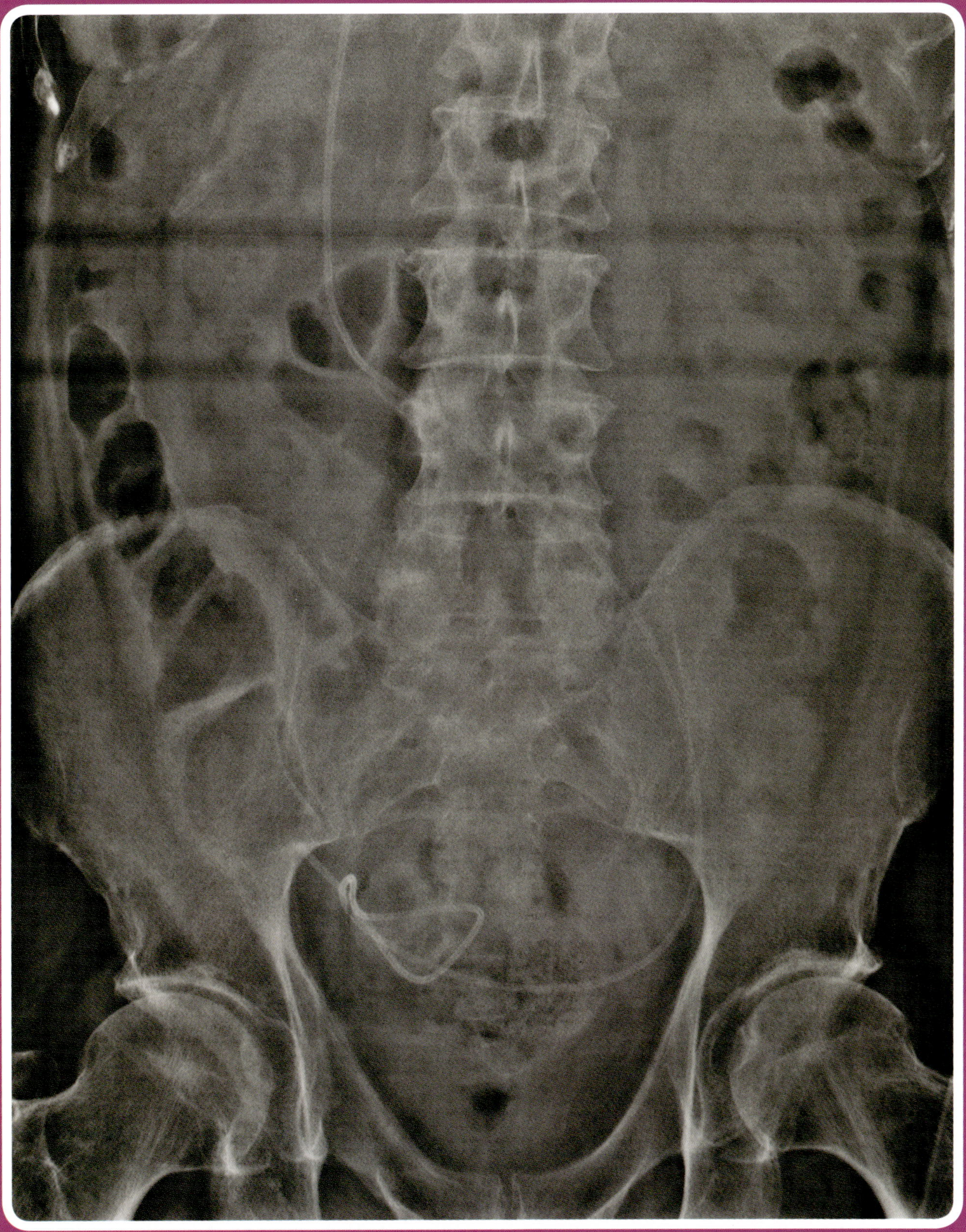

REPORT – VENTRICULOPERITONEAL SHUNT

REPORT
Patient ID: Anonymous.
Projection: AP supine.
Rotation: Adequate.
Penetration: Adequate – the spinous processes are visible.
Coverage: Inadequate – the pubic symphysis and inferior pubic rami have not been included.

BOWEL GAS PATTERN
The bowel gas pattern is normal.

BOWEL WALL
There is no evidence of mural thickening or intramural gas within the large or small bowel.

PNEUMOPERITONEUM
There is no evidence of free intra-abdominal gas.

SOLID ORGANS
The solid organ contours are within normal limits with no solid organ calcification.

VASCULAR
No abnormal vascular calcification.

BONES
There are no abnormalities of the imaged thoracic and lumbar spine, or within the pelvis.

SOFT TISSUES
The psoas muscle outline is visible bilaterally.

The extra-abdominal soft tissues are unremarkable.

OTHER
There is a radiopaque line projecting over the right upper quadrant, crossing the midline and with its tip terminating within the pelvis in keeping with the known VP shunt, which appears intact.

There are no vascular lines, drains or surgical clips.

REVIEW AREAS
Gallstones / Renal calculi: No radiopaque calculi.
Lung bases: Not fully included.
Spine: Normal.
Femoral heads: Normal.

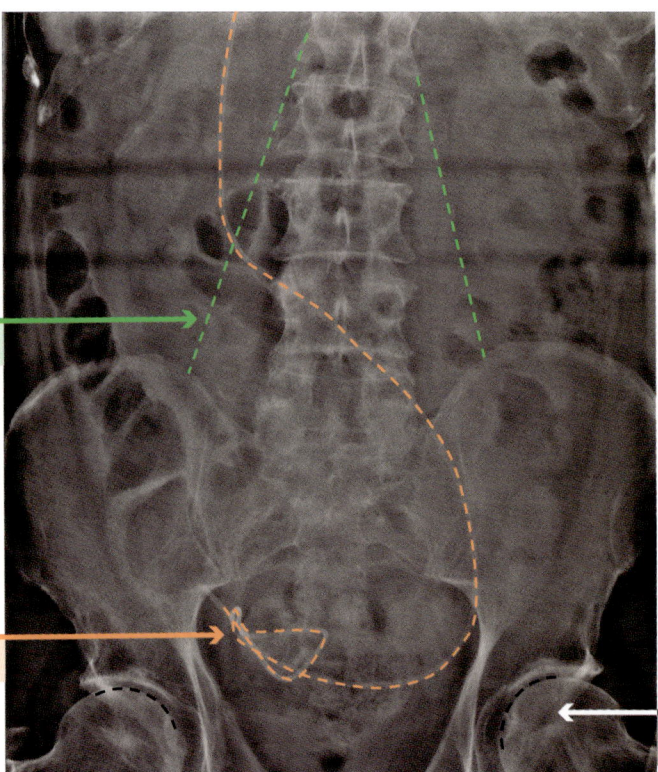

Psoas muscle outlines

VP shunt

Femoral heads normal

SUMMARY
This X-ray demonstrates a VP shunt with its tip projecting within the pelvis, which appears intact. There is no evidence of pneumoperitoneum.

INVESTIGATIONS AND MANAGEMENT
The patient should be resuscitated using an ABCDE approach.

Adequate analgesia and hydration should be provided.

Urgent bloods should be taken including FBC, U&Es, LFTs, amylase, bone profile, blood culture, blood gas, and CRP.

There are no clear findings on the abdominal X-ray to explain the patient's clinical presentation.

An ultrasound scan of the abdomen should be considered in the first instance to exclude gallstones, renal calculi and abdominal/pelvic collections, which may account for the patient's symptoms. The patient is also at risk of a VP shunt infection, so this should be considered as a differential.

SCENARIO 65

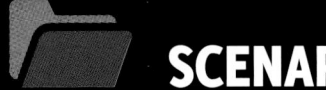

A 3 year old male present to ED with worsening abdominal distension, nausea and vomiting. He has not opened his bowels for the past 24 hours. He has no significant past medical history. On examination, he has saturations of 97% in room air and a temperature of 37.4°C. His HR is 135 bpm and RR is 36. The abdomen is rigid and there is generalised tenderness with tinkling bowel sounds. Urine dipstick is unremarkable.

An abdominal X-ray is requested to assess for possible bowel obstruction.

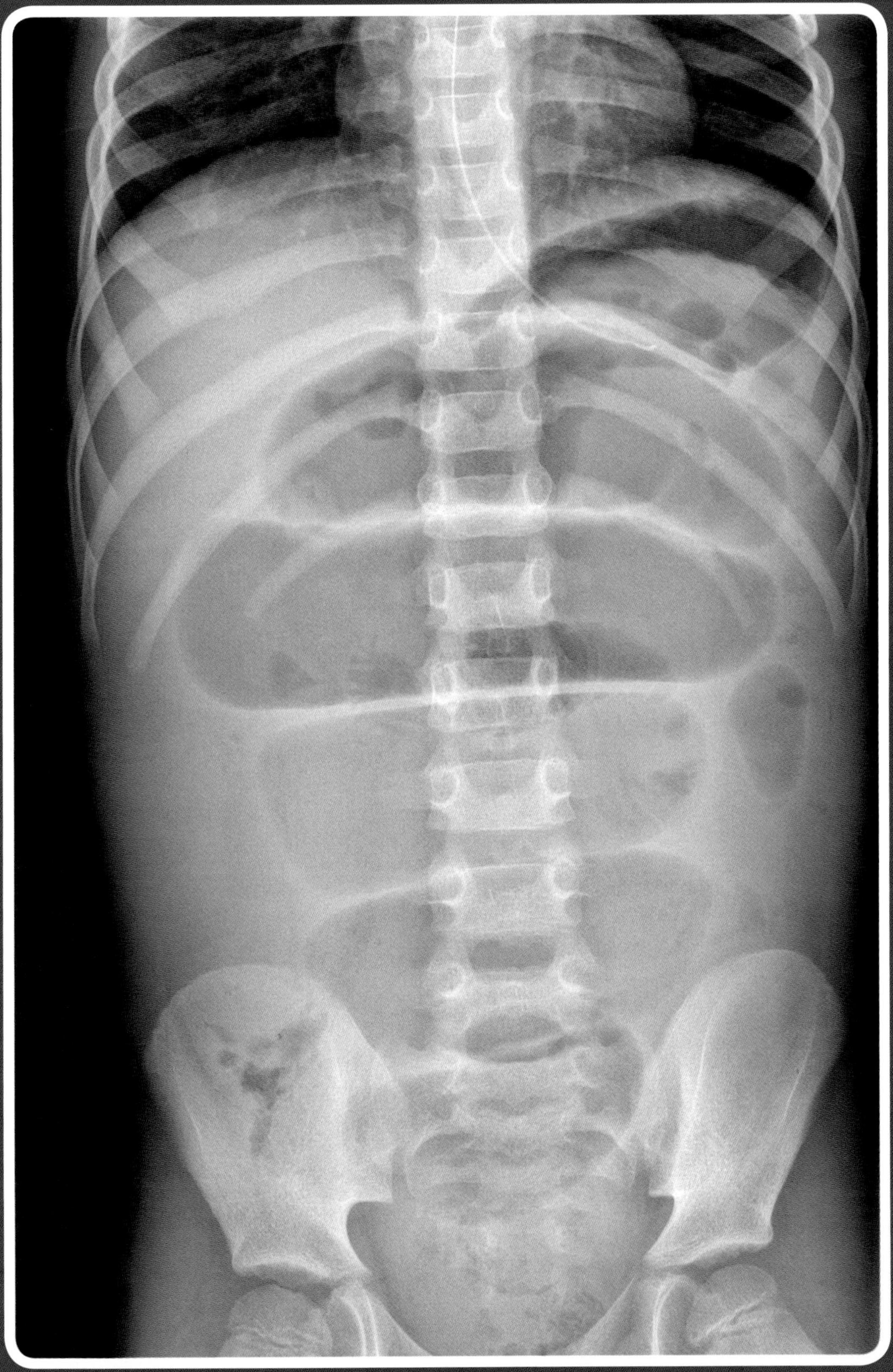

REPORT

Patient ID: Anonymous.
Projection: AP supine.
Rotation: Adequate.
Penetration: Adequate – the spinous processes are visible.
Coverage: Inadequate – the pubic symphysis and inferior pubic rami have not been included.

BOWEL GAS PATTERN

There are multiple loops of dilated bowel seen centrally in the abdomen. Valvulae conniventes are not seen and there is probable mural thickening in keeping with mural oedema. There is a small amount of bowel gas projecting in the right lower quadrant at the caecum and within the lower pelvis in the rectum.

BOWEL WALL

There is mural thickening of the dilated small bowel loops. There is no evidence of intramural gas within the large or small bowel.

PNEUMOPERITONEUM

There is no evidence of free intra-abdominal gas.

SOLID ORGANS

The solid organ contours are within normal limits with no solid organ calcification.

VASCULAR

No abnormal vascular calcification.

BONES

There are no abnormalities of the imaged thoracic and lumbar spine, or within the pelvis.

There are growth plates at the femoral head and acetabulum as the ossification centres have not yet fused, which is a normal finding in a child of this age.

SOFT TISSUES

The psoas muscle outline is not visible bilaterally, which is non-specific, particularly in a child of this age.

The extra-abdominal soft tissues are unremarkable.

OTHER

There is an NG tube in situ with its tip projecting in the left upper quadrant, in the fundus of the stomach.

There are no vascular lines, drains or surgical clips.

REVIEW AREAS

Gallstones / Renal calculi: No radiopaque calculi.
Lung bases: Not fully included.
Spine: Normal.
Femoral heads: Normal – growth plates present.

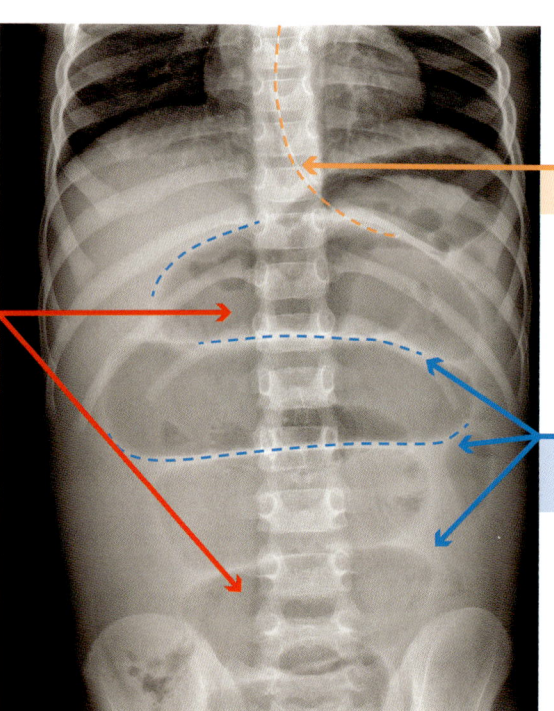

Small bowel dilatation with loss of valvulae conniventes

NG tube

Mural thickening of dilated small bowel loops

Growth plates

SUMMARY

This X-ray demonstrates multiple loops of dilated bowel seen centrally within the abdomen, with loss of the normal pattern of valvulae conniventes, and mural oedema, in keeping with small bowel obstruction, with no cause visible on X-ray. There is an NG tube in situ with its tip in the fundus of the stomach.

INVESTIGATIONS AND MANAGEMENT

The patient should be resuscitated using an ABCDE approach.

Adequate analgesia and hydration should be provided.

The patient should be kept NBM, have their NG tube put on free drainage, and be commenced on IV fluids.

Urgent bloods should be taken, including FBC, U&Es, CRP, LFTs, coagulation, blood gas, and group and save.

The paediatric surgical team should be contacted urgently and further radiological imaging of the abdomen and pelvis should be considered for better visualisation of the anatomy and further assessment.

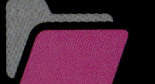

SCENARIO 66

A 59 year old male presents to his doctor with worsening abdominal distension and is transferred to ED by ambulance. He has no significant past medical history and is a non-smoker. On examination, he has saturations of 92% on 4L of oxygen and a temperature of 36.7°C. His HR is 88 bpm, RR is 22 and blood pressure is 130/78 mmHg. The abdomen is peritonitic and there are tinkling bowel sounds. Urine dipstick is unremarkable.

An abdominal X-ray is requested to assess for possible bowel obstruction.

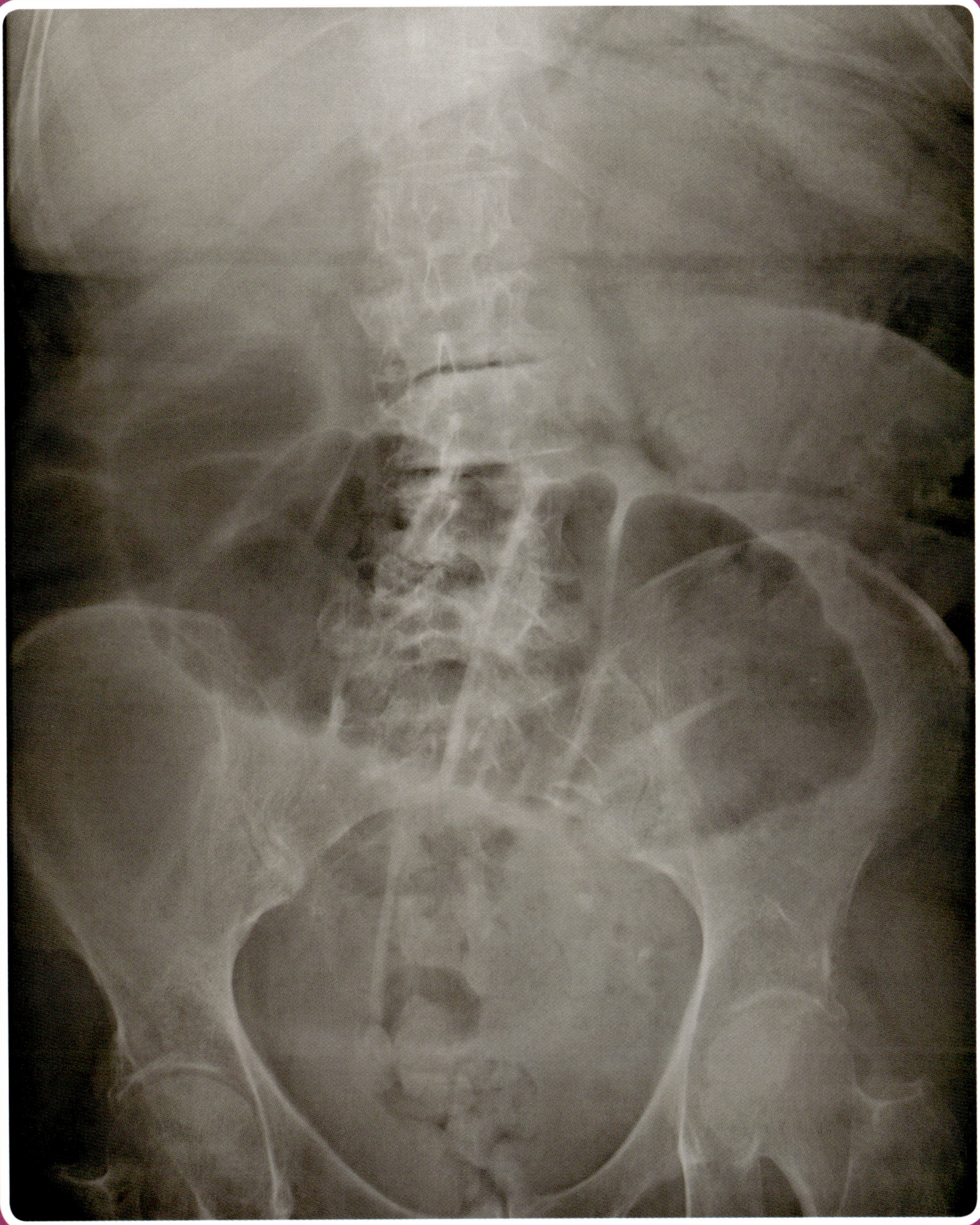

REPORT
Patient ID: Anonymous.
Projection: AP supine.
Rotation: Adequate.
Penetration: Adequate – the spinous processes are visible.
Coverage: Inadequate – the anterior ribs, pubic symphysis and inferior pubic rami have not been fully included.

BOWEL GAS PATTERN
There is a loop of dilated bowel seen centrally within the abdomen demonstrating haustra, suggestive of large bowel obstruction.

BOWEL WALL
There is no evidence of mural thickening or intramural gas within the large or small bowel.

PNEUMOPERITONEUM
There is no evidence of free intra-abdominal gas.

SOLID ORGANS
The solid organ contours are within normal limits with no solid organ calcification.

VASCULAR
No abnormal vascular calcification.

BONES
There is severe degenerative change seen throughout the lower lumbar spine.

There is loss of height of the L5 vertebral body, in keeping with a compression fracture.

The L4 vertebral body demonstrates right-sided loss of height with a wedge shaped appearance suggestive of a probable compression fracture.

There is moderate lumbar scoliosis seen convex to the left, centred on the L4 vertebral body, secondary to degenerative change.

SOFT TISSUES
The psoas muscle outline is not visible bilaterally, which is non-specific.

The extra-abdominal soft tissues are unremarkable.

OTHER
There are no radiopaque foreign bodies.

There are no vascular lines, drains or surgical clips.

REVIEW AREAS
Gallstones / Renal calculi: No radiopaque calculi.
Lung bases: Not fully included.
Spine: Degenerative change in lumbar spine with loss of height of L5 vertebral body and scoliosis.
Femoral heads: Normal.

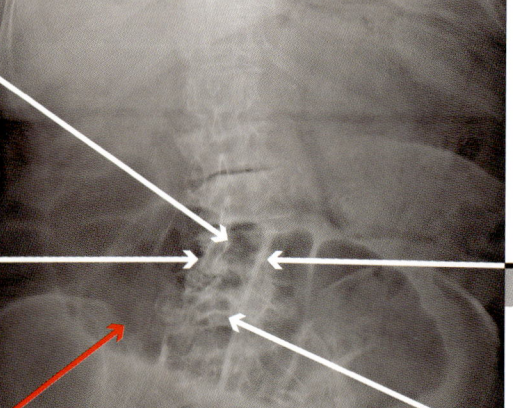

Degenerative change throughout lower lumbar spine

Probable compression fracture of L4 vertebral body

Large bowel dilatation with haustra

Scoliosis

Compression fracture of L5 vertebral body

SUMMARY
This X-ray demonstrates a loop of dilated bowel seen centrally within the abdomen demonstrating haustra, suggestive of large bowel obstruction. There is severe degenerative disease of the lower lumbar spine, with degenerative scoliosis convex to the left centred on the L4 vertebral body and a compression fracture of the L5 vertebral body. There is a further probable L4 compression fracture. Malignancy with secondary bony metastases should be suspected.

INVESTIGATIONS AND MANAGEMENT
The patient should be resuscitated using an ABCDE approach.

Adequate analgesia and hydration should be provided.

The patient should be kept NBM and an NG tube inserted. IV fluids should be commenced.

Urgent bloods should be taken, including FBC, U&Es, CRP, LFTs, coagulation, blood gas, and group and save.

The general surgical team should be contacted urgently and a CT scan of the abdomen/pelvis with IV contrast should be considered for better visualisation of the anatomy and further assessment.

Arthritic changes in the first instance should be managed with lifestyle changes and analgesia, but depending on symptoms, orthopaedic referral may be considered.

Chronic management of vertebral compression fractures may involve lifestyle modification, physiotherapy and pain medication, but further history/examination should be sought, and previous images reviewed.

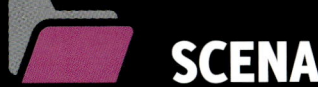

A 67 year old male presents to ED with generalised abdominal pain and distension. He has not passed flatus or opened his bowels for over 24 hours. He has no significant past medical history and is a non-smoker. On examination, he has saturations of 94% in room air and a temperature of 37.2°C. His HR is 90 bpm, RR is 28 and blood pressure is 120/68 mmHg. The abdomen is soft with central tenderness and associated lumbar back pain. Bowel sounds are normal and urine dipstick is unremarkable.

An abdominal X-ray is requested to assess for possible bowel obstruction.

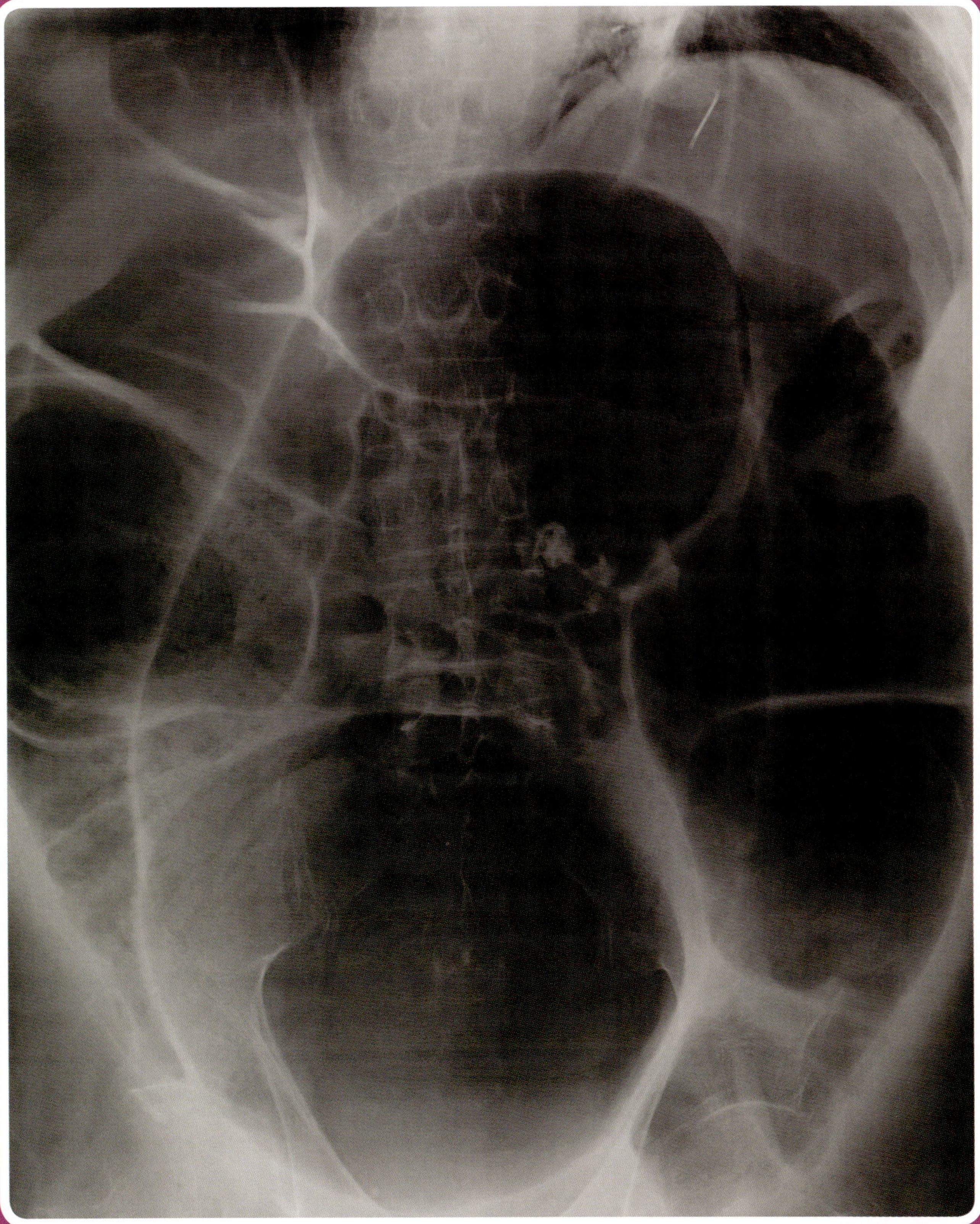

REPORT – SIGMOID VOLVULUS

REPORT
Patient ID: Anonymous.
Projection: AP supine.
Rotation: Adequate.
Penetration: Adequate – the spinous processes are visible.
Coverage: Inadequate – the anterior ribs, pubic symphysis and inferior pubic rami have not been included.

BOWEL GAS PATTERN
There is a large gas filled loop of bowel centrally in the abdomen demonstrating haustra, arising from the pelvis, with its tip pointing towards the upper abdomen, in keeping with sigmoid volvulus. There are further loops of dilated bowel seen peripherally in the abdomen, demonstrating haustra, in keeping with large bowel dilatation.

BOWEL WALL
There is no evidence of mural thickening or intramural gas within the large or small bowel.

PNEUMOPERITONEUM
There is no evidence of free intra-abdominal gas.

SOLID ORGANS
The solid organ contours are within normal limits with no solid organ calcification.

VASCULAR
No abnormal vascular calcification.

BONES
There is mild to moderate degenerative change seen throughout the lower lumbar spine.

There is mild osteoarthritic change seen within both hip joints with joint space narrowing and subchondral sclerosis.

There is diffuse osteopenia of the bones.

SOFT TISSUES
The psoas muscle outline is not visible bilaterally, which is non-specific.

The extra-abdominal soft tissues are unremarkable.

OTHER
There is a radiopacity projecting in the epigastrium, which likely represents film artefact.

There are no radiopaque foreign bodies.

There are no vascular lines, drains or surgical clips.

REVIEW AREAS
Gallstones / Renal calculi: No radiopaque calculi.
Lung bases: Not fully included.
Spine: Degenerative change in lower lumbar spine.
Femoral heads: Mild osteoarthritic change.

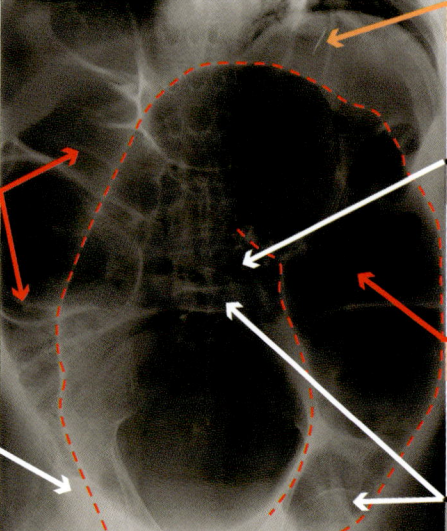

Film artefact

Degenerative change of axial skeleton

Large bowel dilatation with haustra

Sigmoid volvulus

Osteoarthritis of hip joints

Diffuse osteopenia

SUMMARY
This X-ray demonstrates a large gas filled loop of bowel centrally within the abdomen displaying haustra, in keeping with sigmoid volvulus. There are further dilated large bowel loops seen peripherally in keeping with large bowel obstruction secondary to the volvulus. The mild to moderate lower lumbar spine degenerative changes, mild osteoarthritic hip changes and diffuse osteopenia are incidental findings.

INVESTIGATIONS AND MANAGEMENT
The patient should be resuscitated using an ABCDE approach.

Adequate analgesia and hydration should be provided.

The patient should be kept NBM and an NG tube inserted on free drainage. IV fluids should be commenced.

Urgent bloods should be taken, including FBC, U&Es, bone profile, CRP, LFTs, coagulation, blood gas, and group and save.

The general surgical team should be contacted urgently.

Urgent decompression with sigmoidoscopy is required to relieve the obstruction, with a flatus tube left in situ. Elective sigmoidectomy with primary anastomosis may then be undertaken to prevent reoccurrence.

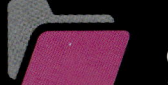

SCENARIO 68

A 50 year old female is currently admitted on the urology ward with longstanding dysuria and the inability to pass urine over the last 12 hours. She has no other significant past medical history and is a non-smoker. On examination, she has saturations of 95% in room air and a temperature of 37.0°C. Her HR is 84 bpm, RR is 14 and blood pressure is 118/80 mmHg. The abdomen is soft and there is tenderness in both flanks with normal bowel sounds. Urine dipstick shows blood ++.

An abdominal X-ray is requested to assess for possible renal calculi.

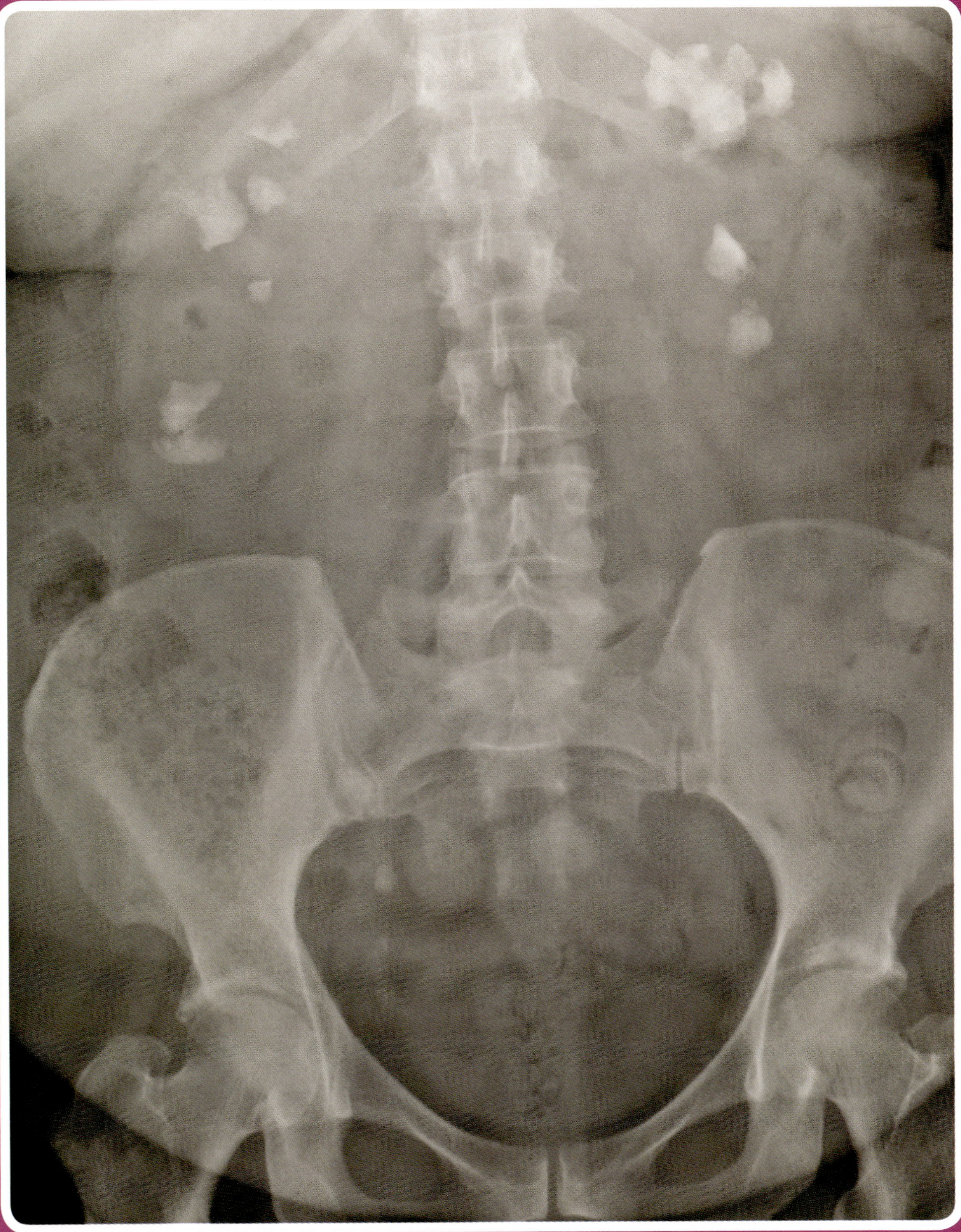

REPORT
Patient ID: Anonymous.
Projection: AP supine.
Rotation: Adequate.
Penetration: Adequate – the spinous processes are visible.
Coverage: Adequate – the anterior ribs are visible superiorly and the inferior pubic rami are visible.

BOWEL GAS PATTERN
There is a paucity of bowel gas but no bowel dilatation is visible.

There is a small to moderate volume of faecal residue present throughout the large bowel.

BOWEL WALL
There is no evidence of mural thickening or intramural gas within the large or small bowel.

PNEUMOPERITONEUM
There is no evidence of free intra-abdominal gas.

SOLID ORGANS
There are multiple large irregular radiopaque densities projected over the regions of both kidneys. The largest density is projecting over the left upper pole conforming to the shape of the renal calyces in keeping with a staghorn calculus.

VASCULAR
No abnormal vascular calcification.

BONES
There are no abnormalities of the imaged thoracic and lumbar spine, or within the pelvis.

SOFT TISSUES
The psoas muscle outline is visible bilaterally.

The extra-abdominal soft tissues are unremarkable.

OTHER
There are no radiopaque foreign bodies.

There are no vascular lines, drains or surgical clips.

REVIEW AREAS
Gallstones / Renal calculi: Likely staghorn calculus in the upper pole of the left kidney with multiple bilateral smaller calculi or renal tissue calcifications in the region of both kidneys.
Lung bases: Not fully included.
Spine: Normal.
Femoral heads: Normal.

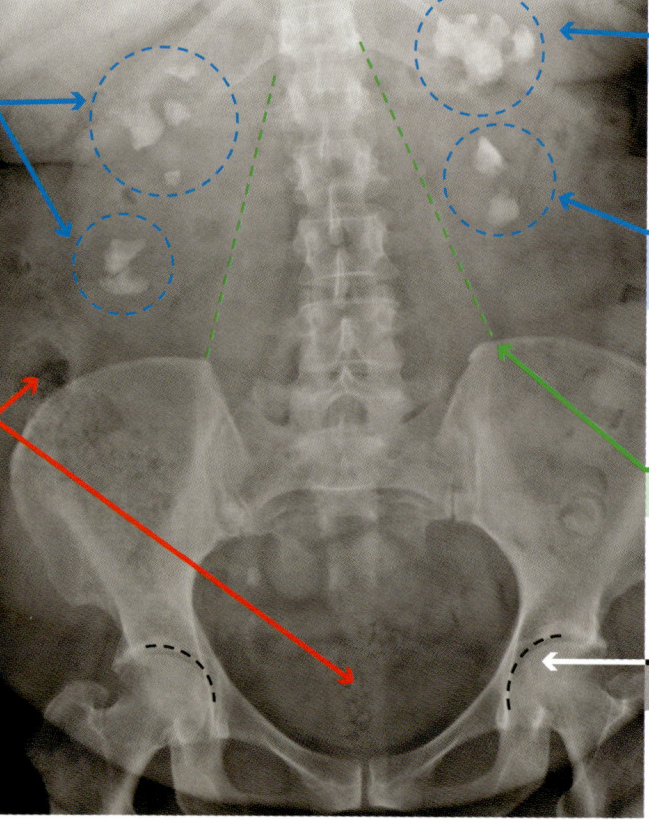

Staghorn calculus

Calcific densities over region of right kidney

Calcific densities over region of left kidney

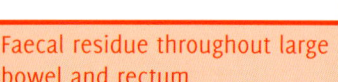
Faecal residue throughout large bowel and rectum

Psoas muscle outlines

Femoral heads normal

SUMMARY
This X-ray demonstrates multiple radiopaque densities projected over the regions of both kidneys, in keeping with medullary nephrocalcinosis with an associated staghorn calculus in the left upper pole.

INVESTIGATIONS AND MANAGEMENT
Adequate analgesia and hydration should be provided.

Urgent bloods should be taken, including FBC, U&Es, CRP, LFTs, blood gas, and bone profile.

The patient should be assessed for acute kidney injury, and if present, an ultrasound of the urinary tract in the first instance would be beneficial in assessing for hydronephrosis. A CT scan of the kidneys, ureters and bladder may be useful for better visualisation of the anatomy.

The patient should be discussed with the urology team for further assessment of the medullary nephrocalcinosis.

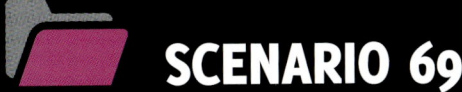

SCENARIO 69

A 20 year old male presents to ED with generalised abdominal pain. He has no significant past medical history and is a non-smoker. On examination, he has saturations of 99% in room air and a temperature of 38.0°C. His HR is 106 bpm, RR is 22 and blood pressure is 120/65 mmHg. The abdomen is rigid and there is generalised tenderness with normal bowel sounds. Urine dipstick is unremarkable.

An abdominal X-ray is requested to assess for possible bowel obstruction.

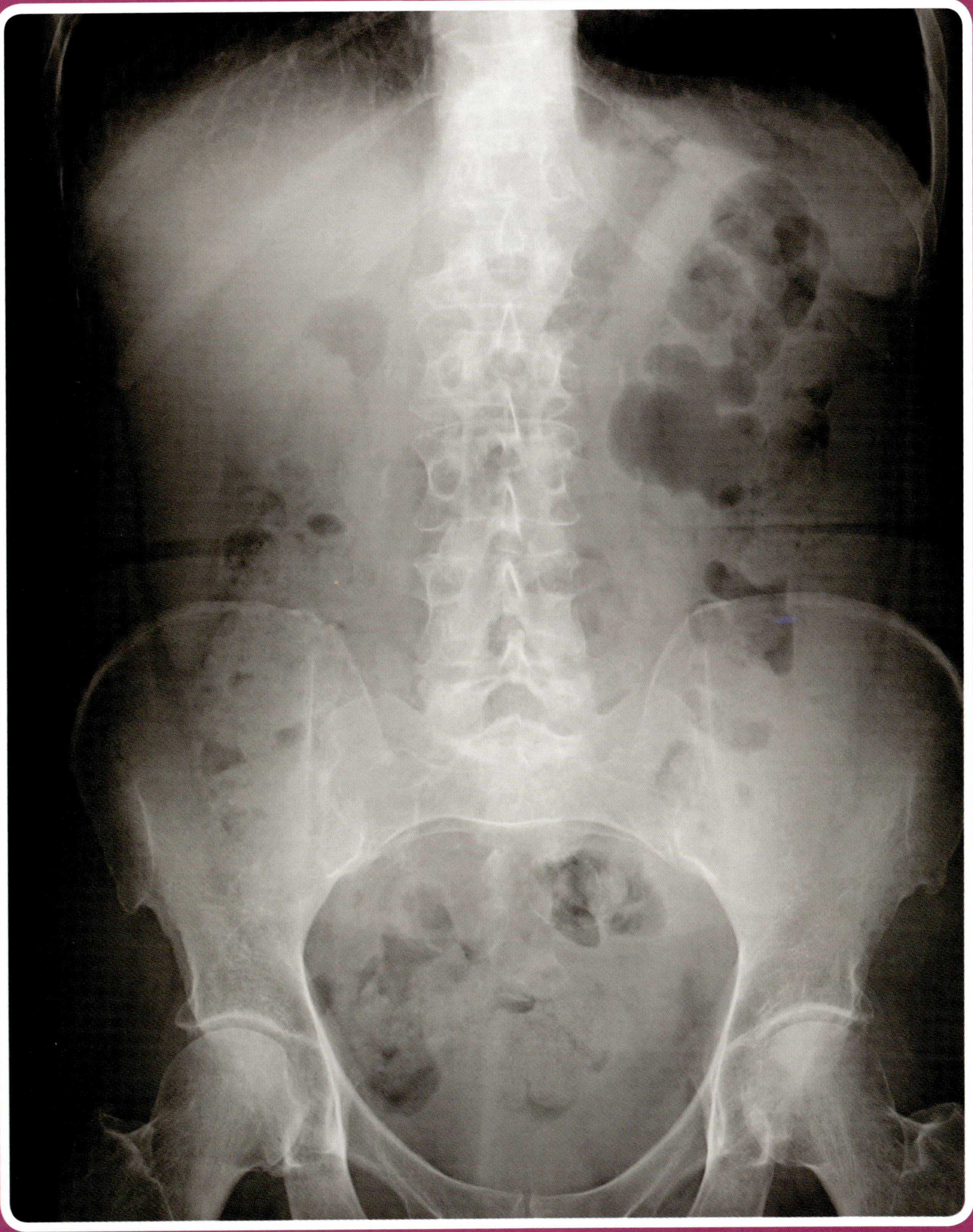

REPORT
Patient ID: Anonymous.
Projection: AP supine.
Rotation: Adequate.
Penetration: Adequate – the spinous processes are visible.
Coverage: Inadequate – the pubic symphysis and inferior pubic rami have not been fully included.

BOWEL GAS PATTERN
The bowel gas pattern is normal.

There is a mild to moderate volume of faecal residue throughout the colon and rectum.

BOWEL WALL
There is no evidence of mural thickening or intramural gas within the large or small bowel. There is mild faecal loading throughout the large bowel and within the rectum.

PNEUMOPERITONEUM
There is no evidence of free intra-abdominal gas.

SOLID ORGANS
The right lobe of the liver extends inferiorly beyond the lower margin of the right kidney, with a tongue-like appearance, in keeping with a Riedel's lobe.

VASCULAR
No abnormal vascular calcification.

BONES
There are no abnormalities of the imaged thoracic and lumbar spine, or within the pelvis.

SOFT TISSUES
The psoas muscle outline is visible bilaterally.

The extra-abdominal soft tissues are unremarkable.

OTHER
There are no radiopaque foreign bodies.

There are no vascular lines, drains or surgical clips.

REVIEW AREAS
Gallstones / Renal calculi: No radiopaque calculi.
Lung bases: Normal.
Spine: Normal.
Femoral heads: Normal.

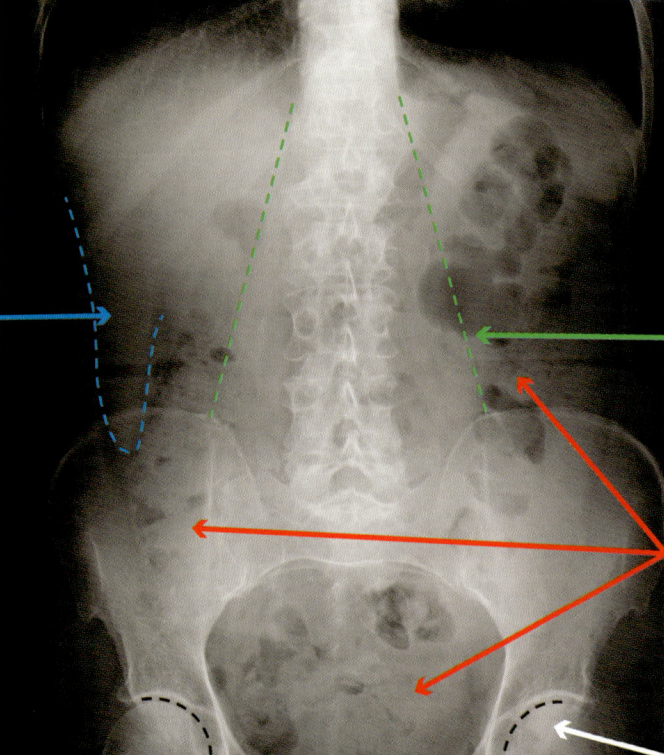

Reidel's lobe of the liver

Psoas muscle outlines

Faecal residue throughout colon and rectum

Femoral heads normal

SUMMARY
This X-ray demonstrates a normal abdominal appearance with no evidence of bowel obstruction or pneumoperitoneum. There is an incidental Riedel's lobe of the liver, which is a normal anatomical variant.

INVESTIGATIONS AND MANAGEMENT
The patient should be resuscitated using an ABCDE approach.

Adequate analgesia and hydration should be provided.

Bloods should be taken, including FBC, U&Es, LFTs, amylase, bone profile, blood gas, blood cultures, group and save and CRP.

The sepsis 6 pathway should be started immediately, including administration of oxygen, IV broad spectrum antibiotics and consideration of a fluid bolus as well as measurement of lactate and urinary output and blood cultures.

The patient should be made NBM and started on IV fluids.

There are no clear findings on the abdominal X-ray to explain the patient's clinical presentation. An ultrasound scan of the abdomen and pelvis should be considered in the first instance for further assessment.

SCENARIO 70

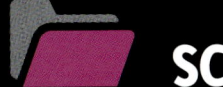

A 6 day old baby girl is currently admitted on NICU, having had bowel surgery on day 5 of life for Hirschsprung's disease. On examination, she has saturations of 98% in room air and a temperature of 36.6°C. Her HR is 160 bpm and RR is 42. The abdomen is soft with normal bowel sounds.

You are asked to review her post operative X-ray.

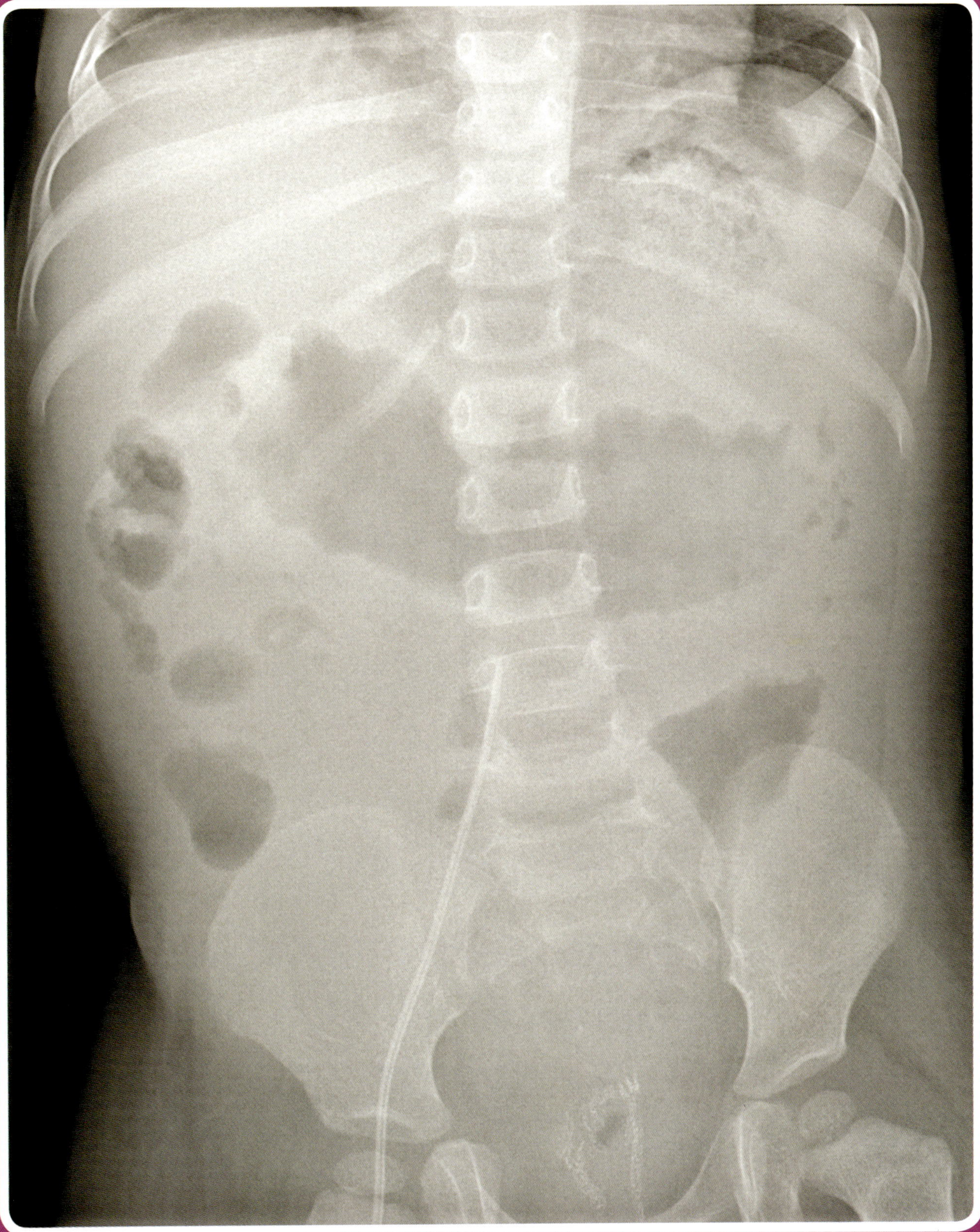

REPORT

Patient ID: Anonymous.
Projection: AP supine.
Rotation: Asymmetrical appearances of the pelvis in keeping with mild patient rotation.
Penetration: Adequate – the spine is visible.
Coverage: Inadequate – the pubic symphysis and inferior pubic rami have not been included.

BOWEL GAS PATTERN

There is prominence of the transverse colon, which is non-specific.

There is a paucity of bowel gas seen within the distal descending and sigmoid colon, but there is gas in the rectum.

BOWEL WALL

There is evidence of mural thickening of the transverse colon in the left and right upper quadrants of the abdomen with evidence of 'thumbprinting', in keeping with mural oedema.

There is no evidence of intramural gas within the large or small bowel.

PNEUMOPERITONEUM

There is no evidence of free intra-abdominal gas.

SOLID ORGANS

The solid organ contours are within normal limits with no solid organ calcification.

VASCULAR

No abnormal vascular calcification.

BONES

There are no abnormalities of the imaged thoracic and lumbar spine, or within the pelvis.

There are growth plates at the femoral head and acetabulum as the ossification centres have not yet fused, which is a normal finding in a child of this age.

There is cartilage seen between the vertebrae, which is a normal finding in a child of this age.

SOFT TISSUES

The psoas muscle outline is not visible bilaterally, which is non-specific, particularly in a child of this age.

The extra-abdominal soft tissues are unremarkable.

OTHER

There is a radiopaque line seen projected over the region of the right hemi-pelvis with its tip projecting at the level of the right L4 vertebral pedicle, in keeping with a right sided femoral venous catheter appropriately sited in the inferior vena cava.

There are radiopaque surgical sutures seen within the rectum, in keeping with previous bowel surgery.

REVIEW AREAS

Gallstones / Renal calculi: No radiopaque calculi.
Lung bases: Normal.
Spine: Normal – cartilage between vertebrae.
Femoral heads: Normal – growth plates present.

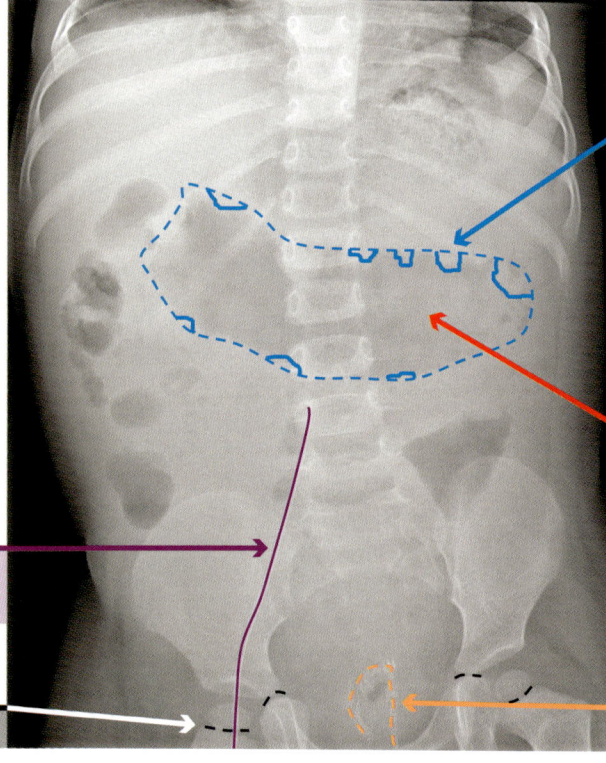

Mural thickening of transverse colon with thumbprinting

Dilated transverse colon

Right-sided femoral venous catheter

Surgical sutures in rectum

Growth plates

SUMMARY

This X-ray demonstrates dilatation of the transverse colon with mural thickening. Given the history of Hirschprung's disease and recent rectal surgery, findings may represent residual colitis in the transverse colon.

INVESTIGATIONS AND MANAGEMENT

Appearances are within normal post-operative limits, however there is possible residual colitis in the transverse colon.

Current management should continue and correlation with clinical findings and biochemical markers should guide further management.

The patient should remain NBM and on TPN, with careful monitoring of fluid balance, broad spectrum antibiotics, and electrolytes.

Regular surgical review is required until discharge.

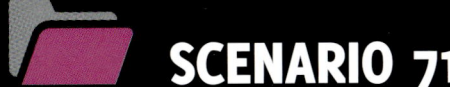
A 60 year old male on the general surgical ward develops severe abdominal pain, vomiting and abdominal distention. His past medical history is significant for recent drainage of an abdominal abscess. On examination, he has saturations of 93% in room air and a temperature of 38.3°C. His HR is 100 bpm and RR is 25. The abdomen is rigid and there is generalised tenderness with normal bowel sounds. Urine dipstick is unremarkable.

An abdominal X-ray is requested to assess for possible bowel obstruction.

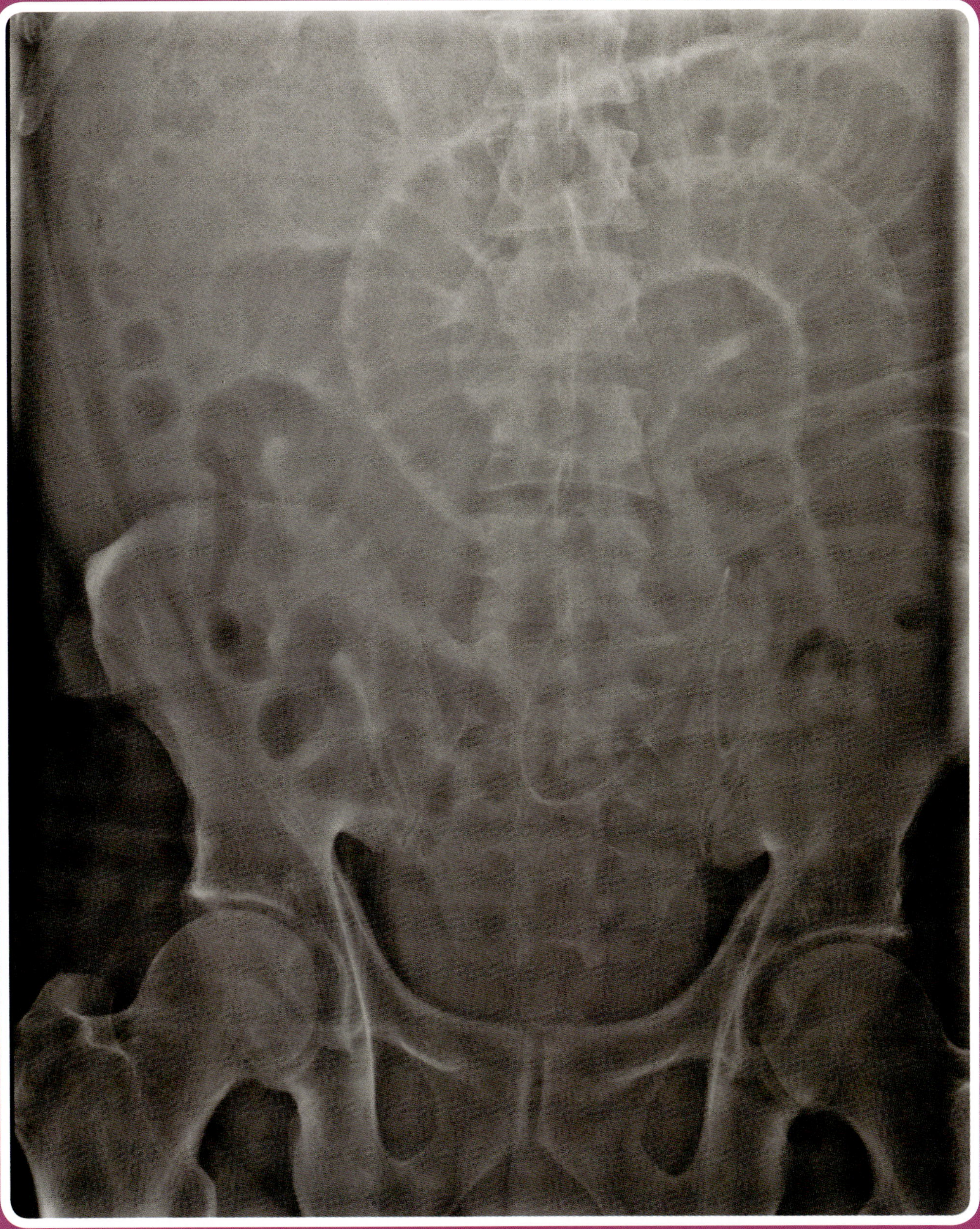

REPORT – SMALL BOWEL OBSTRUCTION WITH MURAL THICKENING

REPORT
Patient ID: Anonymous.
Projection: AP supine.
Rotation: Adequate.
Penetration: Adequate.
Coverage: Inadequate – left and right hemidiaphragms not included.

BOWEL GAS PATTERN
There are multiple loops of prominent small bowel seen centrally in the abdomen demonstrating valvulae conniventes, in keeping with small bowel obstruction.

BOWEL WALL
There is mural thickening of the dilated small bowel loops. There is no evidence of intramural gas within the large or small bowel.

PNEUMOPERITONEUM
There is no evidence of free intra-abdominal gas.

SOLID ORGANS
The solid organ contours are within normal limits with no solid organ calcification.

VASCULAR
No abnormal vascular calcification.

BONES
There are no abnormalities of the imaged thoracic and lumbar spine, or within the pelvis.

SOFT TISSUES
The psoas muscle outline is not visible bilaterally, which is non-specific.

Extra-abdominal soft tissues are unremarkable.

OTHER
There are no radiopaque foreign bodies.

There is a radiopaque line in the lower left quadrant with its tip projecting over the left sacroiliac joint, which likely represents an abdominal drain.

There are no surgical clips.

REVIEW AREAS
Gallstones / Renal calculi: No radiopaque calculi.
Lung bases: Not fully included.
Spine: Normal.
Femoral heads: Normal.

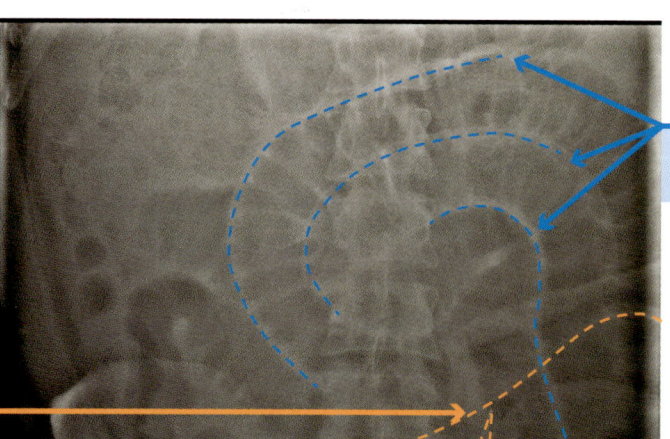
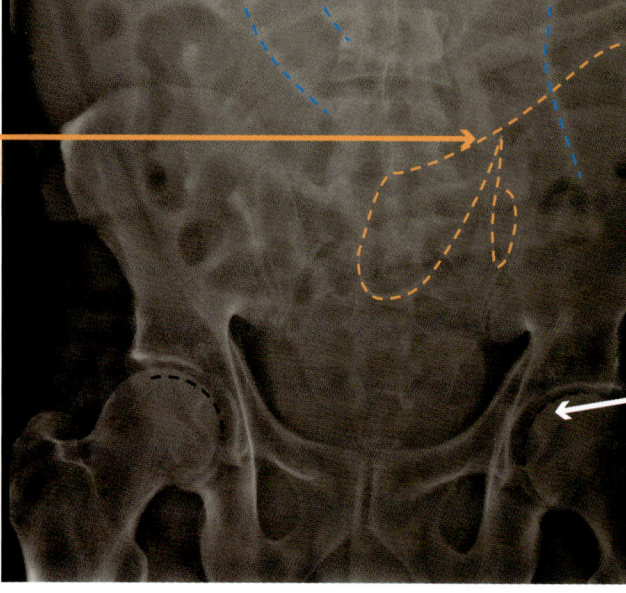

Mural thickening of dilated small bowel loops

Abdominal drain

Femoral heads normal

SUMMARY
This X-ray demonstrates dilatation of small bowel loops, which demonstrate mural thickening in keeping with small bowel obstruction and related inflammatory changes. No cause is visible, although ileus is most likely given the recent abdominal drainage. There is an abdominal drain in situ with its tip projecting over the left sacroiliac joint.

INVESTIGATIONS AND MANAGEMENT
The patient should be resuscitated using an ABCDE approach.

The sepsis 6 pathway should be started immediately, including administration of oxygen, IV broad spectrum antibiotics and consideration of a fluid bolus as well as measurement of lactate, urinary output and blood cultures.

The patient should be made NBM and started on IV fluids, and have an NG tube inserted.

Urgent bloods should be taken, including FBC, U&Es, CRP, bone profile, LFTs, coagulation, blood cultures, blood gas, and group and save.

A CT scan of the abdomen/pelvis with IV contrast should be considered for further evaluation of the abdomen and the general surgical team should be involved.

SCENARIO 72

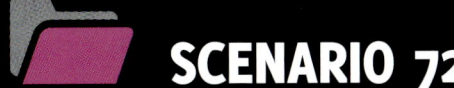

A 60 year old female presents to ED with abdominal pain, vomiting, and severe abdominal distention. She has no significant past medical history. On examination, She has saturations of 94% in room air and a temperature of 37.4°C. Her HR is 100 bpm and RR is 25. The abdomen is soft and distended, with generalised tenderness and normal bowel sounds. Urine dipstick is unremarkable.

An abdominal X-ray is requested to assess for possible bowel obstruction.

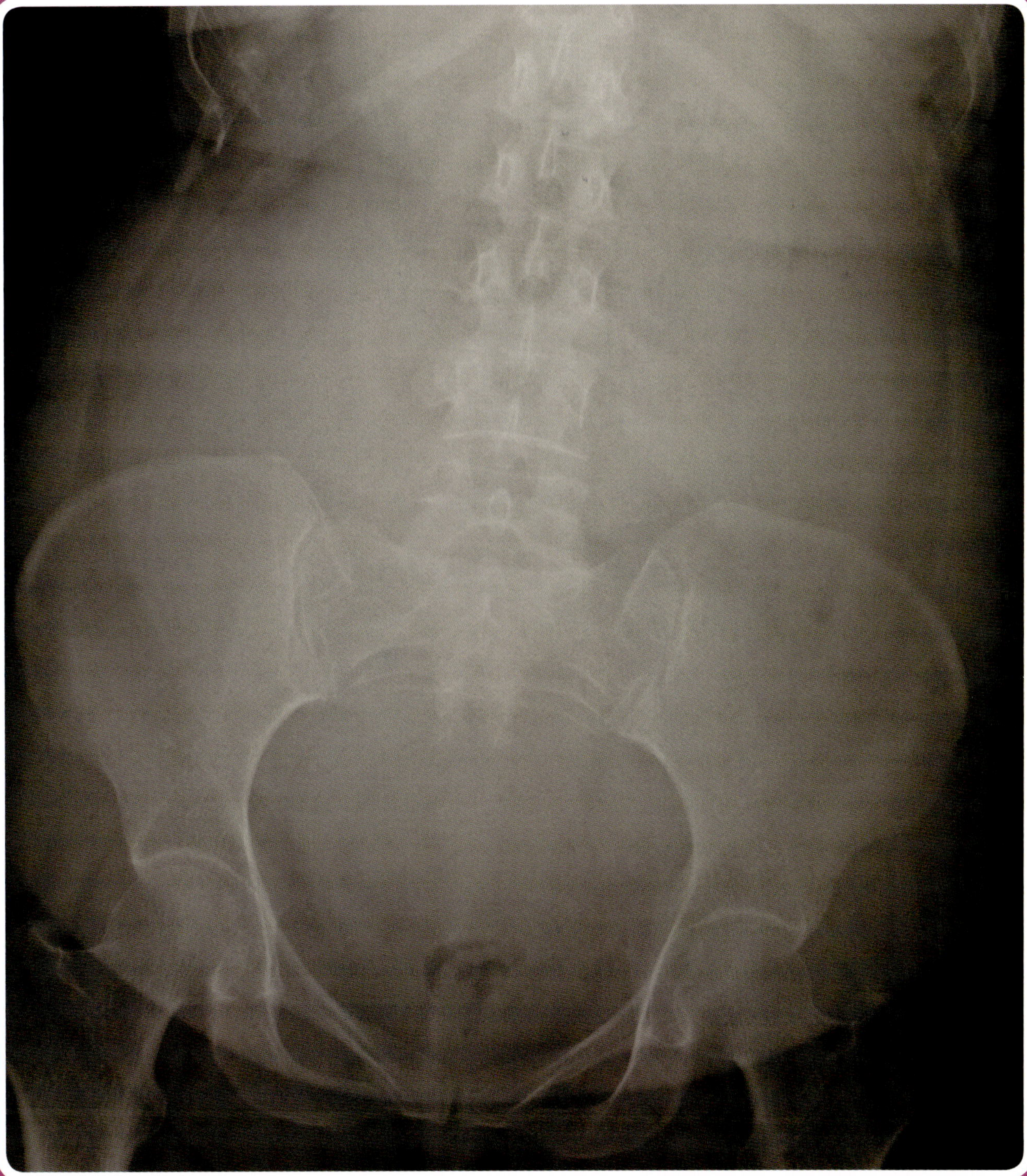

REPORT
Patient ID: Anonymous.
Projection: AP supine.
Rotation: Adequate.
Penetration: Adequate – the spinous processes are visible.
Coverage: Inadequate - the upper abdomen is not fully included.

BOWEL GAS PATTERN
There is a generalised paucity of bowel gas. Gas is seen in the rectum.

BOWEL WALL
There is no evidence of mural thickening or intramural gas within the large or small bowel.

PNEUMOPERITONEUM
There is no evidence of free intra-abdominal gas.

SOLID ORGANS
The solid organs are poorly defined due to diffusely increased density of the abdomen.

VASCULAR
No abnormal vascular calcification.

BONES
There are no abnormalities of the imaged thoracic and lumbar spine, or within the pelvis.

SOFT TISSUES
The psoas muscle outline is not visible bilaterally due to diffusely increased density of the abdomen.

Bulging of the flanks is seen.

OTHER
There are no radiopaque foreign bodies.

There are no vascular lines, drains or surgical clips.

REVIEW AREAS
Gallstones / Renal calculi: No radiopaque calculi.
Lung bases: Not fully included.
Spine: Normal.
Femoral heads: Normal.

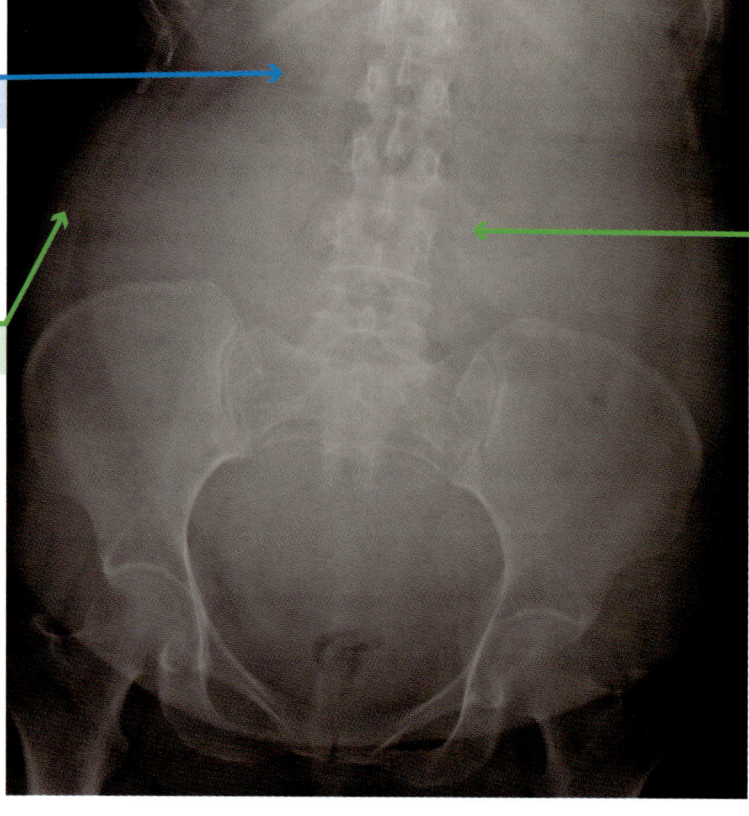

Poorly defined solid organs

Bulging flanks

Psoas muscle shadow obscured by diffusely increased density of abdomen

SUMMARY
This X-ray demonstrates diffuse increased density of the abdomen, with poor definition of the solid organs and other soft tissues including the psoas muscle shadow with bulging at the flanks in keeping with a large volume intra-abdominal ascites. There is no evidence of pneumoperitoneum.

INVESTIGATIONS AND MANAGEMENT
The patient should be resuscitated using an ABCDE approach.

Adequate analgesia, anti-emetics and hydration should be provided.

Urgent bloods should be taken, including FBC, U&Es, CRP, LFTs, TFTs, blood gas, and bone profile.

An USS-guided diagnostic aspiration of the ascitic fluid should be considered to determine the cause. Therapeutic ascitic drain insertion should be considered if clinically appropriate.

Further imaging may be required depending on the underlying cause (e.g. cirrhosis, malignancy).

ADVANCED

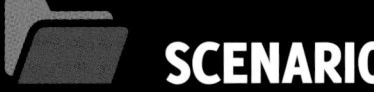

A 75 year old female presents to ED with worsening abdominal pain, abdominal distension, nausea and vomiting. She has no significant past medical history and is a non-smoker. On examination, she has saturations of 94% in room air and a temperature of 37.2°C. Her HR is 98 bpm, RR is 26 and blood pressure is 100/62 mmHg. The abdomen is soft and there is generalised abdominal tenderness with tinkling bowel sounds. Urine dipstick is unremarkable.

An abdominal X-ray is requested to assess for possible bowel obstruction.

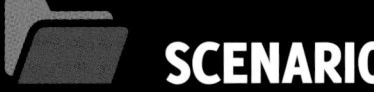

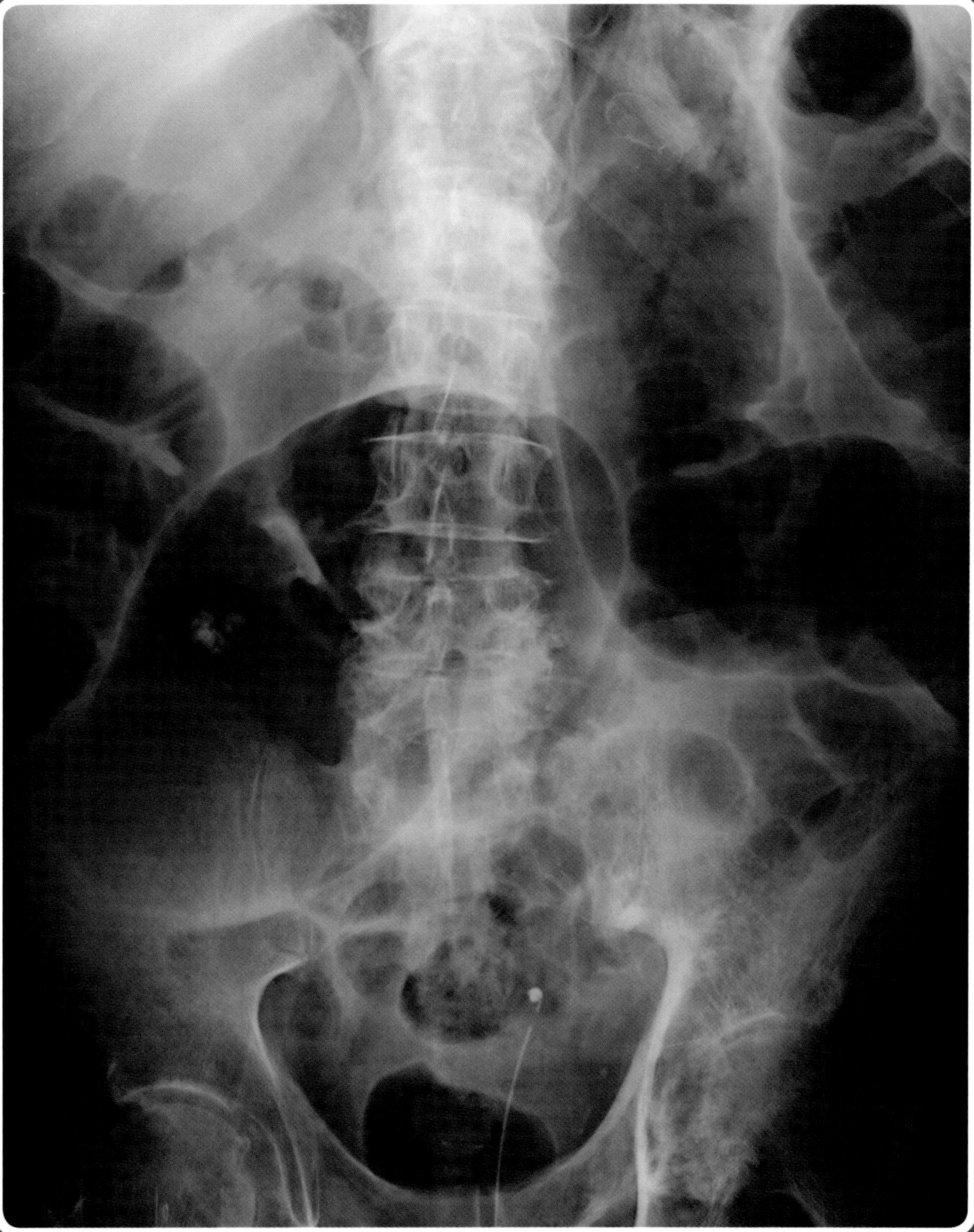

REPORT
Patient ID: Anonymous.
Projection: AP supine.
Rotation: Adequate.
Penetration: Adequate – the spinous processes are visible.
Coverage: Inadequate – the pubic symphysis, inferior pubic rami, and upper abdomen have not been fully included.

BOWEL GAS PATTERN
There are multiple loops of dilated bowel seen centrally and peripherally in the abdomen demonstrating haustra, in keeping with large bowel obstruction.

BOWEL WALL
There is no evidence of mural thickening or intramural gas within the large or small bowel.

PNEUMOPERITONEUM
There is no evidence of free intra-abdominal gas.

SOLID ORGANS
The solid organ contours are within normal limits with no solid organ calcification.

VASCULAR
There is splenic artery calcification in the left upper quadrant.

BONES
There is moderate degenerative change seen in the lower lumbar spine.

There is a mixed lucent and sclerotic architecture of the left hemi-pelvis.

There is mild expansion of the left hemi-pelvis compared to the right hemi-pelvis and coarsening of the trabeculae with cortical thickening of the left ilioischial line.

SOFT TISSUES
The psoas muscle outline is visible bilaterally.

The extra-abdominal soft tissues are unremarkable.

OTHER
There is a urinary catheter in situ within the urinary bladder.

There is an irregular radiopaque area of calcification within the right lower quadrant of the abdomen in keeping with mesenteric lymph node calcification.

There are no vascular lines, drains or surgical clips.

REVIEW AREAS
Gallstones / Renal calculi: No radiopaque calculi.
Lung bases: Not fully included.
Spine: Degenerative change throughout the lower lumbar spine.
Femoral heads: Mixed lucent and sclerotic architecture.

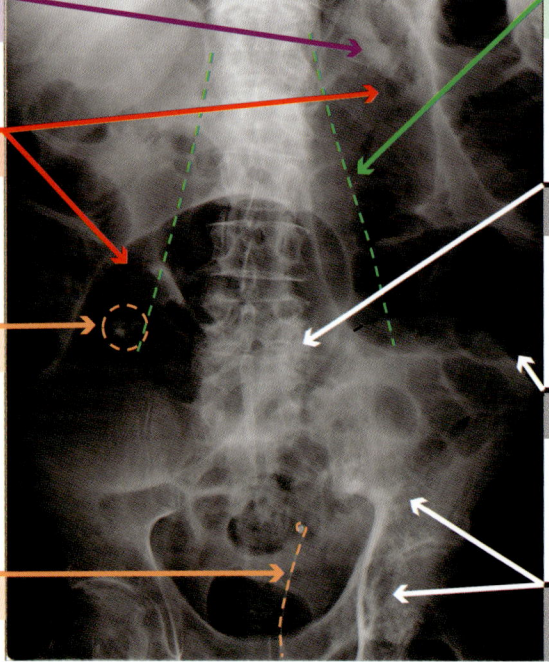

Splenic artery calcifaction

Large bowel dilatation with haustra

Calcification

Urinary catheter

Psoas muscle outlines

Degenerative change

Mild expansion of left hemi-pelvis

Mixed lucent and sclerotic architecture of left hemi-pelvis

SUMMARY
This X-ray demonstrates multiple loops of dilated bowel demonstrating haustra, in keeping with large bowel obstruction. The cause for this is not demonstrated. The left hemi-pelvis bony expansion with coarsening of trabeculae and mixed lucent and sclerotic architecture is in keeping with Paget's disease. There is a urinary catheter in situ.

INVESTIGATIONS AND MANAGEMENT
The patient should be resuscitated using an ABCDE approach.

Adequate analgesia and hydration should be provided.

The patient should be kept NBM and an NG tube inserted on free drainage. IV fluids should be commenced.

Urgent bloods should be taken, including FBC, U&Es, bone profile, CRP, LFTs, coagulation, blood gas, and group and save.

The general surgical team should be contacted urgently and a CT scan of the abdomen/pelvis with IV contrast should be considered for better visualisation of the anatomy and further assessment.

Once the bowel obstruction has been resolved, the patient should be seen in rheumatology clinic for review of her Paget's disease. Arthritic changes in the first instance should be management with lifestyle changes and analgesia, depending on symptoms.

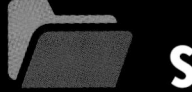

A 40 year old female presents to ED with abdominal pain, having not passed flatus or opened her bowels for over 48 hours. Her past medical history is significant for a previous laparoscopic appendicectomy 6 years ago, and an IVC insertion for recurrent PEs. She is a smoker. On examination, she has saturations of 97% in room air and a temperature of 37.5°C. Her HR is 132 bpm, RR is 25 and blood pressure is 142/86 mmHg. The abdomen is rigid and there is generalised tenderness with tinkling bowel sounds. Urine dipstick is unremarkable and a pregnancy test is negative.

An abdominal X-ray is requested to assess for possible bowel obstruction.

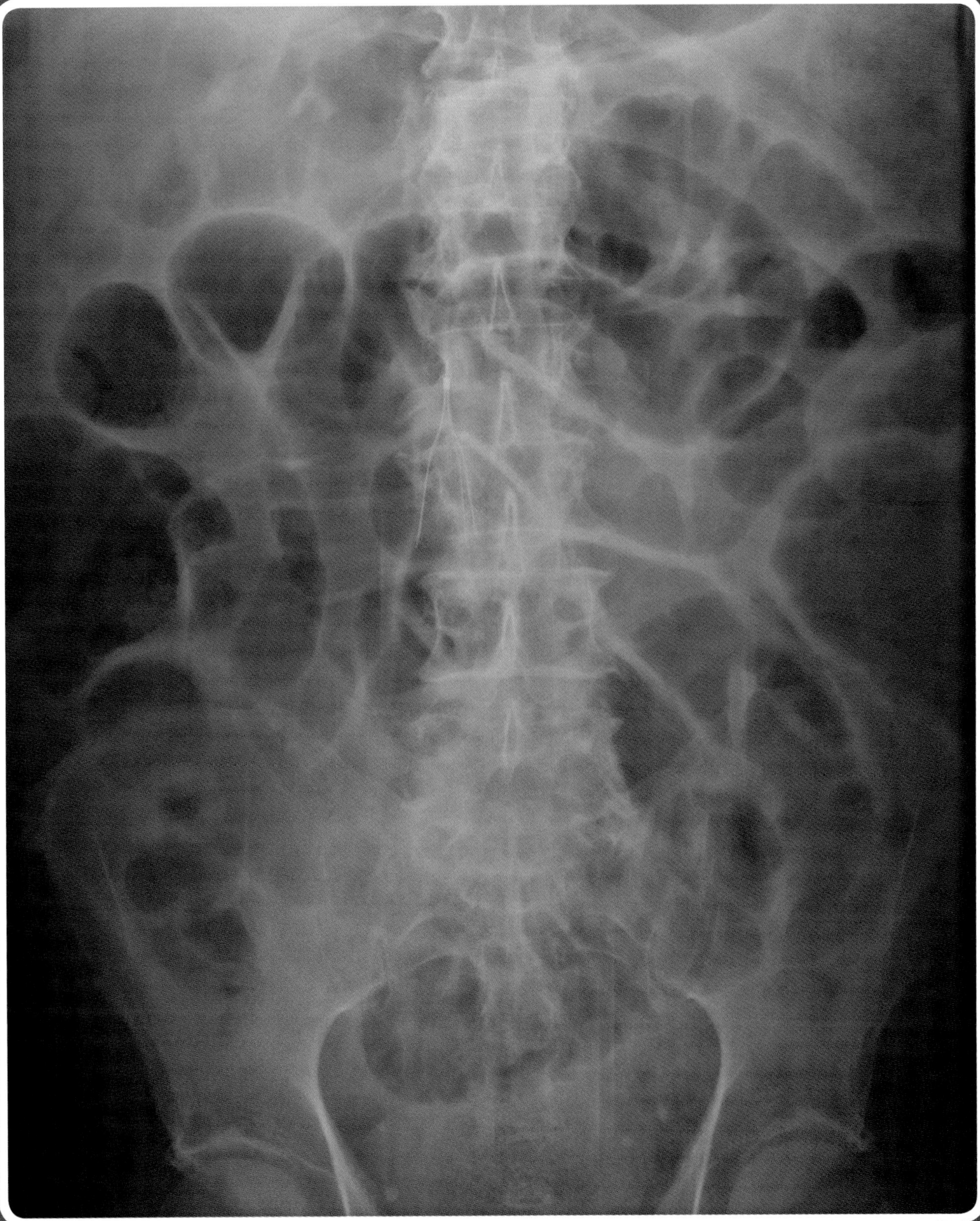

REPORT – SMALL BOWEL OBSTRUCTION AND INFERIOR VENA CAVA FILTER

REPORT
Patient ID: Anonymous.
Projection: AP supine.
Rotation: Adequate.
Penetration: Adequate – the spinous processes are visible.
Coverage: Inadequate – the pubic symphysis and inferior pubic rami have not been included.

BOWEL GAS PATTERN
There are multiple loops of dilated bowel seen centrally in the abdomen, which demonstrate valvulae conniventes in keeping with small bowel dilatation.

There is a small volume of faeces seen in the rectum.

BOWEL WALL
There is no evidence of mural thickening or intramural gas within the large or small bowel.

PNEUMOPERITONEUM
There is no evidence of free intra-abdominal gas.

SOLID ORGANS
The solid organ contours are within normal limits with no solid organ calcification.

VASCULAR
No abnormal vascular calcification.

BONES
There is moderate degenerative change seen in the spine with osteophyte formation.

SOFT TISSUES
The psoas muscle outline is not visible bilaterally, which is non-specific.

The extra-abdominal soft tissues are unremarkable.

OTHER
There is an IVC filter projected over the right pedicles of L2 and L3, within the region of the abdominal inferior vena cava.

There are multiple rounded radiopaque densities projected over the region of the pelvis, most likely phleboliths.

There are no vascular lines, drains or surgical clips.

REVIEW AREAS
Gallstones / Renal calculi: No radiopaque calculi.
Lung bases: Not fully included.
Spine: Moderate degenerative change.
Femoral heads: Normal.

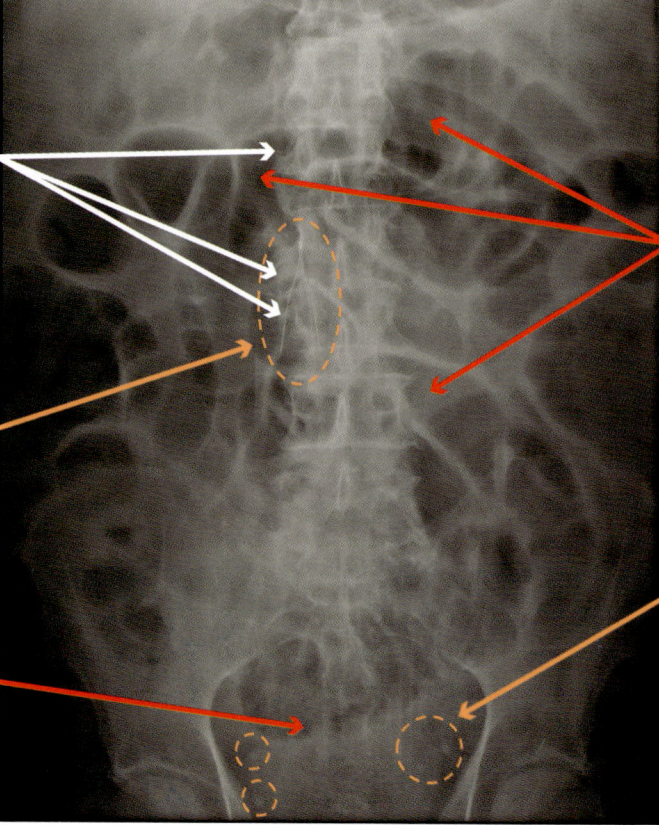

Degenerative change in the spine

Small bowel dilatation

IVC filter

Phleboliths

Faeces in rectum

SUMMARY
This X-ray demonstrates multiple loops of dilated bowel seen centrally within the abdomen demonstrating valvulae conniventes, in keeping with small bowel obstruction. The cause for this is not demonstrated, but may relate to adhesions given the previous surgery. There is an IVC filter in situ in a satisfactory position. The moderate degenerative change in the spine and pelvic phleboliths are incidental findings.

INVESTIGATIONS AND MANAGEMENT
The patient should be resuscitated using an ABCDE approach.

Adequate analgesia and hydration should be provided.

The patient should be kept NBM and an NG tube inserted on free drainage to relieve the pressure in the small bowel. IV fluids should be commenced.

Urgent bloods should be taken, including FBC, U&Es, CRP, LFTs, coagulation, blood gas, and group and save.

The general surgical team should be contacted urgently and a CT scan of the abdomen/pelvis with IV contrast should be considered for better visualisation of the anatomy and further assessment.

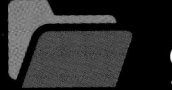
A 10 year old boy presents to the gastroenterology clinic with ongoing constipation. He has a background of chronic constipation, for which he is on laxatives, but no other significant past medical history. A colonic transit study is organised. On examination, he has saturations of 99% in room air and a temperature of 36.5°C. His HR is 88 bpm, RR is 20 and blood pressure is 110/65 mmHg. The abdomen is soft and there is no tenderness with normal bowel sounds.

An abdominal X-ray is requested for day 4 to assess the location of any remaining colonic transit markers.

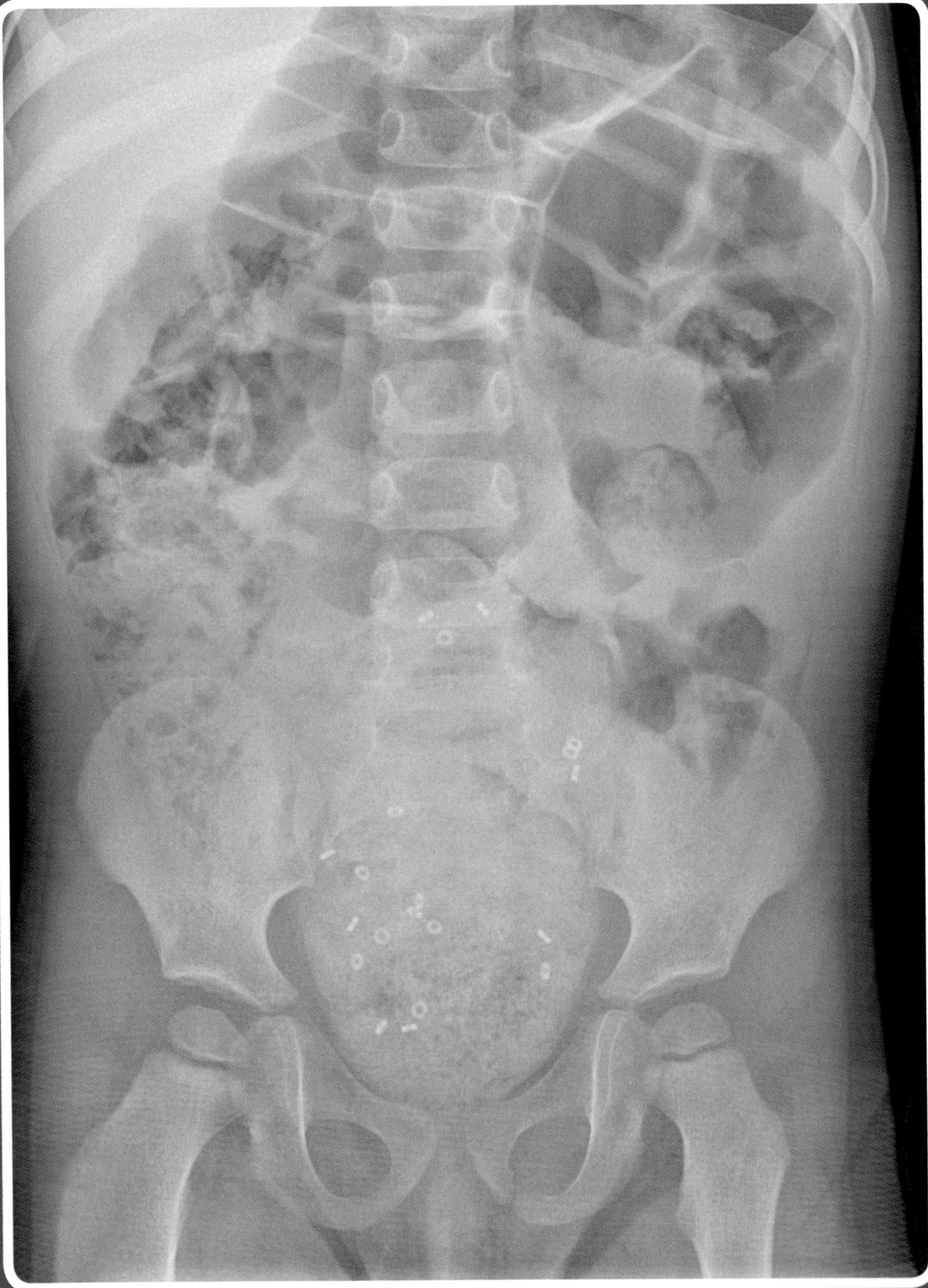

REPORT

Patient ID: Anonymous.
Projection: AP supine.
Rotation: Adequate.
Penetration: Adequate – the spine is visible.
Coverage: Adequate – the anterior ribs are visible superiorly and the pubic rami are visible inferiorly.

BOWEL GAS PATTERN

There are loops of dilated bowel demonstrating haustra seen in the upper abdomen in keeping with large bowel dilatation, predominantly of the transverse colon.

There is a moderate volume of faecal material present throughout the large bowel from the ascending colon to the rectum. The rectum is prominent, containing a significant volume of faeces, which may be impacted.

BOWEL WALL

There is no evidence of mural thickening or intramural gas within the large or small bowel.

PNEUMOPERITONEUM

There is no evidence of free intra-abdominal gas.

SOLID ORGANS

The solid organ contours are within normal limits with no solid organ calcification.

VASCULAR

No abnormal vascular calcification.

BONES

There are no abnormalities of the imaged thoracic and lumbar spine, or within the pelvis.

There are growth plates at the femoral head and acetabulum as the ossification centres have not yet fused, which is a normal finding in a child of this age.

SOFT TISSUES

The psoas muscle outline is visible bilaterally.

The extra-abdominal soft tissues are unremarkable.

OTHER

There are a total of 20 rounded and linear radiopaque densities seen projected over the region of the lower abdomen and pelvis within the sigmoid colon and rectum, in keeping with the known radiopaque transit markers.

There are no vascular lines, drains or surgical clips.

REVIEW AREAS

Gallstones / Renal calculi: No radiopaque calculi.
Lung bases: Not fully included.
Spine: Normal.
Femoral heads: Normal – growth plates present.

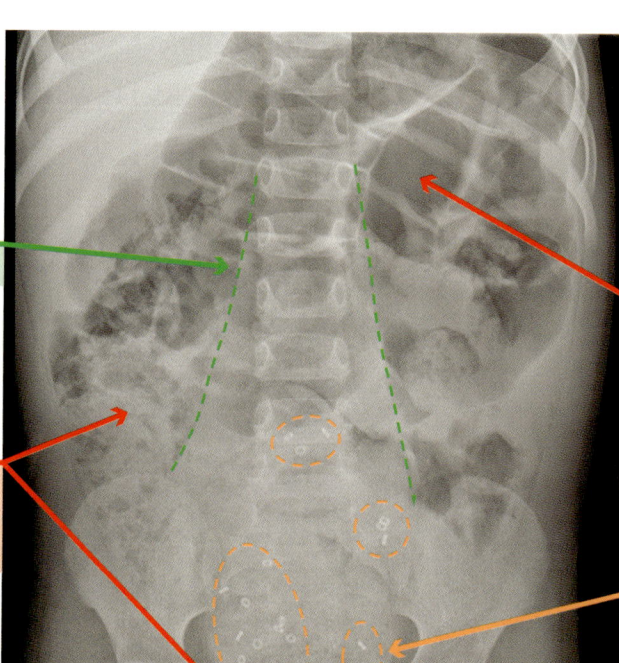

Psoas muscle outlines

Dilated loops of bowel

Faecal residue throughout large bowel, from ascending colon to rectum

Colonic transit markers

Growth plates

SUMMARY

This X-ray demonstrates moderate volume faecal loading throughout the colon with significant faecal impaction in the rectum, which is prominent. There are 20 ingested radiopaque transit markers projecting over the lower abdomen and pelvis, likely within the sigmoid colon and rectum.

INVESTIGATIONS AND MANAGEMENT

The colon transit study should be reviewed and interpreted by a specialist, the results of which will depend on the number of markers ingested and timings of ingestion.

Further investigations should be considered to assess the cause for the patient's ongoing constipation, and in consultation with a gastroenterologist, optimisation of laxatives/enemas and lifestyle advice, including adequate fluid intake, sufficient dietary fibre and exercise is needed.

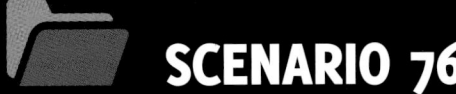

A 73 year old female presents to his primary care physician with a 2 month history of generalised abdominal pain. Her past medical history is significant for chronic renal failure and she is currently on haemodialysis after a failed renal transplant. She is a non-smoker. On examination, she has saturations of 95% in air and a temperature of 37.1°C. Her HR is 78 bpm, RR is 14 and blood pressure is 120/85 mmHg. The abdomen is soft and there is tenderness in the right iliac fossa with normal bowel sounds. Urine dipstick is unremarkable.

An abdominal X-ray is requested to assess for possible bowel obstruction.

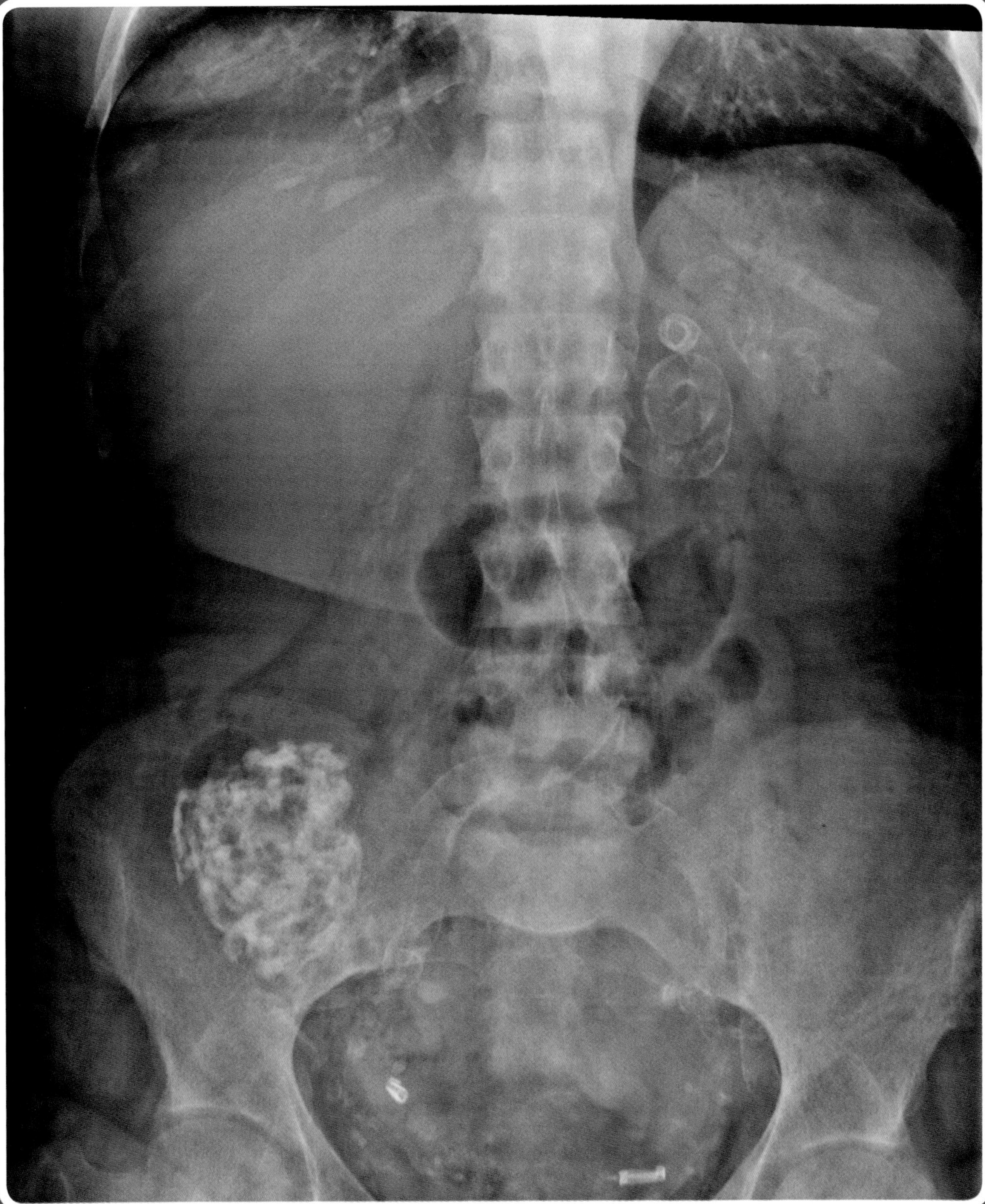

REPORT – FAILED RENAL TRANSPLANT

REPORT
Patient ID: Anonymous.
Projection: AP supine.
Rotation: Adequate
Penetration: Adequate – the spinous processes are visible.
Coverage: Inadequate – the pubic symphysis and inferior pubic rami have not been included.

BOWEL GAS PATTERN
The bowel gas pattern is normal.

BOWEL WALL
There is no evidence of mural thickening or intramural gas within the large or small bowel.

PNEUMOPERITONEUM
There is no evidence of free intra-abdominal gas.

SOLID ORGANS
The solid organ contours are within normal limits with no solid organ calcification.

VASCULAR
There is calcification of the abdominal aorta and iliac arteries with serpiginous calcification in the left upper quadrant in keeping with calcification.

BONES
The vertebral body endplates appear sclerotic, giving the appearance of a 'rugger jersey spine'.

No fractures or destructive bone lesions are visible in the imaged skeleton.

SOFT TISSUES
There is a well-defined radiopaque density projected over the region of the right iliac fossa, which most likely represents a calcified kidney transplant.

The psoas muscle outline is not visible on the left side, which is non-specific.

The extra-abdominal soft tissues are unremarkable.

OTHER
There are two surgical clips projected over the pelvis, possibly related to sterilisation.

There are no vascular lines or drains.

REVIEW AREAS
Gallstones / Renal calculi: No radiopaque calculi.
Lung bases: Normal.
Spine: Sclerotic vertebral body endplates.
Femoral heads: Normal.

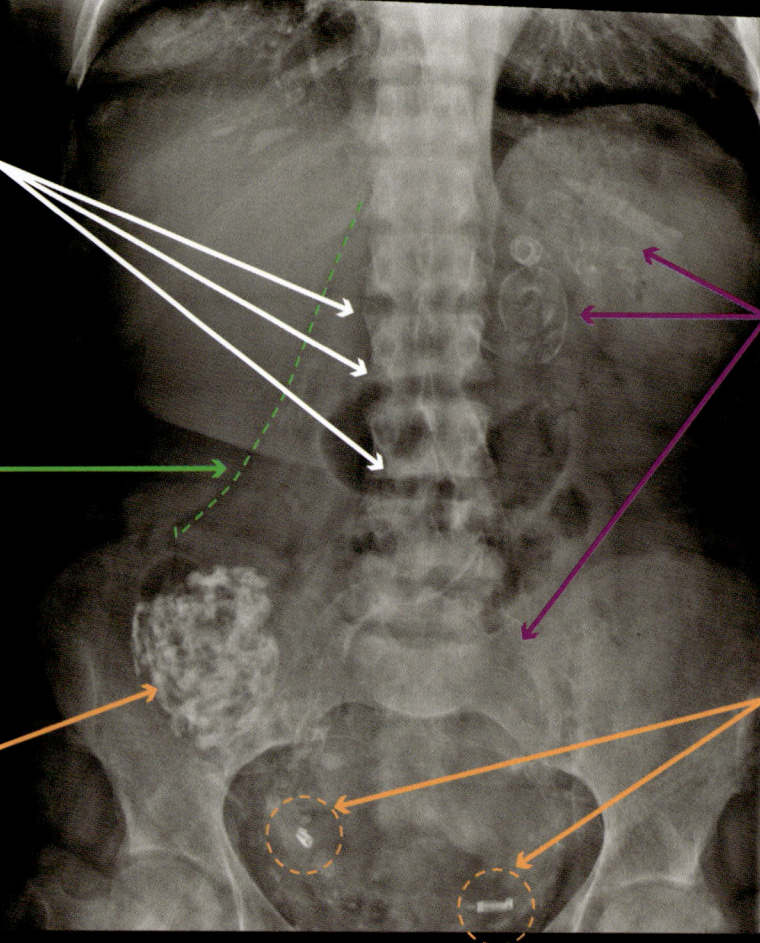

Sclerotic vertebral endplates – 'rugger jersey spine'

Right psoas muscle outline

Failed renal transplant

Vascular calcification

Surgical clips

SUMMARY
This X-ray demonstrates multi-focal vascular calcification as described. It also demonstrates a calcified renal transplant in the right iliac fossa with sclerotic vertebral body endplates, likely related to renal osteodystrophy.

INVESTIGATIONS AND MANAGEMENT
Adequate analgesia and hydration should be provided.

Bloods should be taken including FBC, U&Es, LFTs, bone profile, coagulation, blood gas and CRP.

There are no clear findings on the abdominal X-ray to explain the patient's clinical presentation.

Further imaging may be considered for evaluation of the abdomen and surgical input should be sought. The renal/transplant team may also be required to optimise management of the patient's kidneys.

SCENARIO 77

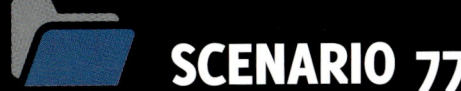

A 75 year old female presents to ED with generalised abdominal pain. Her past medical history is significant for a previous craniectomy and she is a non-smoker. On examination, she has saturations of 95% in air and a temperature of 37.0°C. Her HR is 130 bpm, RR is 21 and blood pressure is 120/85 mmHg. The abdomen is rigid and there is generalised tenderness with normal bowel sounds. Urine dipstick is unremarkable.

An abdominal X-ray is requested to assess for possible bowel obstruction.

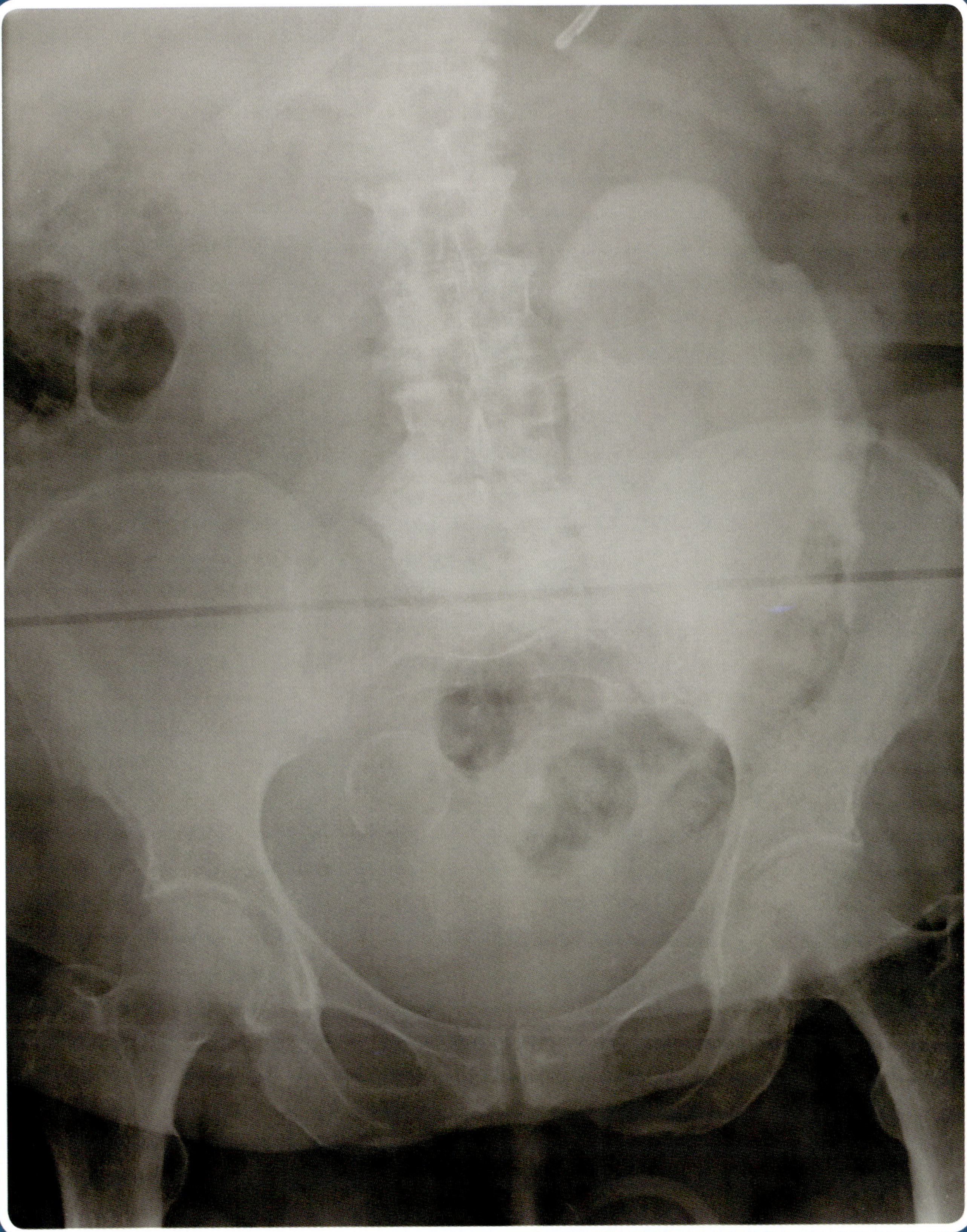

REPORT
Patient ID: Anonymous.
Projection: AP supine.
Rotation: Adequate
Penetration: Adequate – the spinous processes are visible.
Coverage: Inadequate – the upper abdomen and right flank have not been fully imaged.

BOWEL GAS PATTERN
The bowel gas pattern is normal.

BOWEL WALL
There is no evidence of mural thickening or intramural gas within the large or small bowel.

PNEUMOPERITONEUM
There is no evidence of free intra-abdominal gas.

SOLID ORGANS
The solid organ contours are within normal limits with no solid organ calcification.

VASCULAR
There is a curvilinear radiopaque density projecting over the right hemi-pelvis, which may represent calcification of an iliac artery aneurysm.

BONES
There is moderate degenerative change visible in the lumbar spine with bridging osteophyte formation.

No fractures or destructive bone lesions are visible in the imaged skeleton.

SOFT TISSUES
The psoas muscle outline is not visible bilaterally, which is non-specific.

The extra-abdominal soft tissues are unremarkable.

OTHER
There is an NG tube tip projected over the epigastrium likely within the stomach.

There are no vascular lines, drains or surgical clips.

There is a well-defined radiopaque density projected over the left side of the abdomen, which likely represents a craniectomy bone flap being preserved in the abdomen, given the history.

REVIEW AREAS
Gallstones / Renal calculi: No radiopaque calculi.
Lung bases: Not fully included.
Spine: Degenerative change in lumbar spine.
Femoral heads: Normal.

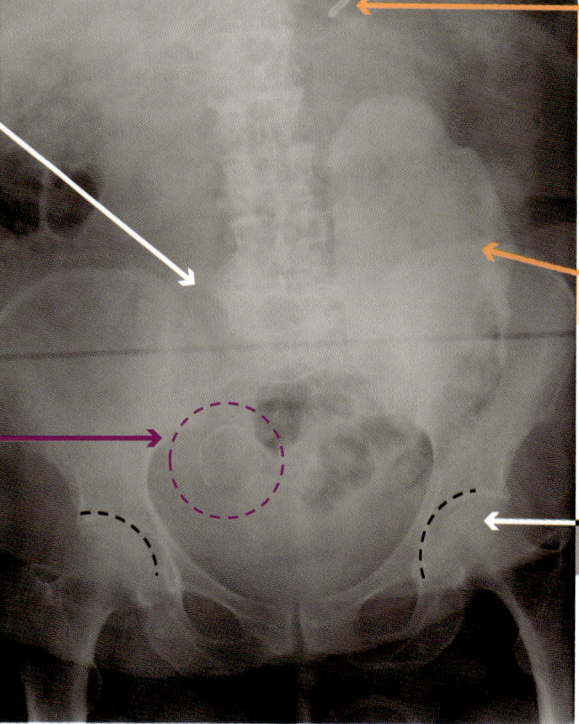

NG tube tip

Degenerative change in lumbar spine with bridging osteophytes

Craniectomy bone flap

Vascular calcification

Femoral heads normal

SUMMARY
This X-ray demonstrates a well-defined radiopaque density projected over the left side of the abdomen, in keeping with a craniectomy bone flap being preserved in the abdomen. There is also a radiopaque curvilinear density projecting over the right hemi-pelvis, which may represent calcification of an iliac artery aneurysm. There is an NG tube tip projecting likely within the stomach. The degenerative change within the lumbar spine is an incidental finding.

INVESTIGATIONS AND MANAGEMENT
The patient should be resuscitated using an ABCDE approach.

Adequate analgesia and hydration should be provided.

Urgent bloods should be taken including FBC, U&Es, bone profile, LFTs, CRP, coagulation, blood gas, and group and save.

Broad spectrum antibiotics should be prescribed.

A CT scan of the abdomen/pelvis with IV contrast may be considered for further evaluation of the abdomen and surgical input should be sought.

Arthritic changes in the first instance should be management with lifestyle changes and analgesia, if they are causing symptoms.

SCENARIO 78

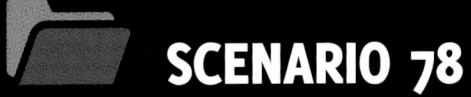

A 50 year old female presents to ED with vomiting, abdominal pain, palpitations and collapse. She has no significant past medical history and is a non-smoker. On examination, she has saturations of 97% in room air and a temperature of 37.2°C. Her HR is 130 bpm, RR is 25 and blood pressure is 92/60 mmHg. Her abdomen is rigid and there is generalised tenderness with normal bowel sounds. Urine dipstick is unremarkable.

An abdominal X-ray is requested to assess for possible bowel obstruction.

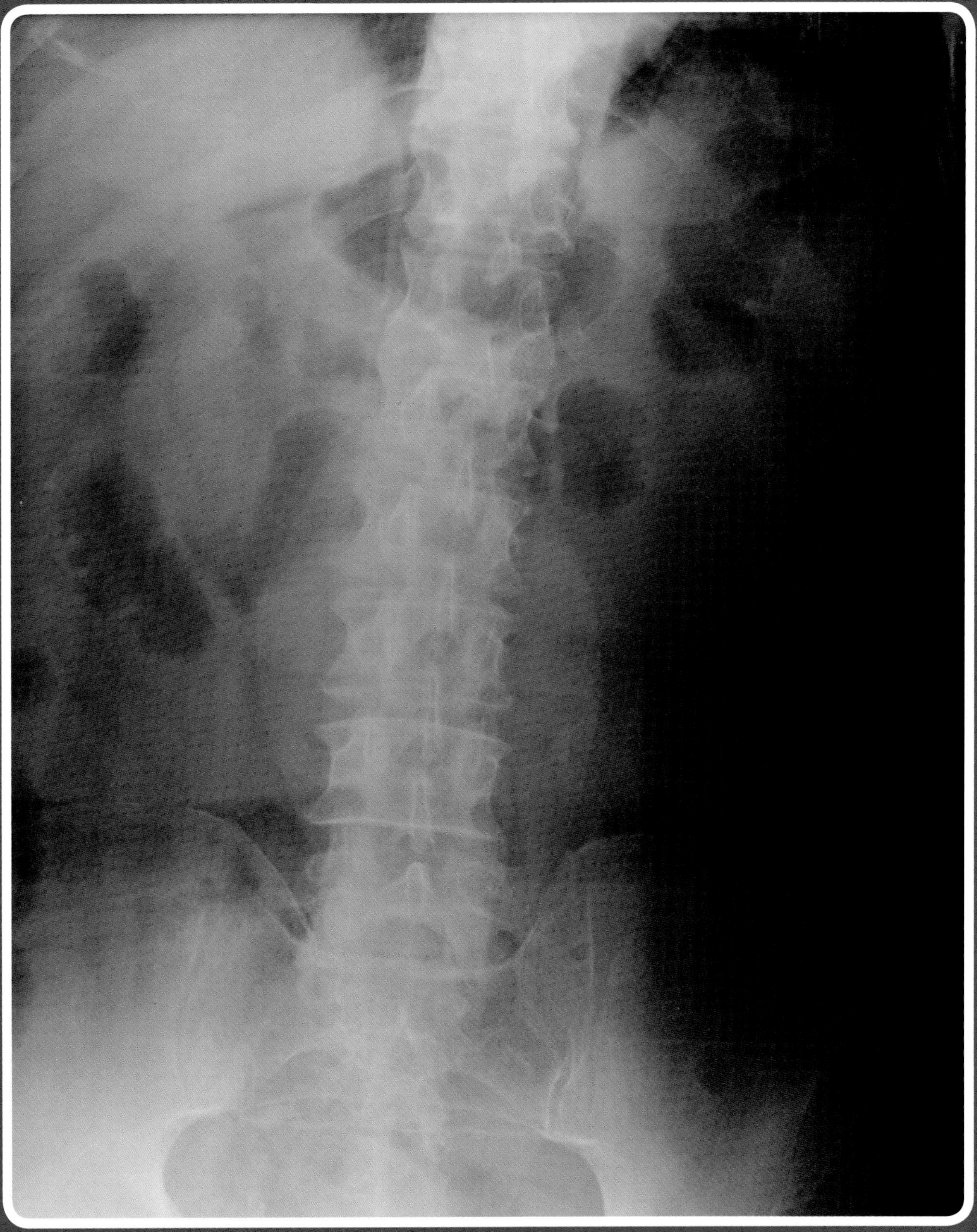

REPORT – ABDOMINAL AORTIC ANEURYSM

REPORT
Patient ID: Anonymous.
Projection: AP supine.
Rotation: Adequate
Penetration: Inadequate – the left side of the X-ray is over-penetrated.
Coverage: Inadequate – the right iliac crest, pubic symphysis and inferior pubic rami have not been fully included.

BOWEL GAS PATTERN
The bowel gas pattern is normal.

BOWEL WALL
There is no evidence of mural thickening or intramural gas within the large or small bowel.

PNEUMOPERITONEUM
There is no evidence of free intra-abdominal gas.

SOLID ORGANS
The right renal contour is clearly seen, which suggests the absence of fluid (haemorrhage) in this region. The left renal contour is not visualised, however this is non-specific.

VASCULAR
The infra-renal abdominal aorta is calcified and demonstrates fusiform aneurysmal dilatation at the level of L3 to S1.

BONES
There are no abnormalities of the imaged thoracic and lumbar spine, or within the pelvis.

SOFT TISSUES
The psoas muscle outline is not visable bilaterally, which is non-specific, however raises the possibility of an abdominal aortic aneurysm leak, especially given the clinical history and low blood pressure.

The extra-abdominal soft tissues are unremarkable.

OTHER
There are no radiopaque foreign bodies.

There are no vascular lines, drains or surgical clips.

REVIEW AREAS
Gallstones / Renal calculi: No radiopaque calculi.
Lung bases: Not fully included.
Spine: Normal.
Femoral heads: Not visualised.

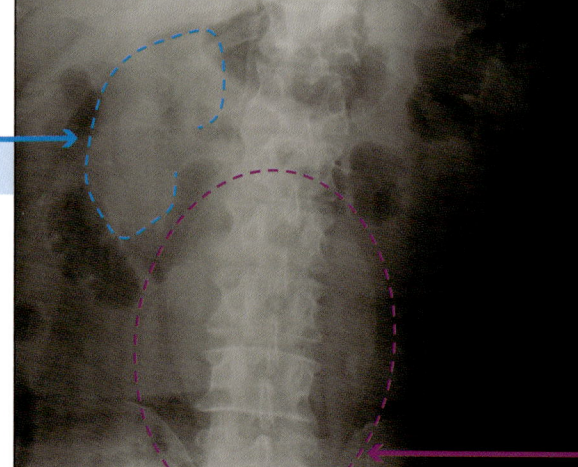

Right renal contour

Calcified abdominal aortic aneurysm

SUMMARY
This X-ray demonstrates fusiform aneurysmal dilatation of the infra-renal abdominal aorta. The psoas muscle outline is not seen bilaterally, which is non-specific however raises the possibility of an abdominal aortic aneurysm leak given the clinical history.

INVESTIGATIONS AND MANAGEMENT
The patient should be resuscitated using an ABCDE approach.

Adequate analgesia and hydration should be provided.

Urgent bloods should be taken including FBC, U&Es, CRP, bone profile, LFTs, coagulation, blood gas, and cross match.

The patient should be made NBM and commenced on IV fluids.

Urgent referral to the vascular surgeons should be made for assessment of an active abdominal aortic aneurysm leak and consideration of repair. A CT scan of the aorta with IV contrast would be useful for better visualisation of the anatomy and to assess for leak.

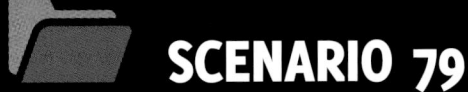
A 69 year old female presents to ED with worsening abdominal distension and difficulty breathing. Her past medical history is significant for treated ovarian cancer and she is a non-smoker. On examination, she has saturations of 93% in room air and a temperature of 36.5°C. Her HR is 98 bpm, RR is 26 and blood pressure is 112/65 mmHg. The abdomen is tense and there is generalised tenderness with normal bowel sounds. Urine dipstick is unremarkable.

An abdominal X-ray is requested to assess for possible bowel obstruction.

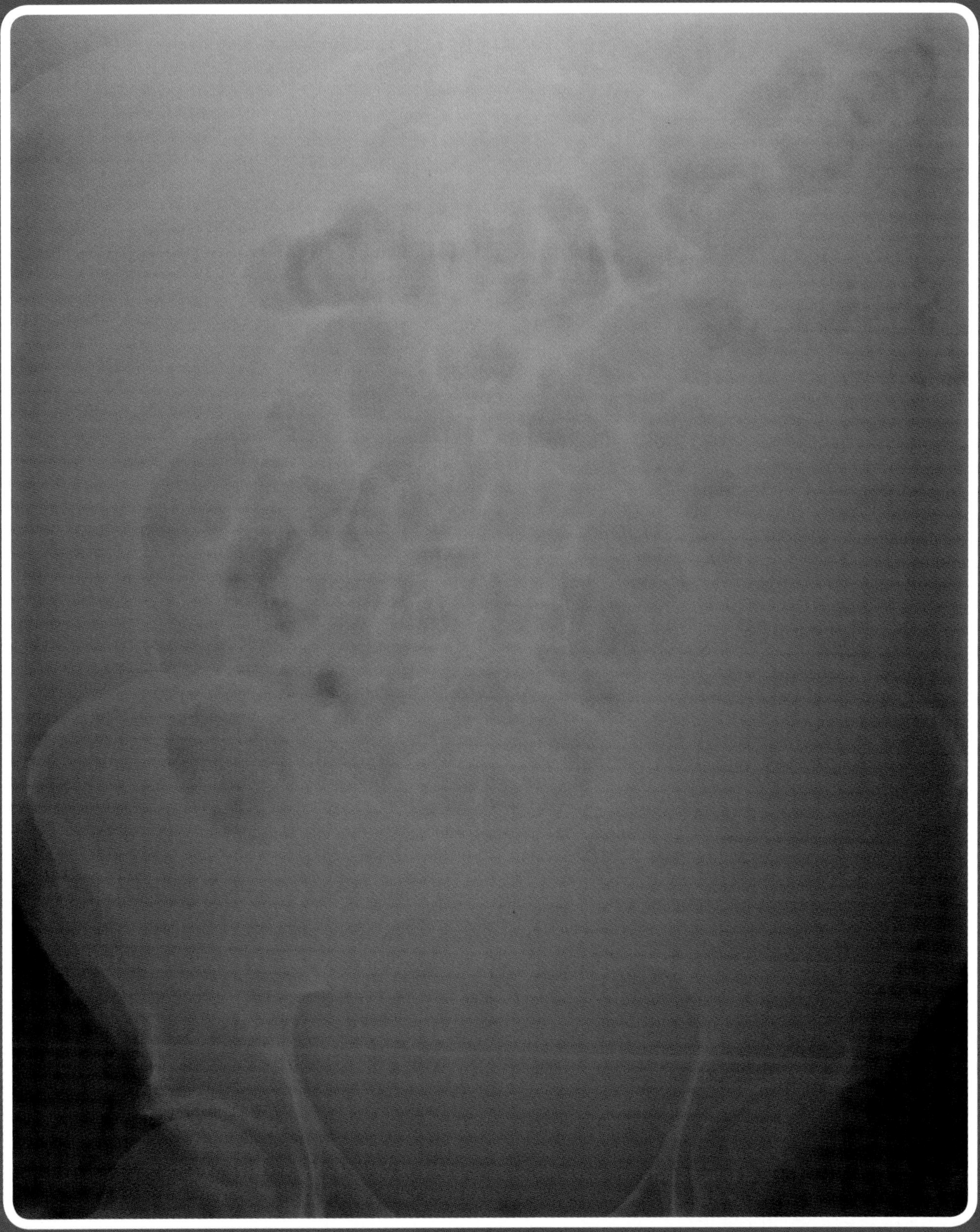

REPORT

Patient ID: Anonymous.
Projection: AP supine.
Rotation: Adequate.
Penetration: Underpenetrated – the spinous processes are not visible.
Coverage: Inadequate – the pubic symphysis, inferior pubic rami and hemi-diaphragms have not been included.

BOWEL GAS PATTERN

There are multiple loops of centrally placed bowel loops with peripheral paucity of bowel gas in the flanks and iliac fossae.

BOWEL WALL

There is no evidence of mural thickening or intramural gas within the large or small bowel.

PNEUMOPERITONEUM

There is no evidence of free intra-abdominal gas.

SOLID ORGANS

There is a diffusely increased density of the abdomen with poor definition of all soft tissue shadows and solid organs.

VASCULAR

No abnormal vascular calcification.

BONES

There are no abnormalities of the imaged thoracic and lumbar spine, or within the pelvis, but the bones are not clearly visualised.

SOFT TISSUES

The psoas muscle outline is not visible bilaterally, related to the presence of ascites.

The extra-abdominal soft tissues are unremarkable.

OTHER

There are no radiopaque foreign bodies.

There are no vascular lines, drains or surgical clips.

REVIEW AREAS

Gallstones / Renal calculi: No radiopaque calculi.
Lung bases: Normal.
Spine: Not visible.
Femoral heads: Normal.

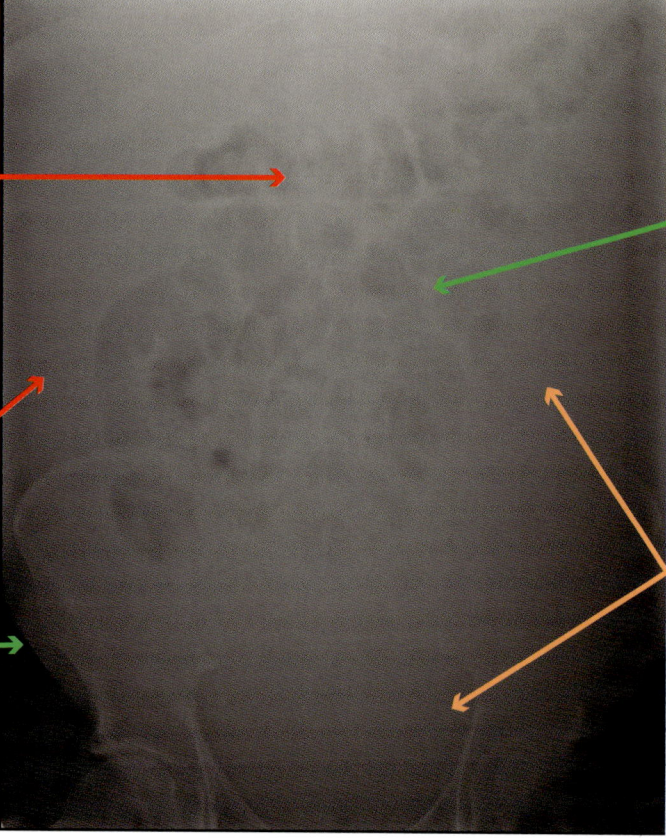

Central placement of loops of bowel

Peripheral paucity of bowel gas

Bulging flanks

Psoas muscle shadow obscured by diffusely increased density of abdomen

Ascites

SUMMARY

This X-ray demonstrates multiple loops of centrally placed bowel within the abdomen, with peripheral paucity of bowel gas in the flanks and iliac fossae and diffusely increased density of the abdomen resulting in poor definition of soft tissues, solid organs and bones. These findings are in keeping with extensive ascites.

INVESTIGATIONS AND MANAGEMENT

The patient should be resuscitated using an ABCDE approach.

Adequate analgesia and hydration should be provided.

Urgent bloods should be taken, including FBC, U&Es, CRP, LFTs, TFTs, blood gas, and bone profile.

If no recent imaging has been performed, a staging CT scan of the chest, abdomen and pelvis with IV contrast should be considered to re-assess the known ovarian cancer for disease recurrence.

If the CT scan confirms disease recurrence, the patient should be referred to oncology services for further management, which may include biopsy and MDT discussion. Treatment, which may include surgery, radiotherapy, chemotherapy, or palliative treatment, will depend on the outcome of the MDT investigations and the patient's wishes.

Ultrasound-guided drainage of the ascites could be performed for symptomatic relief.

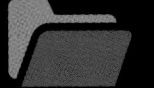

SCENARIO 80

A 2 month old baby boy presents to ED with vomiting and colicky abdominal pain. His past medical history is significant for a recent viral flu-like illness. On examination, he has saturations of 98% in room air and a temperature of 37.8°C. His HR is 170 bpm and RR 60. The abdomen is soft and a sausage-shaped mass is palpable in the right upper quadrant with tinkling bowel sounds. Urine dipstick is unremarkable.

An abdominal X-ray is requested to assess for possible bowel obstruction.

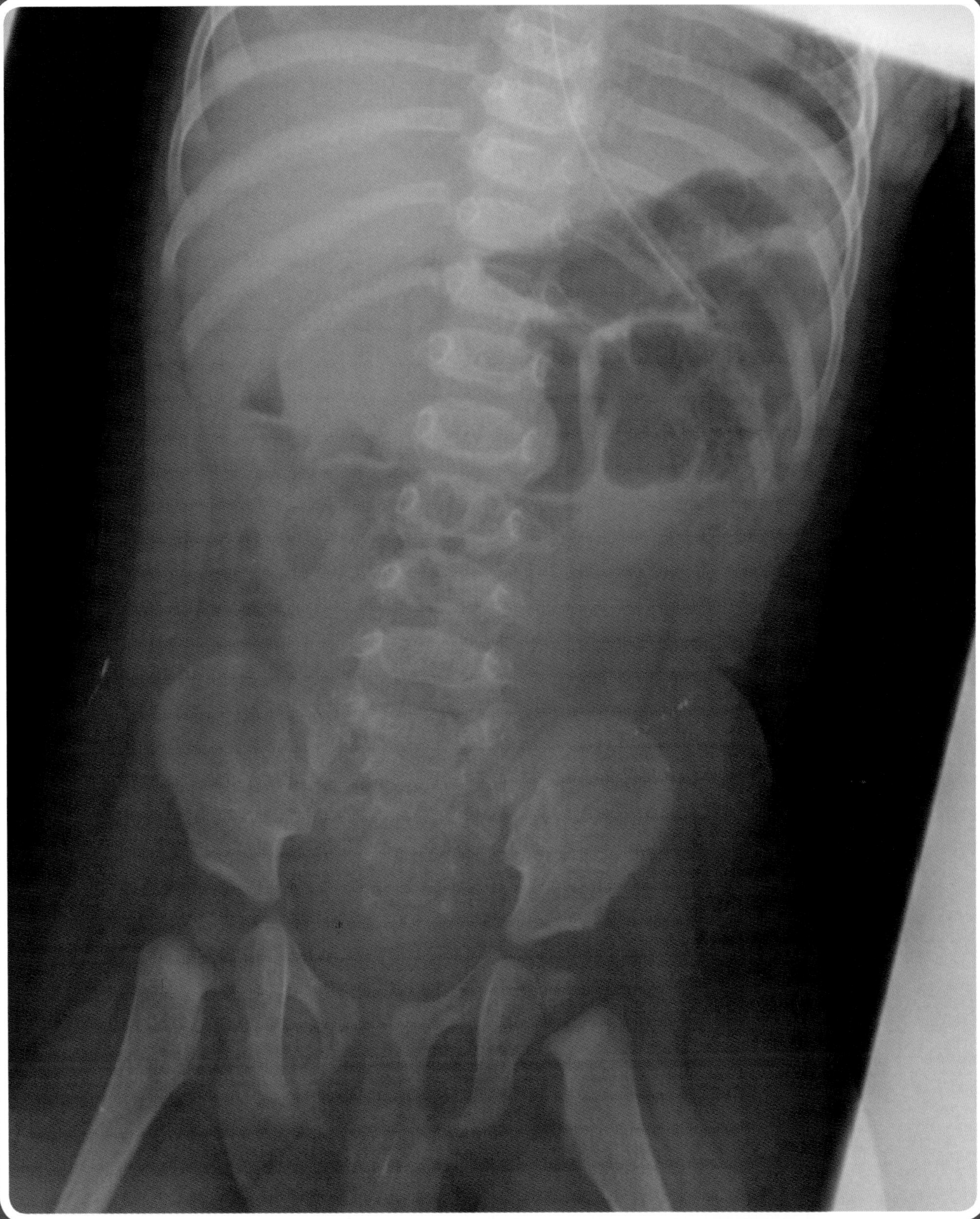

REPORT – INTUSSUSCEPTION

REPORT
Patient ID: Anonymous.
Projection: AP supine.
Rotation: Adequate.
Penetration: Adequate – the spine is visible.
Coverage: Adequate – the anterior ribs are visible superiorly and the inferior pubic rami are visible.

BOWEL GAS PATTERN
There are multiple loops of dilatated bowel in the left upper quadrant of the abdomen. A small volume of gas is seen within the ascending colon.

BOWEL WALL
There is no evidence of mural thickening or intramural gas within the large or small bowel.

PNEUMOPERITONEUM
There is no evidence of free intra-abdominal gas.

SOLID ORGANS
The solid organ contours are within normal limits with no solid organ calcification.

VASCULAR
No abnormal vascular calcification.

BONES
There are no abnormalities of the imaged thoracic and lumbar spine, or within the pelvis.

There is cartilage present between the pelvic bones and femurs as they have not yet fused which is a normal finding in a child of this age.

SOFT TISSUES
There is an elongated soft tissue mass seen in the right upper quadrant of the abdomen.

The psoas muscle outline is not visible bilaterally, which is non-specific, particularly in a child of this age.

The extra-abdominal soft tissues are unremarkable.

OTHER
There is an NG tube in situ, with its tip seen projecting in the left upper quadrant, likely within the stomach.

There are no vascular lines, drains or surgical clips.

REVIEW AREAS
Gallstones / Renal calculi: No radiopaque calculi.
Lung bases: Right lung base not fully included.
Spine: Normal.
Femoral heads: Normal – growth plates present.

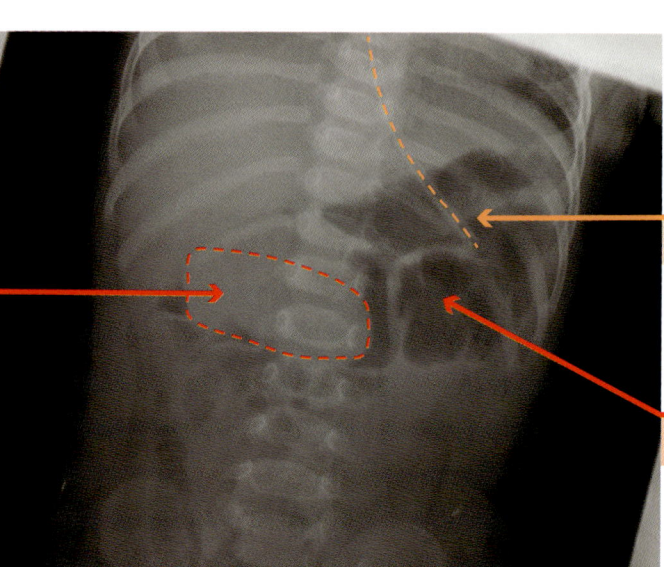

Elongated soft tissue mass

NG tube

Dilated loops of bowel

Cartilage between unfused bones

SUMMARY
This X-ray demonstrates an elongated soft tissue mass in the right upper quadrant, with dilated loops of bowel in the left upper quadrant, which given the clinical history is in keeping with intussusception. There is an NG tube in situ with the tip projecting over the stomach.

INVESTIGATIONS AND MANAGEMENT
The patient should be resuscitated using an ABCDE approach.

Adequate analgesia and hydration should be provided.

The patient should be made NBM and commenced on IV fluids.

Urgent bloods should be taken including FBC, U&Es, blood gas, coagulation, group and save, and CRP.

An urgent abdominal USS should be performed to confirm the diagnosis of intussusception. Surgical input should be sought.

Fluoroscopic air contrast enema or water-soluble contrast enema can assist in diagnosis and in most cases can successfully reduce the intussusception.

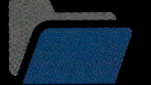

SCENARIO 81

A 40 year old male presents to ED with symptoms of alcohol withdrawal and abdominal pain. His past medical history is significant for alcoholism and he is a non-smoker. On examination, he has saturations of 97% in air, and a temperature of 36.8°C. His HR is 80 bpm, RR is 22 and blood pressure is 120/85 mmHg. The abdomen is soft and there is generalised tenderness with normal bowel sounds. Urine dipstick is unremarkable.

An abdominal X-ray is requested to assess for possible bowel obstruction.

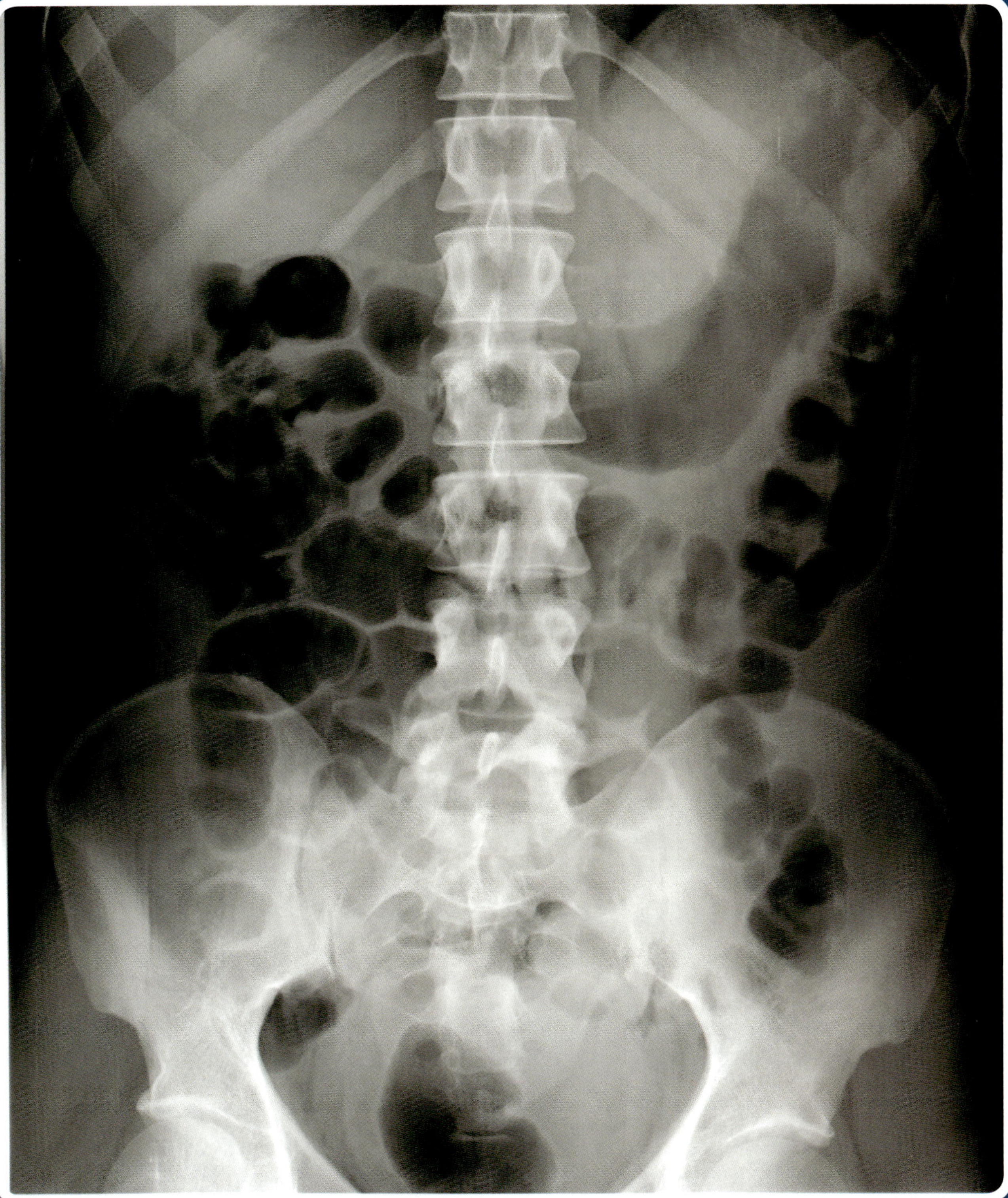

REPORT
Patient ID: Anonymous.
Projection: AP supine.
Rotation: Adequate
Penetration: Adequate – the spinous processes are visible.
Coverage: Inadequate – the pubic symphysis and inferior pubic rami have not been included.

BOWEL GAS PATTERN
The bowel gas pattern is normal.

BOWEL WALL
There is no evidence of mural thickening or intramural gas within the large or small bowel.

PNEUMOPERITONEUM
There is no evidence of free intra-abdominal gas.

SOLID ORGANS
This X-ray demonstrates subtle speckled calcification projecting over the distribution of the pancreas, which given the clinical history may represent pancreatic calcification in keeping with chronic pancreatitis.

VASCULAR
No abnormal vascular calcification.

BONES
There are no abnormalities of the imaged thoracic and lumbar spine, or within the pelvis.

SOFT TISSUES
The psoas muscle outline is visible bilaterally.

The extra-abdominal soft tissues are unremarkable.

OTHER
There are no radiopaque foreign bodies.

There are no vascular lines, drains or surgical clips.

REVIEW AREAS
Gallstones / Renal calculi: No radiopaque calculi.
Lung bases: Normal.
Spine: Normal.
Femoral heads: Normal.

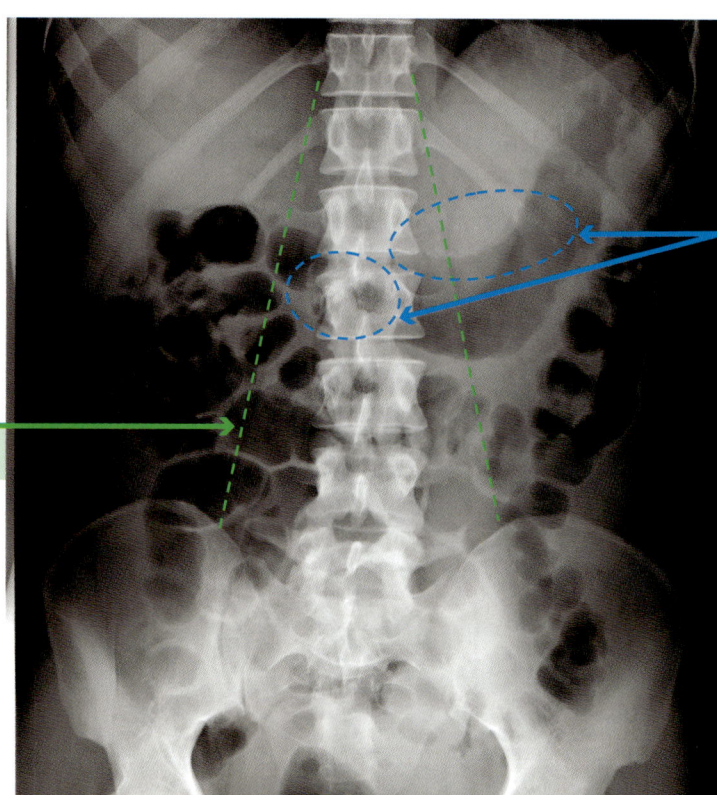

Pancreatic calcification

Psoas muscle outlines

SUMMARY
This X-ray demonstrates subtle speckled calcification projecting over the distribution of the pancreas, which given the clinical history may represent pancreatic calcification in keeping with chronic pancreatitis.

INVESTIGATIONS AND MANAGEMENT
The patient should be resuscitated using an ABCDE approach.

Adequate analgesia and hydration should be provided.

Urgent bloods should be taken including FBC, U&Es, LFTs, amylase, blood gas, bone profile and CRP.

The acute alcohol withdrawal should be treated with thiamine and benzodiazepines.

Referral to gastroenterology should be made for possible chronic pancreatitis. Management may include analgesia and enzymatic supplementation. A CT scan of the abdomen with IV contrast may be considered for further evaluation of the pancreas.

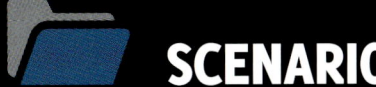

SCENARIO 82

A 52 year old female presents to ED with generalised abdominal pain. She has a complicated past medical history, having had a previous bowel resection with a colostomy in place. She also has a long term congenital bladder defect and she is a non-smoker. On examination, she has saturations of 97% in room air and a temperature of 37.3°C. Her HR is 94 bpm, RR is 20 and blood pressure is 125/72 mmHg. The abdomen is soft and there is generalised tenderness with tinkling bowel sounds. Urine dipstick is unremarkable and a pregnancy test is negative.

An abdominal X-ray is requested to assess for possible bowel obstruction.

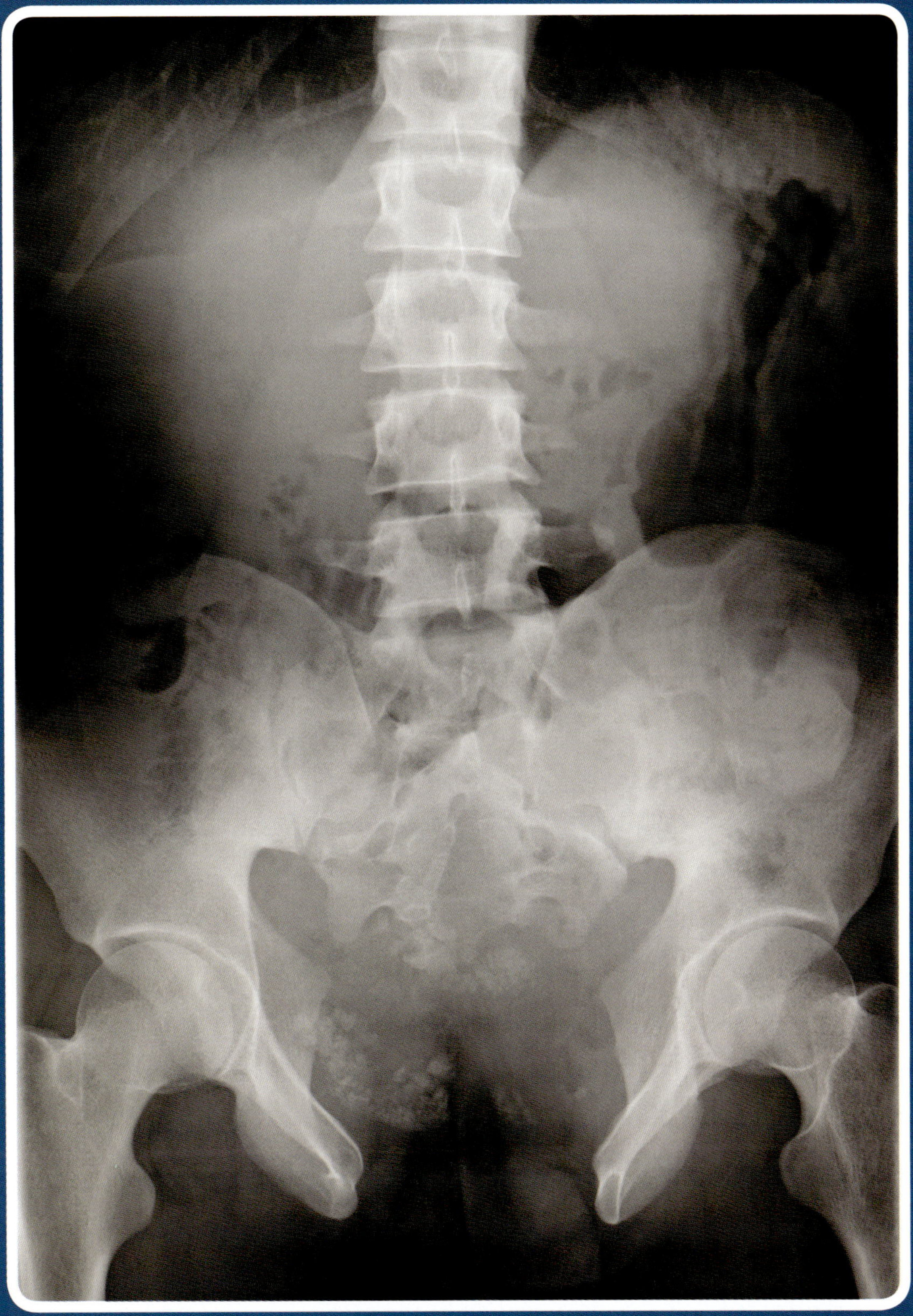

REPORT
Patient ID: Anonymous.
Projection: AP supine.
Rotation: Adequate.
Penetration: Adequate – the spinous processes are visible.
Coverage: Adequate – the anterior ribs are visible superiorly and the inferior pubic rami are visible.

BOWEL GAS PATTERN
The bowel gas pattern is normal.

BOWEL WALL
There is no evidence of mural thickening or intramural gas within the large or small bowel.

PNEUMOPERITONEUM
There is no evidence of free intra-abdominal gas.

SOLID ORGANS
The solid organ contours are within normal limits with no solid organ calcification.

VASCULAR
No abnormal vascular calcification.

BONES
There is a failure of the pubic bones to meet in the midline at the pubic symphysis, termed the 'Manta Ray sign'.

There are no abnormalities of the imaged thoracic and lumbar spine.

SOFT TISSUES
The psoas muscle outline is visible bilaterally.

There appears to be a defect in the extra-abdominal soft tissues in the pelvis, overlying the region of the widened pubic symphysis.

OTHER
There is a rounded radiopaque density projected over the region of the left iliac fossa, in keeping with a colostomy bag external to the patient.

There are several radiopaque calcific densities projected over the region of the abnormally shaped bladder, which represent faceted bladder calculi.

There are no vascular lines, drains or surgical clips.

REVIEW AREAS
Gallstones / Renal calculi: Multiple calculi projecting over the bladder.
Lung bases: Normal.
Spine: Normal.
Femoral heads: Normal.

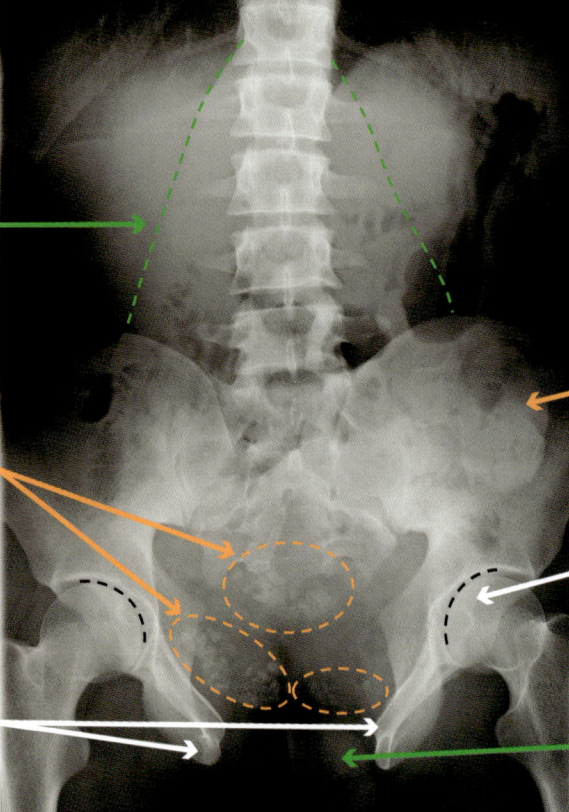

Psoas muscle outlines

Colostomy bag

Bladder calculi

Femoral heads normal

Failure of pubic bones to meet in midline: Manta Ray sign

Defect in extra-abdominal soft tissue

SUMMARY
This X-ray demonstrates a wide separation of the pubic bones termed the 'Manta Ray sign', and a defect in the extra-abdominal soft tissues overlying this region. It also demonstrates several calcific densities projected over the region of an abnormally shaped bladder. Findings are in keeping with bladder exstrophy and vesical calculi formation. Note is also made of the left iliac fossa colostomy.

INVESTIGATIONS AND MANAGEMENT
The patient should be resuscitated using an ABCDE approach.

Adequate analgesia and hydration should be provided.

Urgent bloods should be taken, including FBC, U&Es, LFTs, amylase, bone profile, blood gas, and CRP.

Vesical calculi formation is a known complication following surgery for bladder extrophy. The patient should be referred to the urology team for further management. A CT scan of the kidneys, ureters and bladder might be useful for better visualisation of the anatomy and evaluation of the abdominal pain.

SCENARIO 83

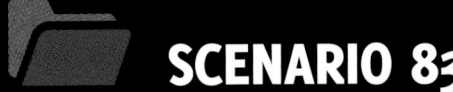

A 6 hour old baby girl has just been admitted to NICU having been born prematurely at 28 weeks. She has been intubated and had an umbilical arterial and venous catheter inserted. On examination, while intubated, she has saturations of 100% on 40% oxygen and a temperature of 36.6°C. Her HR is 176 bpm and RR is 48. The abdomen is soft with normal bowel sounds.

An abdominal X-ray is requested to assess correct positioning of lines.

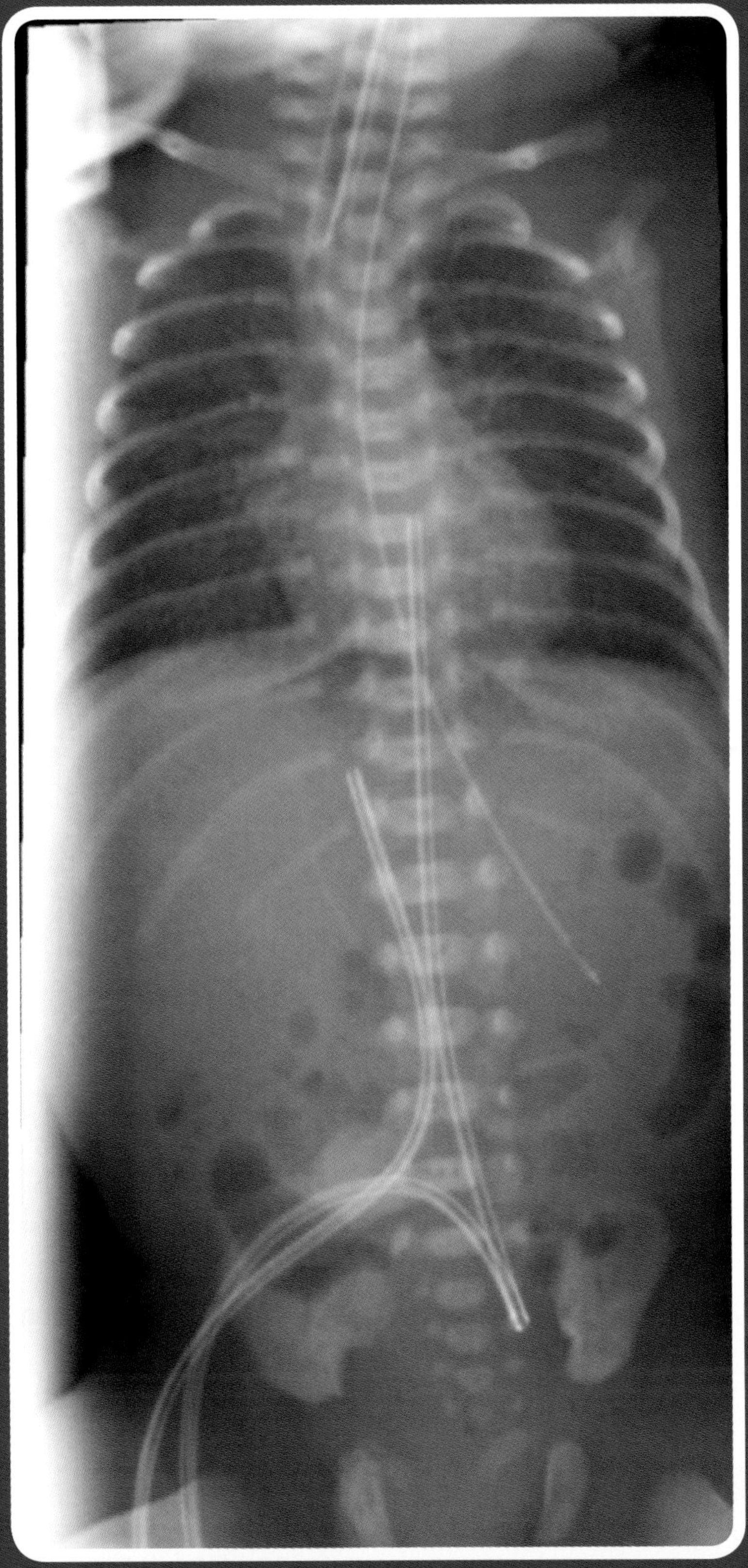

REPORT

Patient ID: Anonymous.
Projection: AP supine 'babygram' of chest and abdomen.
Rotation: Adequate.
Penetration: Adequate – the spine is visible.
Coverage: Adequate – the anterior ribs are visible superiorly and the pubic rami are visible inferiorly.

BOWEL GAS PATTERN

The bowel gas pattern is normal.

BOWEL WALL

There is no evidence of mural thickening or intramural gas within the large or small bowel.

PNEUMOPERITONEUM

There is no evidence of free intra-abdominal gas.

SOLID ORGANS

The solid organs are poorly defined due to diffusely increased density of the abdomen. The lung fields look normal.

VASCULAR

No abnormal vascular calcification.

BONES

There are no abnormalities of the imaged thoracic and lumbar spine, or within the pelvis.

There are growth plates at the femoral head, greater trochanter and acetabulum as the ossification centres have not yet fused, which is a normal finding in a child of this age.

There is cartilage seen between vertebrae, which is a normal finding in a child of this age.

SOFT TISSUES

The psoas muscle outline is not visible bilaterally, which is non-specific, particularly in a child of this age.

The extra-abdominal soft tissues are unremarkable.

OTHER

There is an NG tube in situ, with its tip projecting within the body of the stomach.

There is an ET tube in situ, with its tip at T2.

There is an umbilical artery catheter seen external to the patient, entering the umbilical artery at the umbilicus, travelling inferiorly in the umbilical artery to enter the internal iliac artery where it then travels superiorly up the common iliac artery to the aorta. Its tip is seen appropriately sited above the diaphragm, at the level of T7.

There is an umbilical venous catheter seen external to the patient, with its tip seen at the level of T11 in a slightly low position.

There are no drains or surgical clips.

REVIEW AREAS

Gallstones / Renal calculi: No radiopaque calculi.
Lung bases: Normal.
Spine: Normal – cartilage between vertebrae.
Femoral heads: Normal – cartilage between femur and acetabulum.

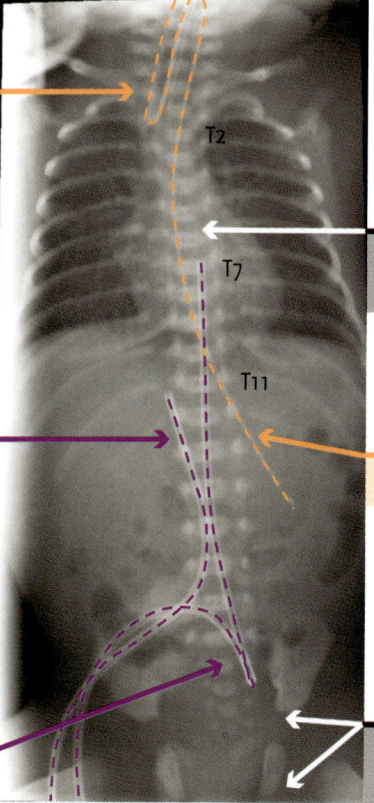

ET tube

T2

Cartilage between unfused vertebrae

T7

Umbilical venous catheter

T11

NG tube

Umbilical artery catheter

Cartilage between unfused bones

SUMMARY

This X-ray demonstrates an NG tube, ET tube and umbilical artery catheter in satisfactory positions. The umbilical venous catheter tip projects at the level of T11.

INVESTIGATIONS AND MANAGEMENT

The umbilical venous catheter is in an abnormally low position. This should be removed, and replaced by another catheter advanced slightly further to approximately T10 to lie within the inferior vena cava at the level of the diaphragm.

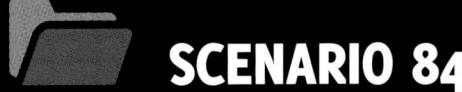
A 35 year old female presents to ED with left flank pain. Her past medical history is significant for ureteric obstruction, for which she has recently undergone placement of bilateral JJ ureteric stents. She has no other significant past medical history and is a non-smoker. On examination, she has saturations of 98% in room air and a temperature of 36.7°C. Her HR is 82 bpm, RR is 16 and blood pressure is 120/68 mmHg. The abdomen is soft and there is tenderness over the left flank with normal bowel sounds. Urine dipstick shows blood ++ and a pregnancy test is negative.

An abdominal X-ray is requested to assess for possible renal calculi.

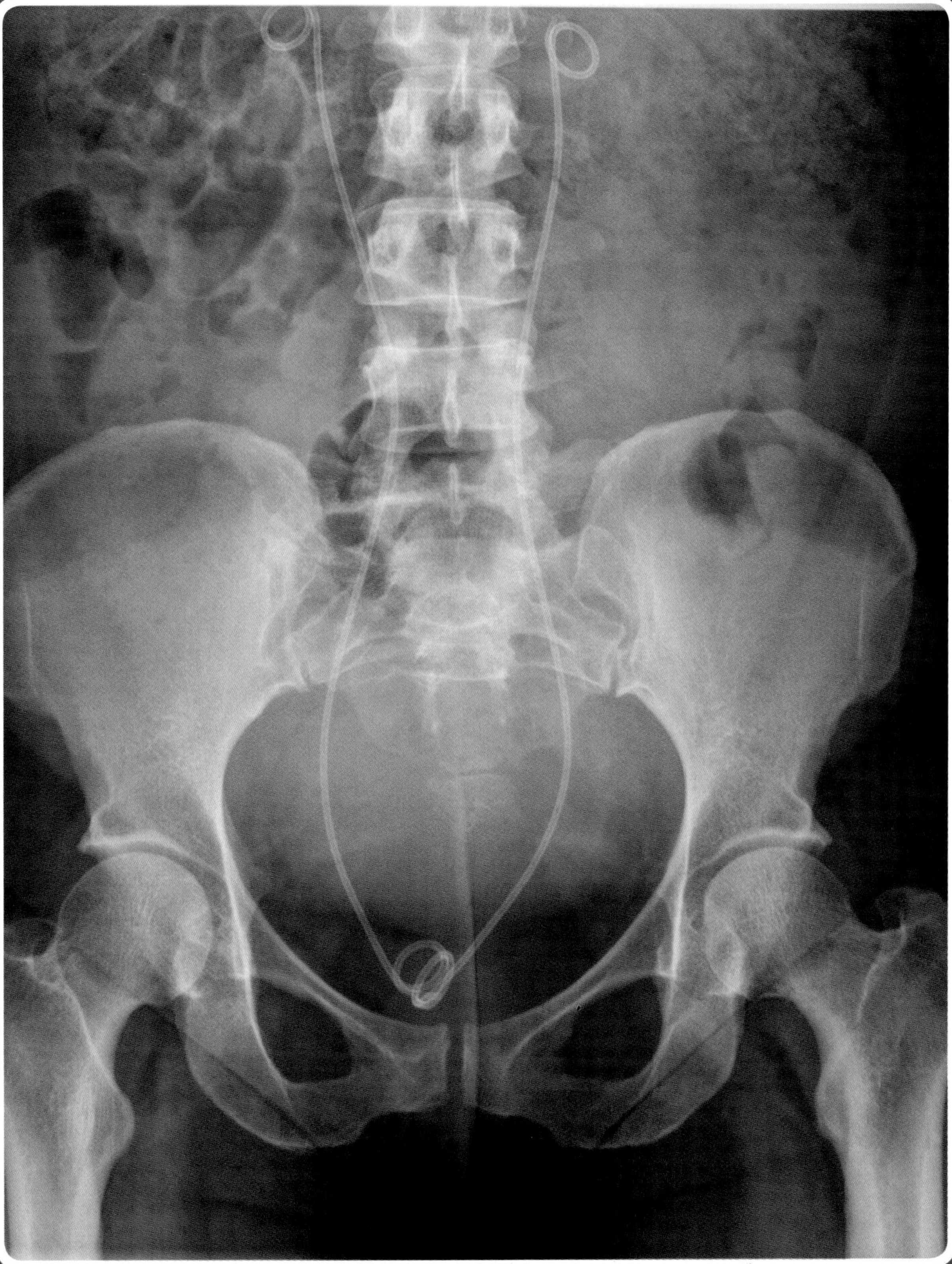

REPORT
Patient ID: Anonymous.
Projection: AP supine.
Rotation: Adequate.
Penetration: Adequate – the spinous processes are visible.
Coverage: Inadequate – the anterior ribs have not been included.

BOWEL GAS PATTERN
The bowel gas pattern is normal.

There is a moderate volume of faecal residue present throughout the transverse and descending colon.

BOWEL WALL
There is no evidence of mural thickening or intramural gas within the large or small bowel.

PNEUMOPERITONEUM
There is no evidence of free intra-abdominal gas.

SOLID ORGANS
There is medial deviation of the proximal ureters bilaterally, which contain JJ stents.

VASCULAR
No abnormal vascular calcification.

BONES
There are no abnormalities of the imaged thoracic and lumbar spine, or within the pelvis.

SOFT TISSUES
The psoas muscle outline is not visible bilaterally.

The extra-abdominal soft tissues are unremarkable.

OTHER
There are bilateral JJ ureteric stents in situ. Both proximal stents are projected over the expected position of the renal pelvises, and both distal stents projected over the urinary bladder, however both stents deviate medially.

There are no vascular lines, drains or surgical clips.

REVIEW AREAS
Gallstones / Renal calculi: No radiopaque calculi.
Lung bases: Not fully included.
Spine: Normal.
Femoral heads: Normal.

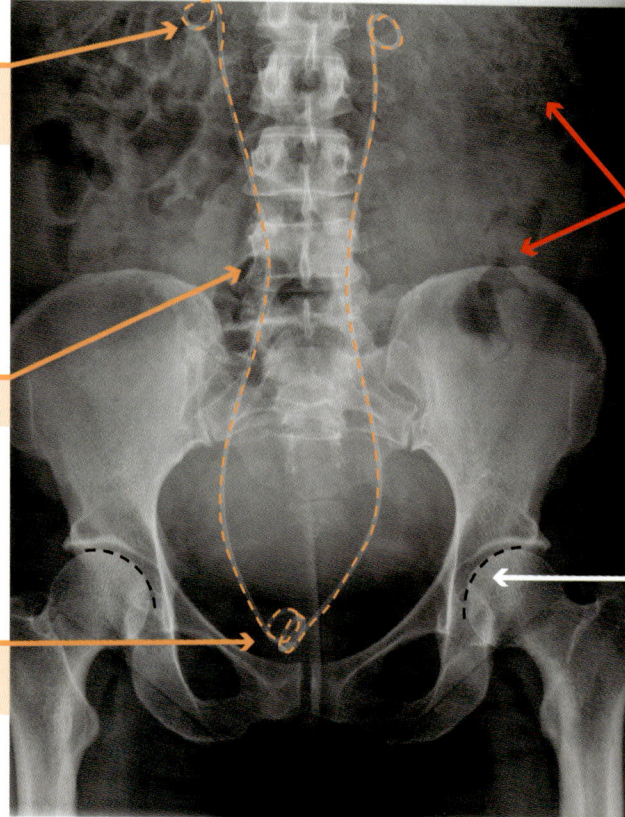

JJ ureteric stents in situ in renal pelvis

JJ ureteric stent coursing medially

JJ ureteric stents in situ in bladder

Faecal residue throughout transverse and descending colon

Femoral heads normal

SUMMARY
This X-ray demonstrates bilateral JJ ureteric stents with medial deviation of the mid ureters, indicating that the ureteric obstruction may be due to retroperitoneal fibrosis. There is a moderate volume of faecal residue throughout the transverse and descending colon.

INVESTIGATIONS AND MANAGEMENT
The patient should be resuscitated using an ABCDE approach.

Adequate analgesia and hydration should be provided.

Referral to the renal/urology team should be made. Urgent bloods should be taken, including FBC, U&Es, CRP, ESR, LFTs, bone profile, blood gas, and tumour markers.

A CT scan of the kidneys, ureters and bladder might be useful for better visualisation of the anatomy, and subsequent consideration of removal/replacement of the ureteric stents if there is evidence that they are blocked.

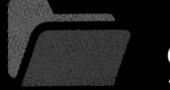

A 70 year old male presents to ED with generalised abdominal pain and vomiting. His past medical history is significant for a stable abdominal aortic aneurysm and previous dynamic hip screw insertion on the right. He has no other significant past medical history and is a non-smoker. On examination, he has saturations of 94% in air and a temperature of 37.2°C. His HR is 98 bpm, RR is 22 and blood pressure is 110/65 mmHg. The abdomen is rigid and there is generalised tenderness with sluggish bowel sounds. Urine dipstick is unremarkable.

An abdominal X-ray is requested to assess for possible bowel obstruction.

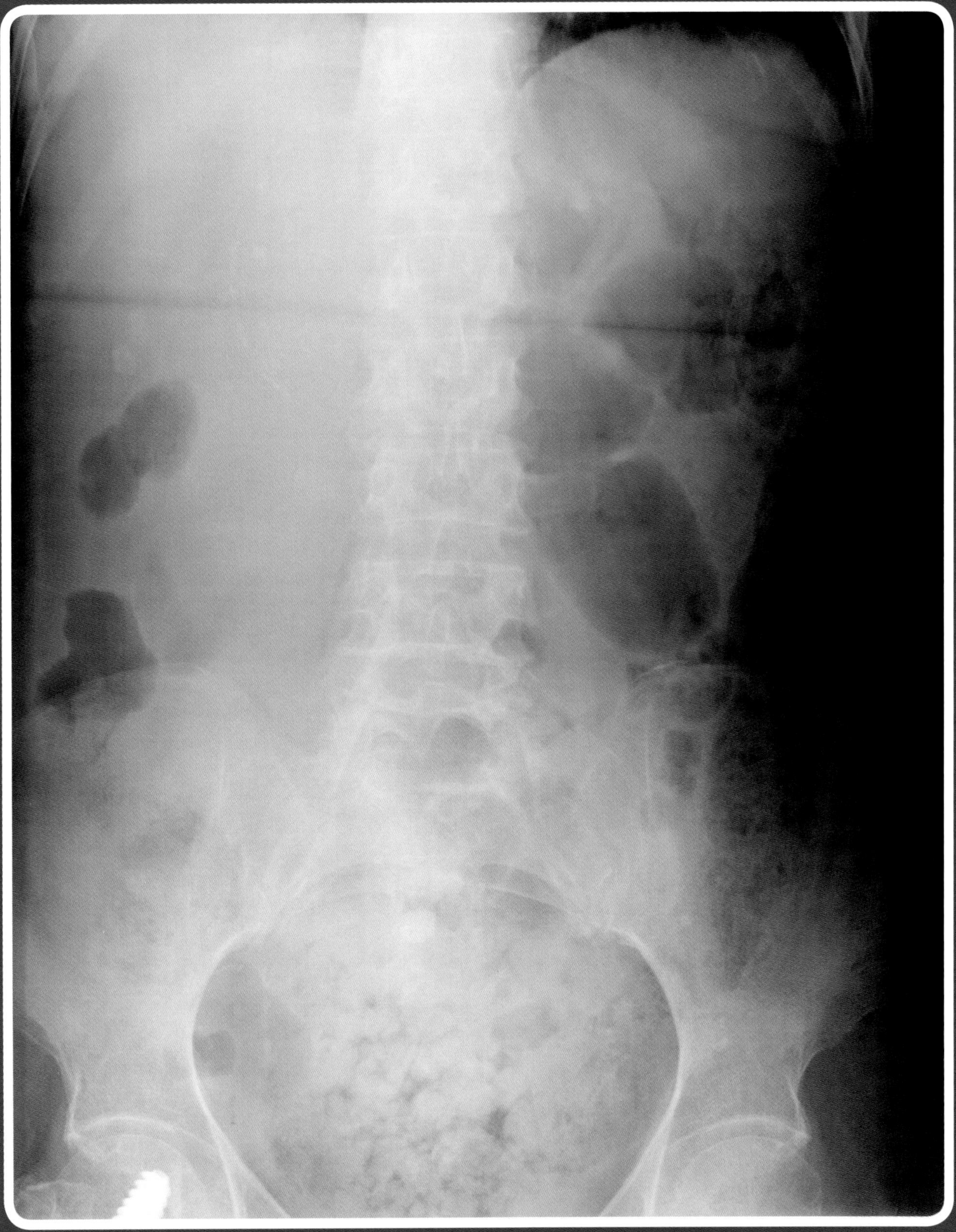

REPORT – ABDOMINAL AORTIC ANEURYSM AND FAECAL RESIDUE

REPORT

Patient ID: Anonymous.
Projection: AP supine.
Rotation: Adequate.
Penetration: Adequate – the spinous processes are visible.
Coverage: Inadequate – the right iliac crest, pubic symphysis and inferior pubic rami have not been fully included.

BOWEL GAS PATTERN

The bowel gas pattern is normal.

There is a significant volume of faecal residue present throughout the descending colon and prominent rectum.

BOWEL WALL

There is a prominent gaseous loop of distal large bowel on the left side of the abdomen.

There is no evidence of intramural gas.

PNEUMOPERITONEUM

There is no evidence of free intra-abdominal gas.

SOLID ORGANS

The solid organ contours are within normal limits with no solid organ calcification.

VASCULAR

The abdominal aorta is calcified and demonstrates fusiform aneurysmal dilatation at the level of T12 to L4.

BONES

There are no abnormalities of the imaged thoracic and lumbar spine, or within the pelvis.

SOFT TISSUES

The right psoas muscle outline is not visible, which is non-specific, however raises the possibility of abdominal aortic aneurysm leak.

The extra-abdominal soft tissues are unremarkable.

OTHER

There is a dynamic hip screw in situ in the right proximal femur. There are no other radiopaque foreign bodies.

There are no vascular lines, drains or surgical clips.

REVIEW AREAS

Gallstones / Renal calculi: No radiopaque calculi.
Lung bases: The right lung base is not visualised.
Spine: Normal.
Femoral heads: Right-sided dynamic hip screw in situ.

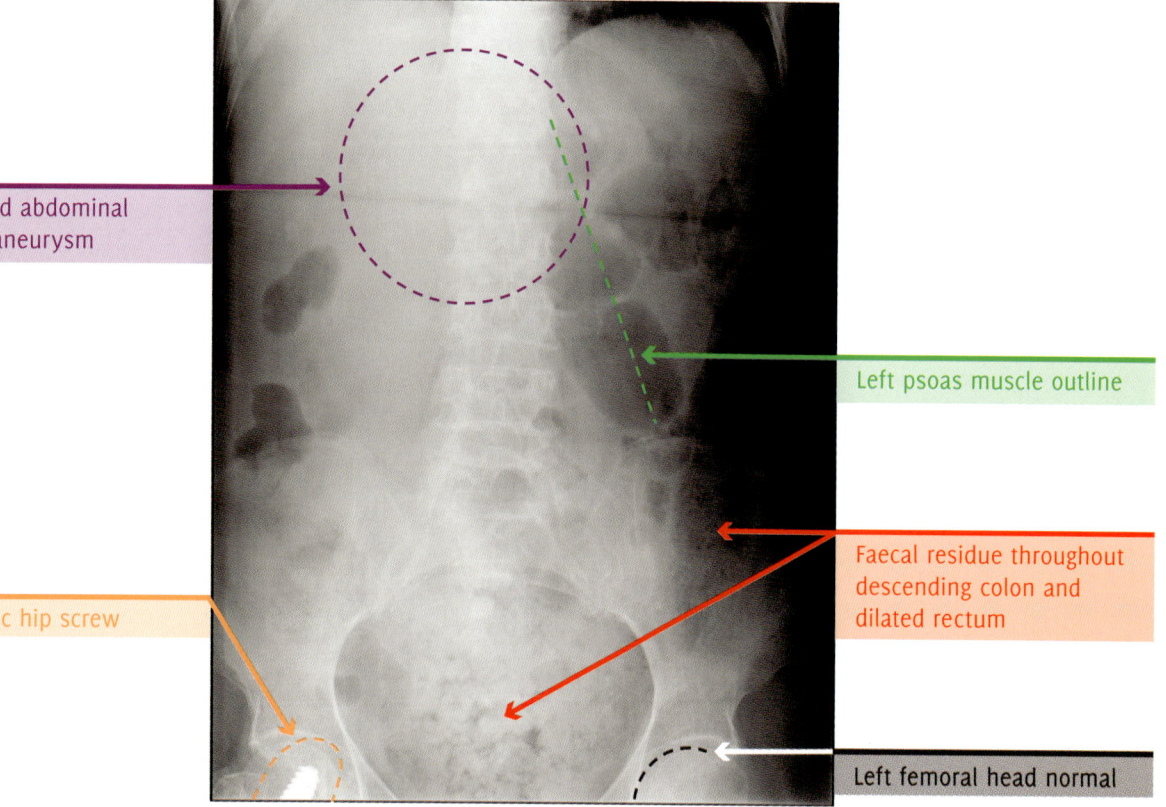

Calcified abdominal aortic aneurysm

Left psoas muscle outline

Faecal residue throughout descending colon and dilated rectum

Dynamic hip screw

Left femoral head normal

SUMMARY

This X-ray demonstrates a non-specific prominent gaseous loop of distal large bowel and significant faecal loading of the descending colon and rectum which is dilated. The X-ray also demonstrates a long-standing large fusiform calcified abdominal aortic aneurysm. The right-sided dynamic hip screw is an incidental finding.

INVESTIGATIONS AND MANAGEMENT

The patient should be resuscitated using an ABCDE approach.

Adequate analgesia and hydration should be provided.

Urgent bloods should be taken including FBC, U&Es, CRP, bone profile, LFTs, coagulation, blood gas and cross match.

The patient should be made NBM and commenced on IV fluids.

The patient should be referred urgently to vascular surgery for assessment and a CT scan of the abdomen/pelvis with IV contrast should be considered to assess for abdominal aortic aneurysm leak, which could be obscuring the psoas outline.

The general surgical team and/or the vascular team may need to be involved depending on the findings of these additional investigations and the clinical picture.

SCENARIO 86

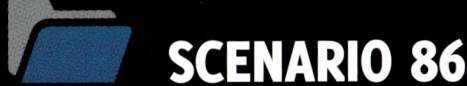

A 60 year old male presents to ED with generalised abdominal pain. He has no significant past medical history and is a smoker. On examination, he has saturations of 94% in air and a temperature of 36.6°C. His HR is 118 bpm, RR is 19 and blood pressure is 110/90 mmHg. The abdomen is rigid and there is generalised tenderness with tinkling bowel sounds. Urine dipstick is unremarkable.

An abdominal X-ray is requested to assess for possible bowel obstruction.

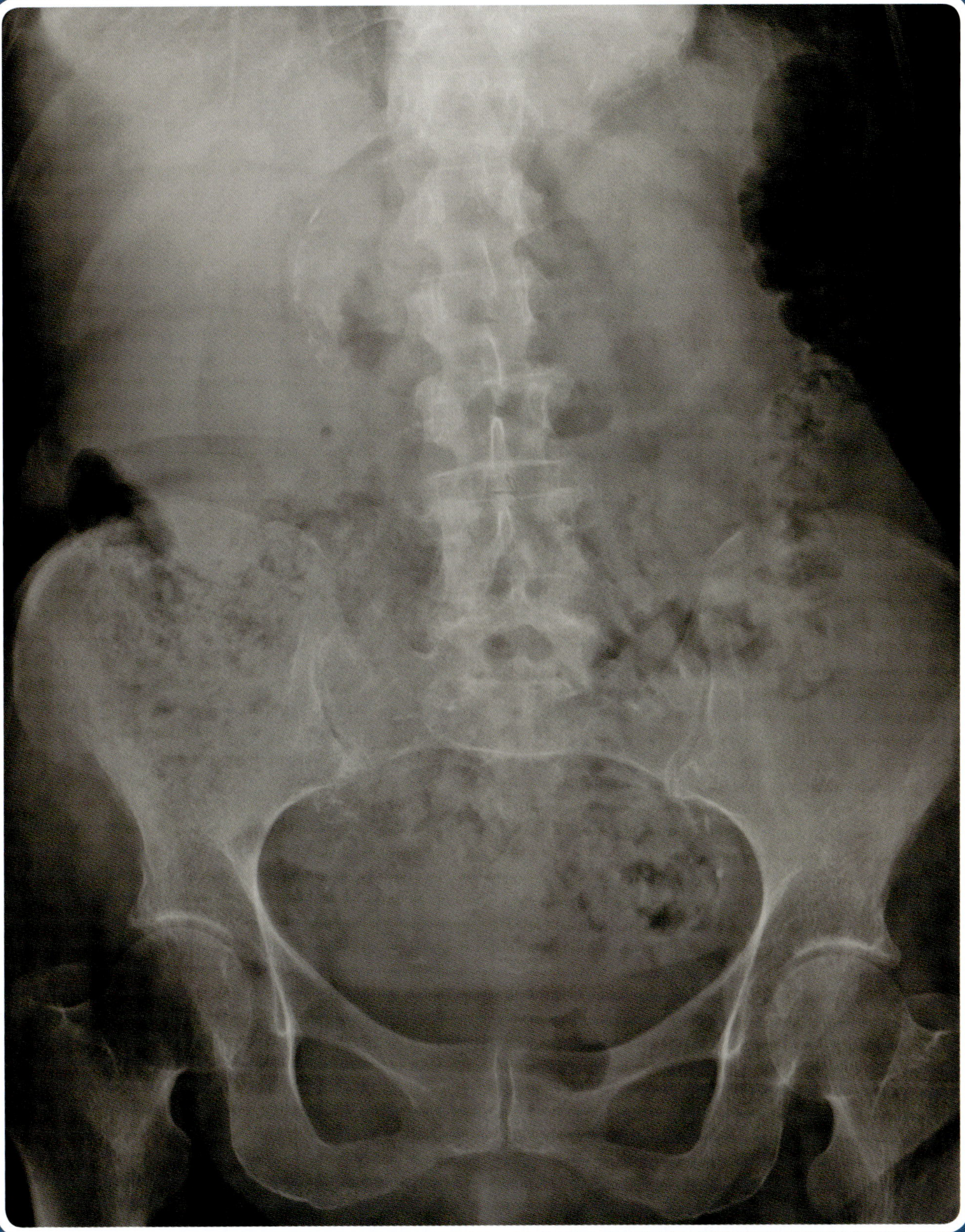

REPORT – ABDOMINAL AORTIC ANEURYSM AND VASCULAR CALCIFICATION

REPORT
Patient ID: Anonymous.
Projection: AP supine.
Rotation: Adequate
Penetration: Adequate – the spinous processes are visible.
Coverage: Adequate – the anterior ribs are visible superiorly and the inferior pubic rami are visible.

BOWEL GAS PATTERN
The bowel gas pattern is normal.

There is a moderate volume of faecal residue present predominantly in the caecum, distal descending and sigmoid colon.

BOWEL WALL
There is no evidence of mural thickening or intramural gas within the large or small bowel.

PNEUMOPERITONEUM
There is no evidence of free intra-abdominal gas.

SOLID ORGANS
The solid organ contours are within normal limits with no solid organ calcification.

VASCULAR
The abdominal aorta is calcified and demonstrates significant fusiform aneurysmal dilatation at the level of T12 to L3. There is calcification of the iliac arteries bilaterally.

BONES
There are no abnormalities of the imaged thoracic and lumbar spine, or within the pelvis.

SOFT TISSUES
The psoas muscle outline is visible bilaterally.

The extra-abdominal soft tissues are unremarkable.

OTHER
There are no radiopaque foreign bodies.

There are no vascular lines, drains or surgical clips.

REVIEW AREAS
Gallstones / Renal calculi: No radiopaque calculi.
Lung bases: Normal.
Spine: Normal.
Femoral heads: Normal.

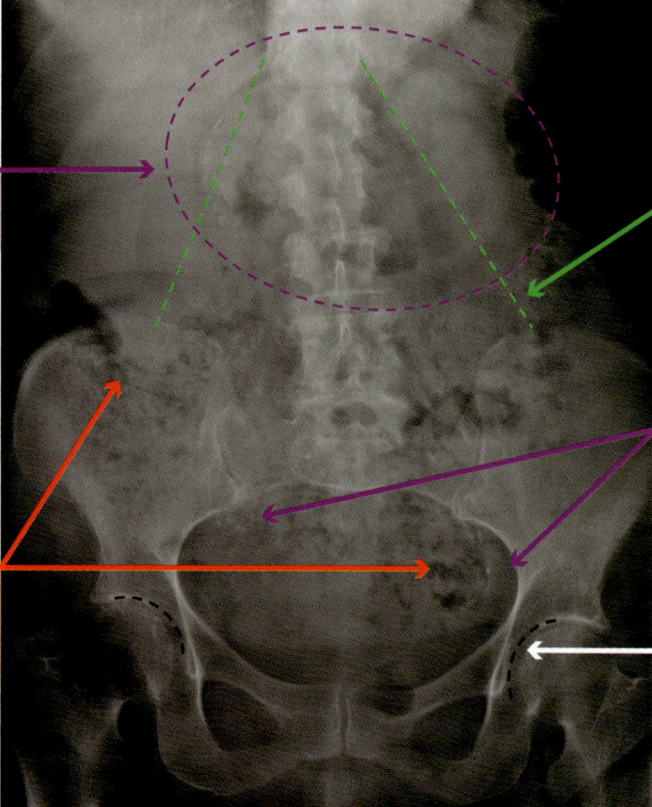

Calcified abdominal aortic aneurysm

Psoas muscle outline

Calcified iliac arteries

Faecal residue in caecum and distal descending/sigmoid colon

Femoral heads normal

SUMMARY
This X-ray demonstrates fusiform aneurysmal dilatation of the abdominal aorta. There is a moderate volume of faecal residue present predominantly in the caecum, distal descending and sigmoid colon, however no evidence of bowel obstruction. The iliac artery calcification is an incidental finding.

INVESTIGATIONS AND MANAGEMENT
The patient should be resuscitated using an ABCDE approach.

Adequate analgesia and hydration should be provided.

Urgent bloods should be taken including FBC, U&Es, bone profile, LFTs, CRP, coagulation, blood gas and crossmatch.

The patient should be made NBM and commenced on IV fluids.

The patient should be referred urgently to vascular surgery for assessment and a CT scan of the abdomen/pelvis with IV contrast to assess for abdominal aortic aneurysm leak should be considered.

The general surgical team and/or the vascular team may need to be involved depending on the findings of these additional investigations and the clinical picture.

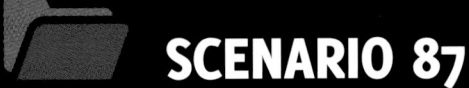

SCENARIO 87

A 40 year old female presents to ED with abdominal pain, nausea and vomiting. She has not opened her bowels for 5 days. She has a complex past medical history having had a previous bowel resection with formation of an ileostomy for Crohn's disease. She is a non-smoker. On examination, she has saturations of 98% in room air and a temperature of 36.5°C. Her HR is 100 bpm, RR is 24 and blood pressure is 118/64 mmHg. The abdomen is rigid and there is generalised tenderness with normal bowel sounds. Urine dipstick is unremarkable and a pregnancy test is negative.

An abdominal X-ray is requested to assess for possible bowel obstruction.

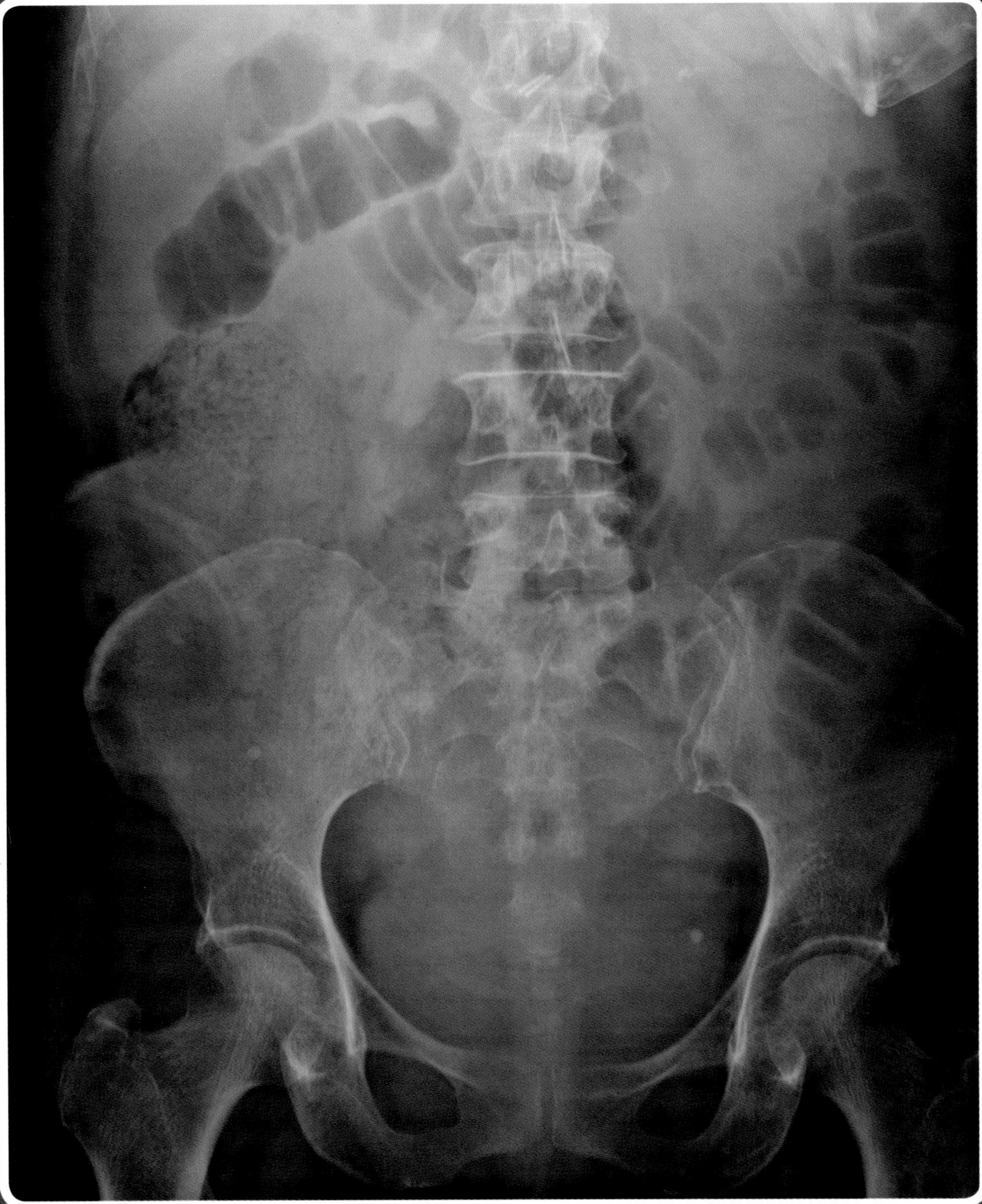

REPORT – ILEOSTOMY WITH DILATED SMALL BOWEL

REPORT
Patient ID: Anonymous.
Projection: AP supine.
Rotation: Adequate.
Penetration: Adequate – the spinous processes are visible.
Coverage: Adequate – the anterior ribs are visible superiorly and the pubic rami are visible inferiorly.

BOWEL GAS PATTERN
There are multiple loops of dilated bowel seen predominantly centrally in the abdomen. Valvulae conniventes are present, which appear separated with trapped gas in-between in keeping with small bowel dilatation.

BOWEL WALL
There is no evidence of mural thickening or intramural gas within the large or small bowel.

PNEUMOPERITONEUM
There is no evidence of free intra-abdominal gas.

SOLID ORGANS
The solid organ contours are within normal limits with no solid organ calcification.

VASCULAR
No abnormal vascular calcification.

BONES
There are mild degenerative changes in the hip joints with osteophyte formation.

SOFT TISSUES
The psoas muscle outline is visible bilaterally.

The extra-abdominal soft tissues are unremarkable.

OTHER
There is a rounded radiopaque density seen projected over the region of the right iliac fossa, in keeping with an ileostomy bag external to the patient. There is a moderate volume of faecal material in the area surrounding the ileostomy bag.

There is a small rounded radiopaque density projected over the region of the pelvis, which most likely represents a phlebolith.

There are surgical clips projected over the epigastrium.

There are no vascular lines or drains.

REVIEW AREAS
Gallstones / Renal calculi: No radiopaque calculi.
Lung bases: Not fully included.
Spine: Normal.
Femoral heads: Normal.

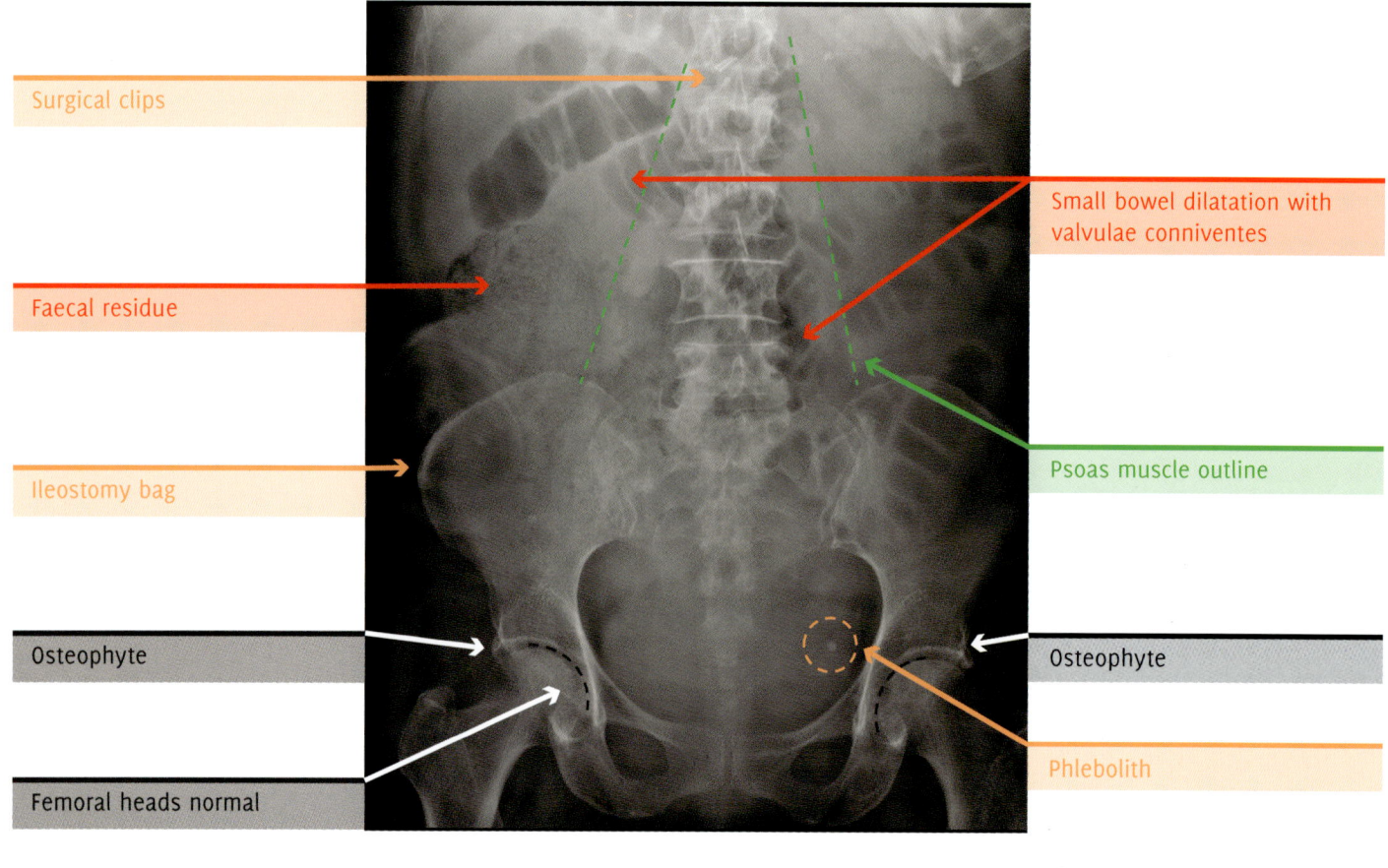

Surgical clips

Faecal residue

Ileostomy bag

Osteophyte

Femoral heads normal

Small bowel dilatation with valvulae conniventes

Psoas muscle outline

Osteophyte

Phlebolith

SUMMARY
This X-ray demonstrates predominantly centrally located bowel dilatation with valvulae conniventes, in keeping with small bowel obstruction. It also demonstrates an ileostomy bag projecting over the right iliac fossa with moderate volume faecal material seen in and surrounding the bag. Findings may be related to adhesions, recurrence of a Crohn's stricture or faecal impaction.

INVESTIGATIONS AND MANAGEMENT
The patient should be resuscitated using an ABCDE approach.

Adequate analgesia and hydration should be provided. The stoma should be assessed for patency.

The patient should be kept NBM, an NG tube inserted on free drainage to relieve the pressure in the small bowel, and IV fluids started.

Urgent bloods should be taken, including FBC, U&Es, CRP, LFTs, coagulation, blood gas, and group and save.

The general surgical team should be contacted urgently and a CT scan of the abdomen/pelvis with IV contrast considered.

SCENARIO 88

A 27 year old male presents to the gastroenterology outpatient clinic with worsening abdominal pain and a recent history of loss of weight. He has no significant past medical history and is a non-smoker. On examination, he has saturations of 97% in room air and a temperature of 39.2°C. His HR is 112 bpm, RR is 26 and blood pressure is 140/78 mmHg. The abdomen is rigid and there is severe generalised tenderness and guarding with normal bowel sounds. Urine dipstick is unremarkable.

An abdominal X-ray is requested to assess for possible perforation.

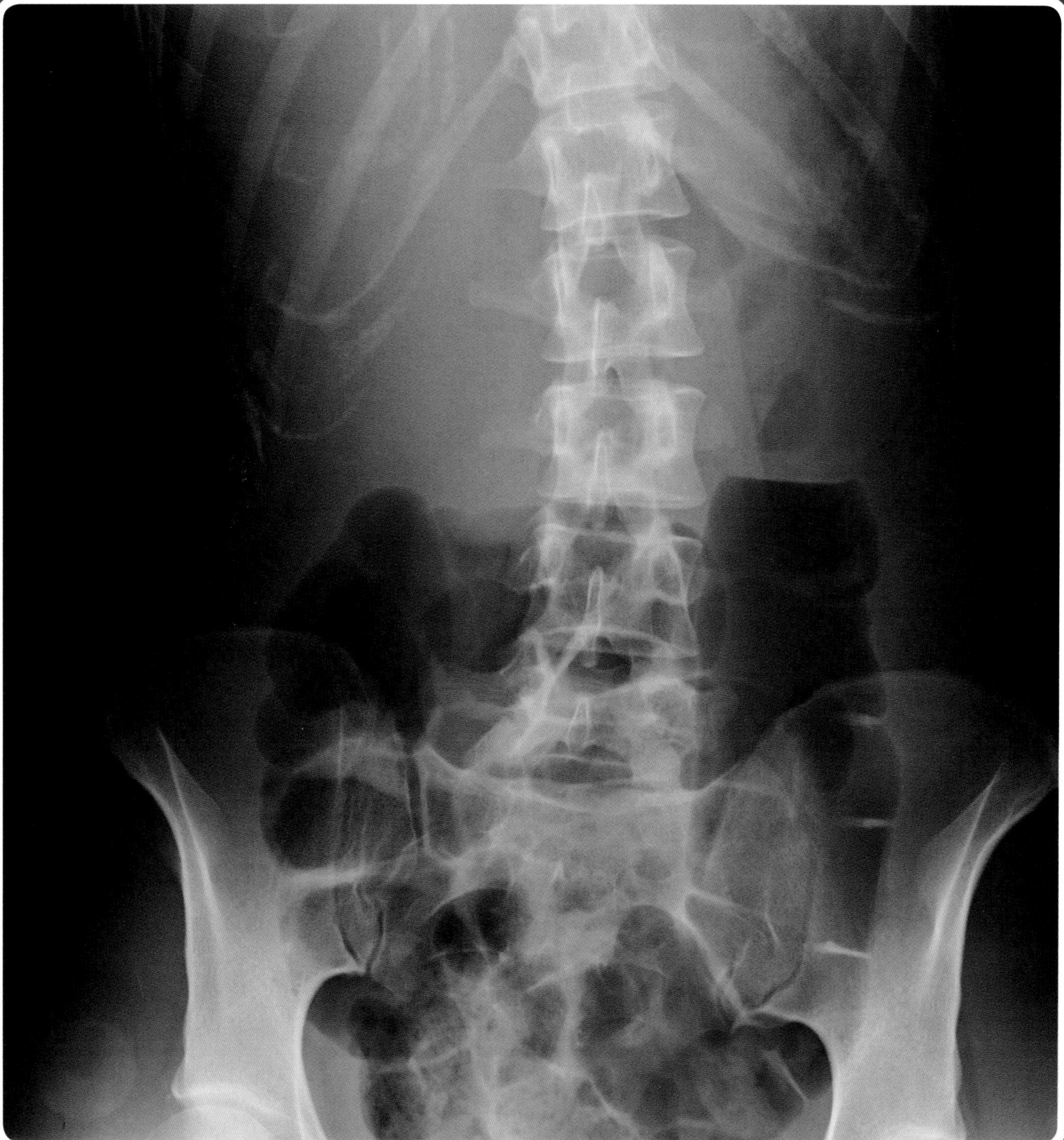

REPORT – RETROPERITONEAL MASS

REPORT
Patient ID: Anonymous.
Projection: AP supine.
Rotation: Adequate.
Penetration: Adequate – the spinous processes are visible.
Coverage: Inadequate – the pubic symphysis, inferior pubic rami and hip joints have not been fully included.

BOWEL GAS PATTERN
The large bowel is displaced inferiorly towards the pelvis, implying there is possibly a large soft tissue mass in the upper abdomen.

BOWEL WALL
There is no evidence of mural thickening or intramural gas within the large or small bowel.

PNEUMOPERITONEUM
There is no evidence of free intra-abdominal gas.

SOLID ORGANS
The solid organ contours are within normal limits with no solid organ calcification.

VASCULAR
No abnormal vascular calcification.

BONES
There is mild lumbar scoliosis convex to the left, centred at the L2/L3 level.

There are no other abnormalities of the imaged thoracic and lumbar spine, or within the pelvis.

SOFT TISSUES
The psoas muscle outline is not preserved on the right side which may relate to the presence of an abdominal mass.

The extra-abdominal soft tissues are unremarkable.

OTHER
There is a large homogeneous opacification seen in the upper abdomen, which is displacing the large bowel down into the pelvis.

There are no vascular lines, drains or surgical clips.

REVIEW AREAS
Gallstones / Renal calculi: No radiopaque calculi.
Lung bases: Normal.
Spine: Lumbar scoliosis seen convex to the left, centred on the L2/L3 vertebral bodies.
Femoral heads: Not visible.

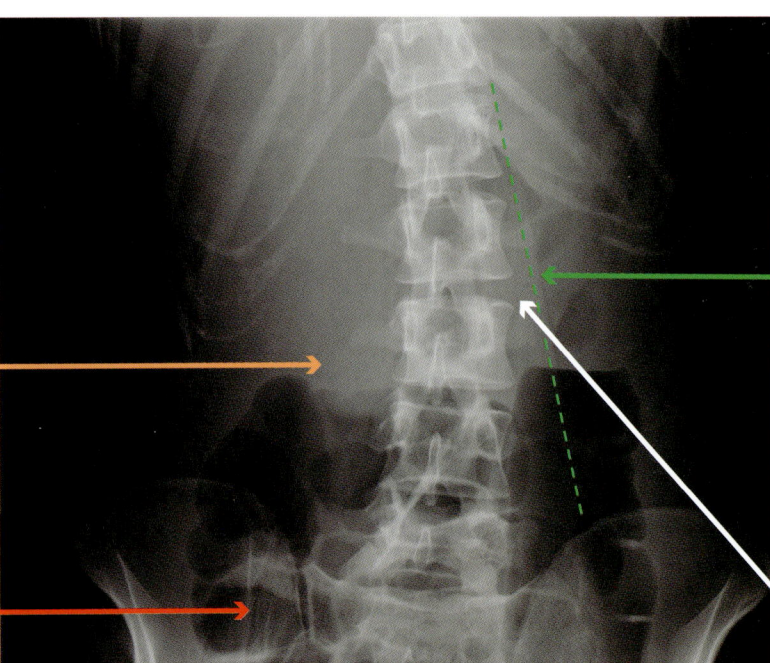

Large homogeneous opacification: possible psoas abscess or retroperitoneal collection

Inferior displacement of large bowel towards pelvis

Only left psoas muscle outline visible

Scoliosis

SUMMARY
This X-ray demonstrates a large homogeneous opacification in the upper abdomen, which is displacing the large bowel inferiorly into the pelvis and obscuring the right psoas muscle outline. Given the clinical history, findings are suggestive of a large abdominal mass, which is probably retroperitoneal due to the loss of the right psoas muscle outline. The mild lumbar scoliosis is likely relative to this.

INVESTIGATIONS AND MANAGEMENT
The patient is clinically unwell and should be resuscitated using an ABCDE approach.

Adequate analgesia and hydration should be provided.

Urgent bloods should be taken including FBC, U&Es, LFTs, amylase, bone profile, CRP, blood gas, and blood cultures.

The sepsis 6 pathway should be started immediately, including administration of oxygen, IV broad spectrum antibiotics and consideration of a fluid bolus as well as measurement of lactate and urinary output and blood cultures.

A CT scan of the abdomen/pelvis with IV contrast would be useful for better visualisation of the anatomy and the general surgical team should be involved.

A 52 year old male is currently admitted on the surgical ward following cardiothoracic surgery. He has not opened his bowels for 5 days. His past medical history is significant for aortic stenosis and type II diabetes mellitus. He is an ex-smoker. On examination, he has saturations of 98% in room air and a temperature of 37.1°C. His HR is 75 bpm, RR is 13 and blood pressure is 120/65 mmHg. The abdomen is soft and there is no tenderness with normal bowel sounds. Urine dipstick is unremarkable.

An abdominal X-ray is requested to assess for possible bowel obstruction.

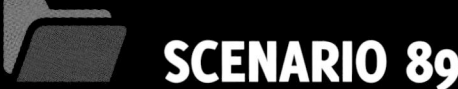

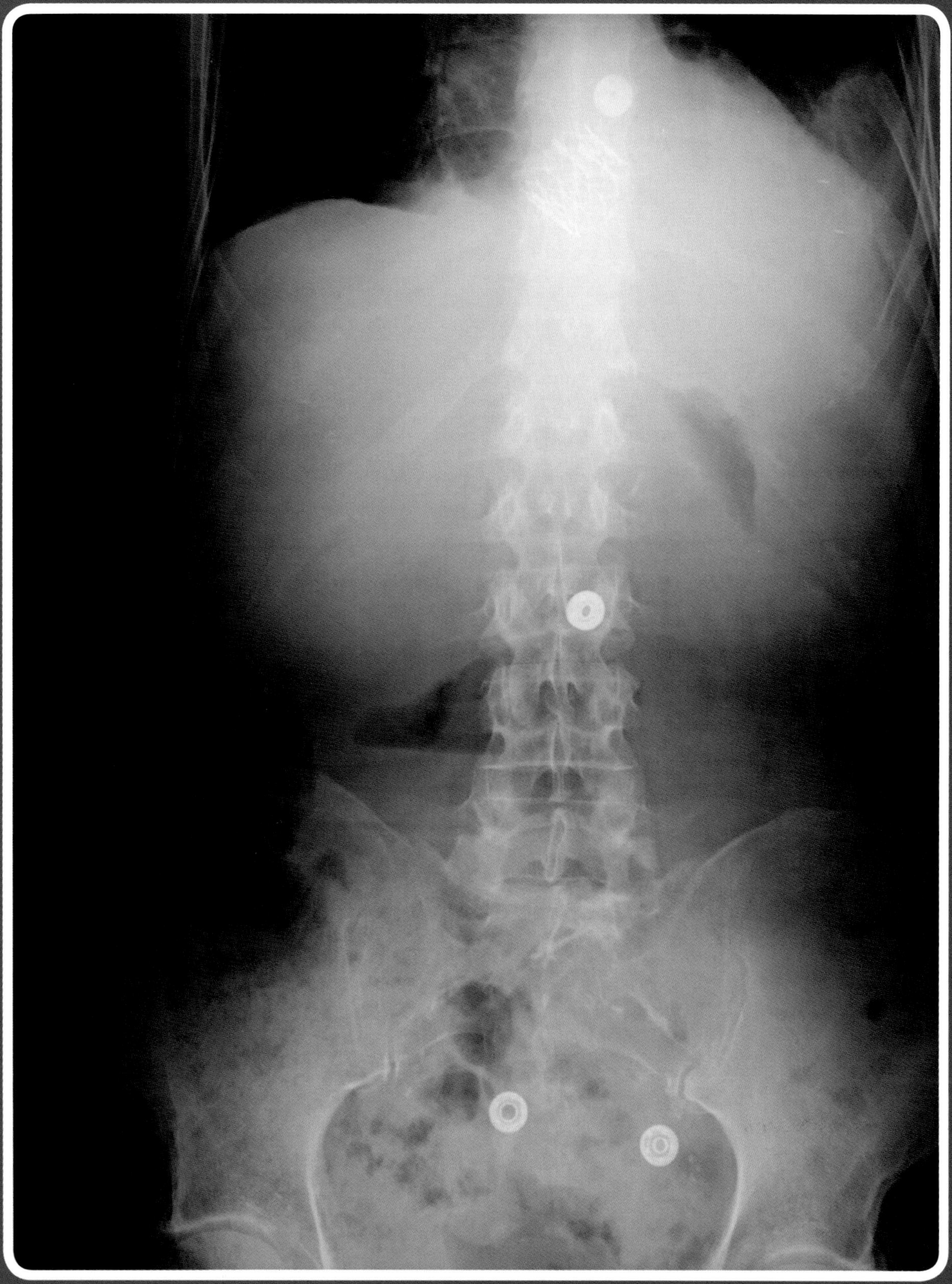

REPORT

Patient ID: Anonymous.
Projection: AP supine.
Rotation: Adequate.
Penetration: Adequate – the spinous processes are visible.
Coverage: Inadequate – the pubic symphysis, inferior pubic rami and hip joints have not been fully included.

BOWEL GAS PATTERN

The bowel gas pattern is normal. There is a moderate volume of faecal residue in the caecum.

BOWEL WALL

There is no evidence of mural thickening or intramural gas within the large or small bowel.

PNEUMOPERITONEUM

There is no evidence of free intra-abdominal gas.

SOLID ORGANS

There is a triangular opacity projecting in the left retrocardiac area in keeping with left lower lobe collapse.

There is also hetrogenous opacification at the base of the left lung in keeping with possible consolidation/effusion.

VASCULAR

No abnormal vascular calcification.

BONES

There are no abnormalities of the imaged thoracic and lumbar spine, or within the pelvis.

SOFT TISSUES

The psoas muscle outline is not visible bilaterally, which is non-specific.

The extra-abdominal soft tissues are unremarkable.

OTHER

There are two surgical clips projecting over the left cardiac border with a further surgical clip projecting over the mediastinum.

There is a radiopaque density projected over the mediastinum in the midline, in keeping with a transcatheter aortic valve implantation.

There are 4 small rounded radiopaque densities projected in the midline from the chest to the pelvis external to the patient, most likely popper fastenings on a cardigan.

There are no vascular lines or drains.

REVIEW AREAS

Gallstones / Renal calculi: No radiopaque calculi.
Lung bases: Left lower lobe collapse with possible consolidation/effusion
Spine: Normal.
Femoral heads: Normal.

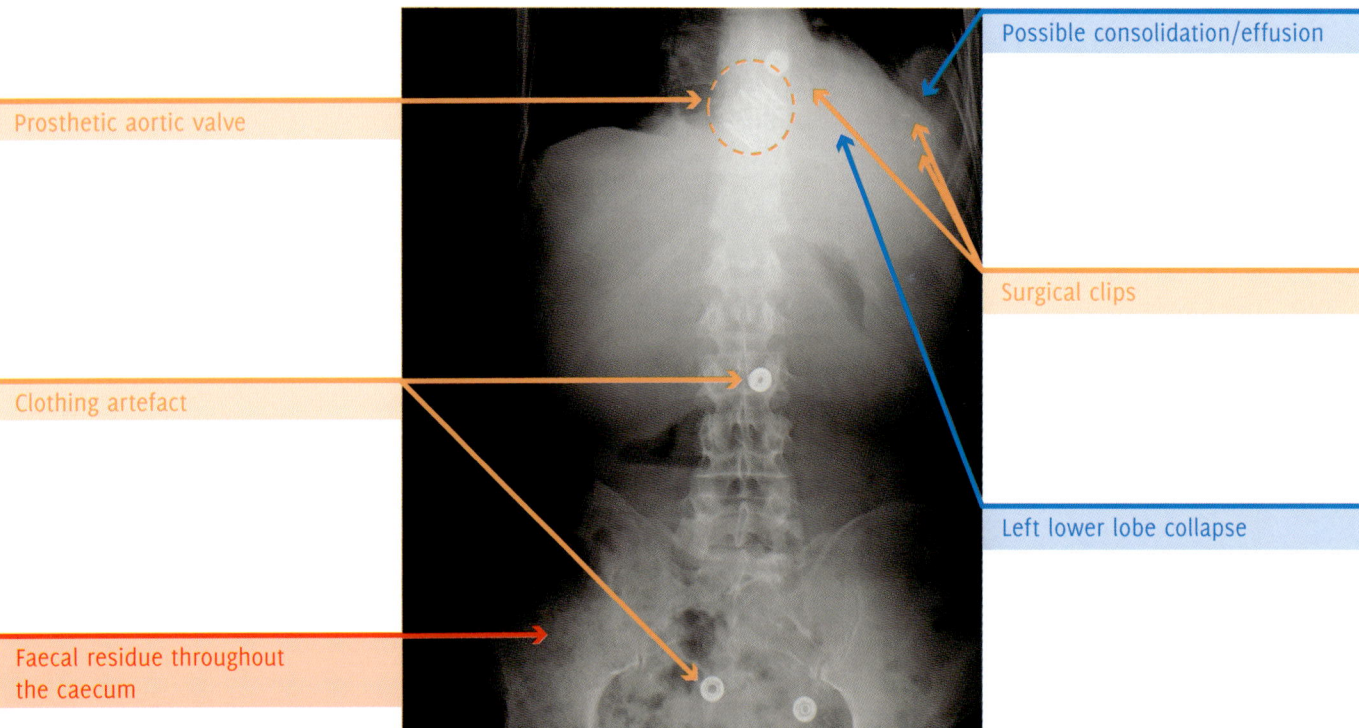

Possible consolidation/effusion

Prosthetic aortic valve

Surgical clips

Clothing artefact

Left lower lobe collapse

Faecal residue throughout the caecum

SUMMARY

This X-ray demonstrates a prosthetic aortic valve in situ. There is left lower lobe collapse with possible left basal consolidation/effusion. There is a moderate volume of faecal residue in the caecum.

INVESTIGATIONS AND MANAGEMENT

Adequate analgesia and hydration should be provided.

A formal CXR would be helpful, as would an ultrasound to quantify the size of any effusion.

Urgent bloods should be taken, including FBC, U&Es, LFTs, blood gas, blood culture and CRP.

The patient should be commenced on antibiotics for a hospital acquired pneumonia. Laxatives should be considered for constipation.

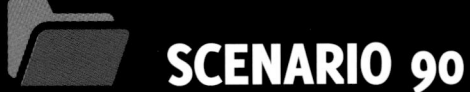

SCENARIO 90

A 6 hour old newborn currently admitted on the postnatal ward develops vomiting and abdominal distension. His past medical history is significant for Down's syndrome. On examination, he has saturations of 98% in room air and a temperature of 36.9°C. His HR is 170 bpm and RR is 60. The abdomen is grossly distended and bowel sounds are absent.

An abdominal X-ray is requested to assess for possible bowel obstruction.

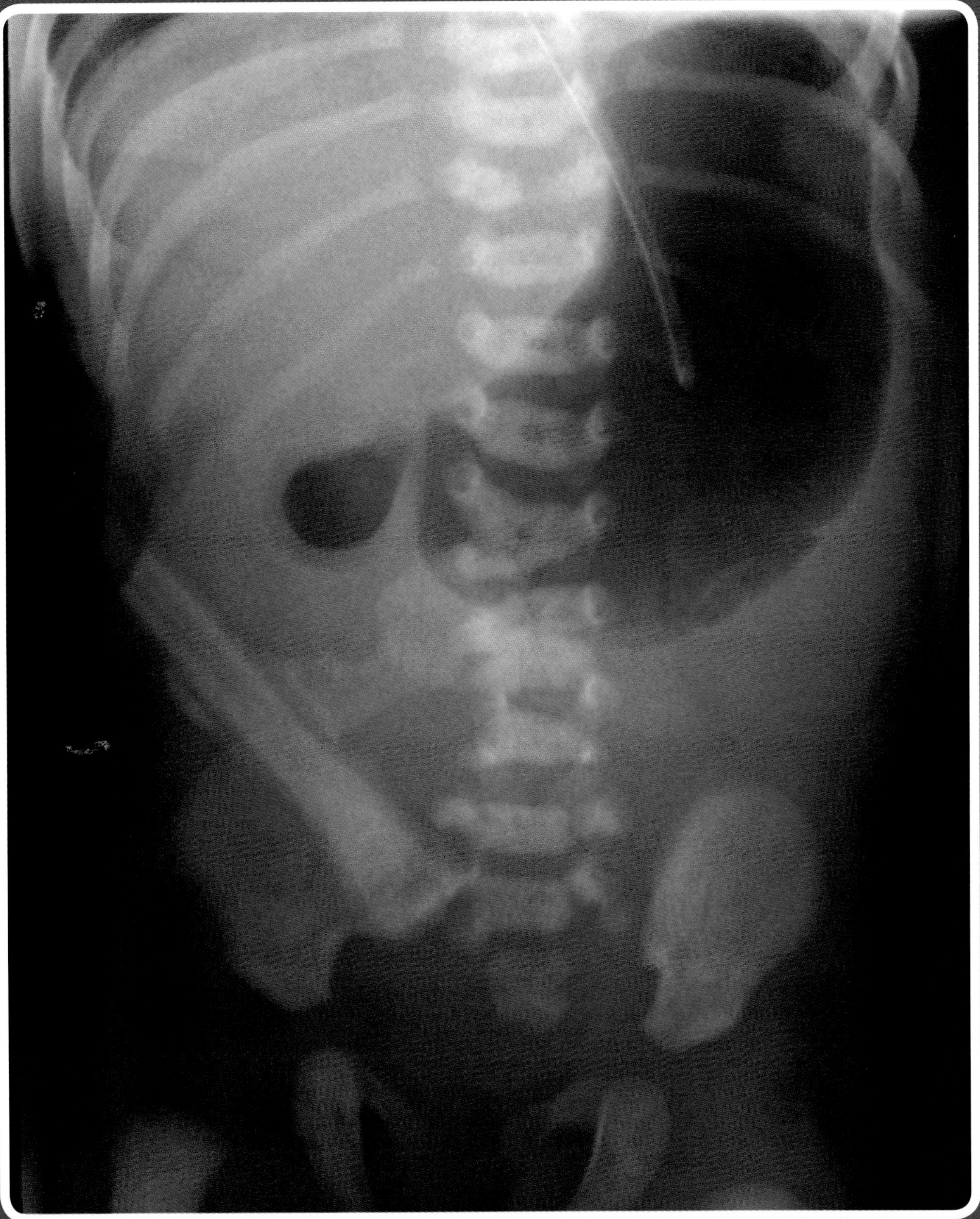

REPORT
Patient ID: Anonymous.
Projection: AP supine.
Rotation: Asymmetrical appearance of the pelvis due to patient rotation to the right.
Penetration: Adequate – the spine is visible.
Coverage: Adequate – the anterior ribs are visible superiorly and the inferior pubic rami are visible.

BOWEL GAS PATTERN
There is distension of the stomach and proximal duodenum which are filled with gas and separated by the pyloric sphincter, creating a 'double-bubble' sign.

There is absence of bowel gas seen distal to the duodenum.

BOWEL WALL
There is no evidence of mural thickening or intramural gas within the large or small bowel.

PNEUMOPERITONEUM
There is no evidence of free intra-abdominal gas.

SOLID ORGANS
The solid organ contours are within normal limits with no solid organ calcification.

VASCULAR
No abnormal vascular calcification.

BONES
There are segmentation abnormalities of the lumbar spine, which may be part of an underlying syndrome.

SOFT TISSUES
The psoas muscle outline is not visible bilaterally, which is non-specific, particularly in a child of this age.

The extra-abdominal soft tissues are unremarkable.

OTHER
There is a NG tube in situ, with its tip seen in the left upper quadrant, within the body of the stomach.

There is a clamp seen projecting external to the patient on the right side of the abdomen in keeping with an umbilical cord clamp.

There are no vascular lines, drains or surgical clips.

REVIEW AREAS
Gallstones / Renal calculi: No radiopaque calculi.
Lung bases: Not fully included.
Spine: Normal – cartilage between vertebrae.
Femoral heads: Normal – growth plates present.

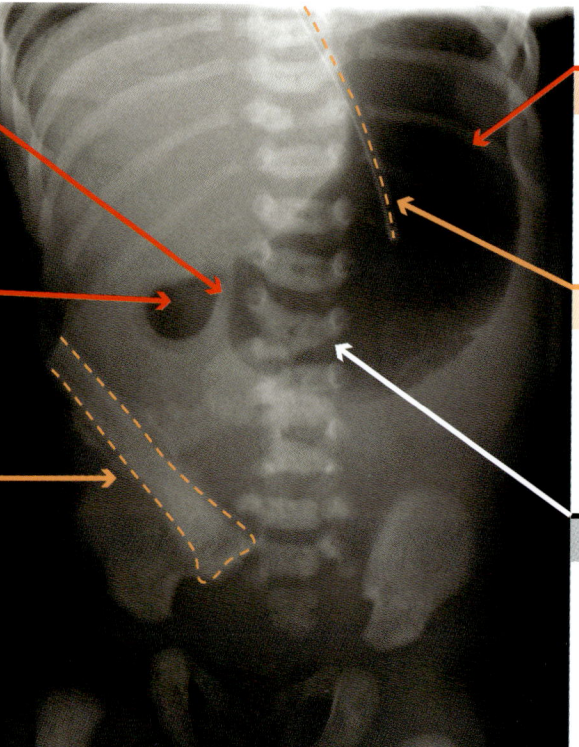

Pyloric sphincter

Distended proximal duodenum

Umbilical cord clamp

Distended stomach

NG tube

Segmentation abnormality

SUMMARY
This X-ray demonstrates gaseous distension of the stomach and proximal duodenum with absence of bowel gas distal to this point, in keeping with duodenal atresia. There is an NG tube in situ in satisfactory position within the stomach and the umbilical cord is clamped.

INVESTIGATIONS AND MANAGEMENT
The baby should be resuscitated using an ABCDE approach.

The baby should be commenced on broad spectrum antibiotics, IV fluids and be made NBM.

Urgent bloods should be taken including FBC, U&Es, blood culture, blood gas, and CRP.

The patient should be referred urgently to the neonatal surgeons for operative intervention. Given the vertebral abnormalities, associated defects should be looked for i.e. VACTERL (anal atresia, cardiac defects, tracheo-esophageal fistula, renal anomalies, and limb abnormalities).

SCENARIO 91

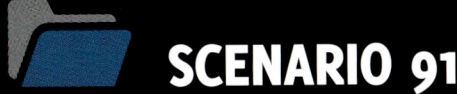

A 2 day old baby boy, currently admitted on NICU after being born at 29 weeks, develops abdominal distension, bile-stained vomitus, and is feeding poorly. On examination, he has saturations of 100% whilst intubated on 40% oxygen, and a temperature of 37.8°C. His HR is 180 bpm and RR is 65. The abdomen is rigid and bowel sounds are absent.

An abdominal X-ray is requested to assess for possible necrotising enterocolitis.

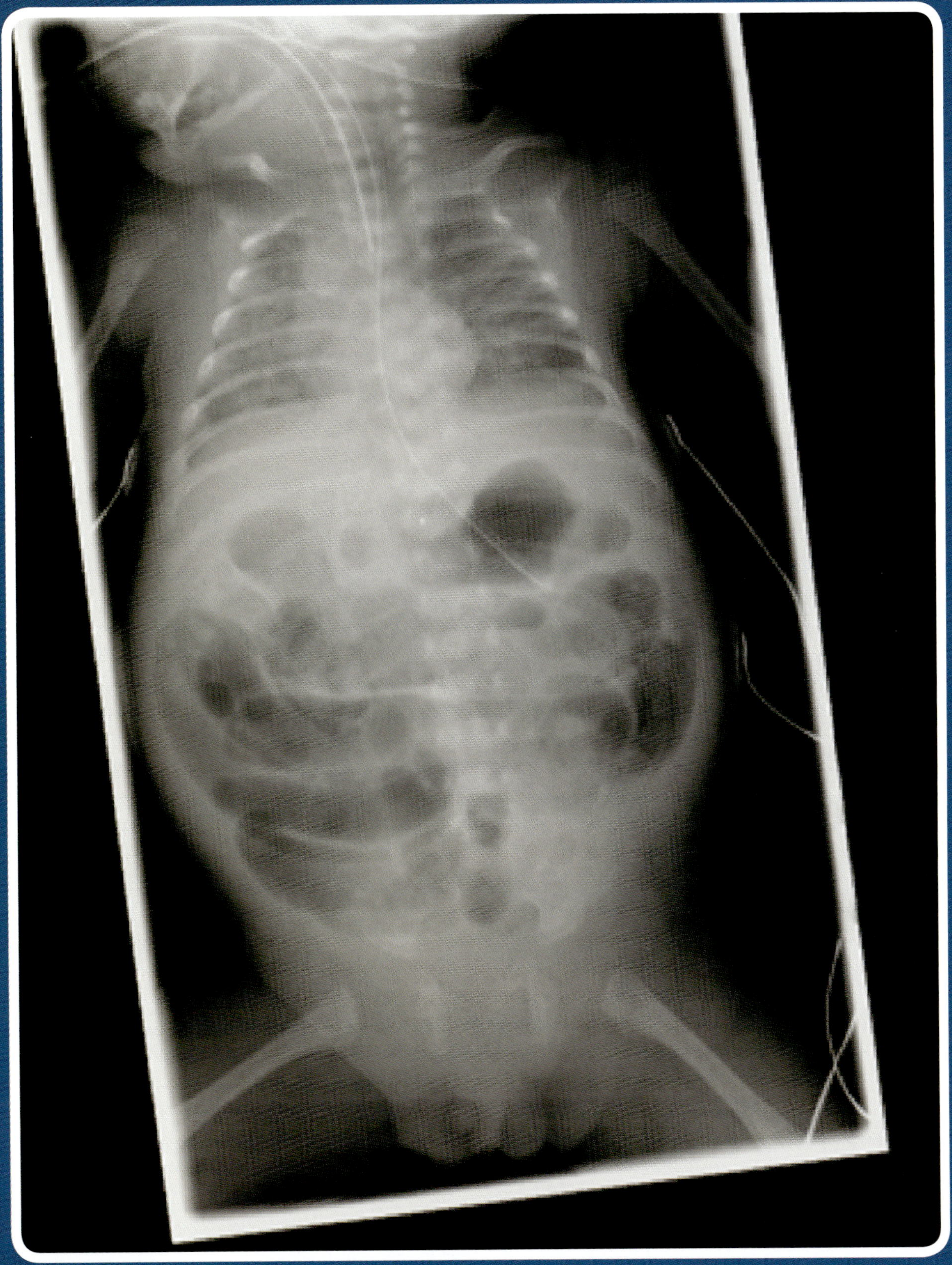

REPORT – BOWEL OBSTRUCTION AND PNEUMOPERITONEUM

REPORT

Patient ID: Anonymous.

Projection: AP supine 'babygram' of chest and abdomen.

Rotation: Asymmetrical appearances of the pelvis with deviation of the spine to the left due to patient rotation to the right.

Penetration: Adequate – the spine is visible.

Coverage: Adequate – the anterior ribs are visible superiorly and the inferior pubic rami are visible.

BOWEL GAS PATTERN

There are multiple, predominantly small bowel loops of dilated bowel seen throughout the abdomen. These demonstrate a 'featureless' appearance in keeping with inflammation.

BOWEL WALL

There is no evidence of mural thickening or intramural gas within the large or small bowel.

PNEUMOPERITONEUM

There is evidence of free intra-abdominal gas, in keeping with pneumoperitoneum.

Rigler's sign can be seen (double wall sign), in keeping with air present on both the luminal and peritoneal sides of the bowel wall.

SOLID ORGANS

Lung fields show bilateral heterogeneous opacification. Abdominal organs are difficult to visualise.

VASCULAR

No abnormal vascular calcification.

BONES

There are no abnormalities of the imaged thoracic and lumbar spine, or within the pelvis.

There is cartilage present between the pelvic bones and femurs as they have not yet fused, which is a normal finding in a child of this age.

SOFT TISSUES

The psoas muscle outline is not visible bilaterally, which is non-specific, particularly in a child of this age.

The extra-abdominal soft tissues are unremarkable.

OTHER

There is an NG tube in situ, with its tip seen in the left upper quadrant of the abdomen, within the body of the stomach.

There is an ET tube in situ, with its tip seen in the midline, just proximal to the carina.

There are three electrodes and leads external to the patient, in keeping with cardiopulmonary monitoring.

There are no vascular lines, drains or surgical clips.

REVIEW AREAS

Gallstones / Renal calculi: No radiopaque calculi.

Lung bases: Normal.

Spine: Normal.

Femoral heads: Normal – growth plates present.

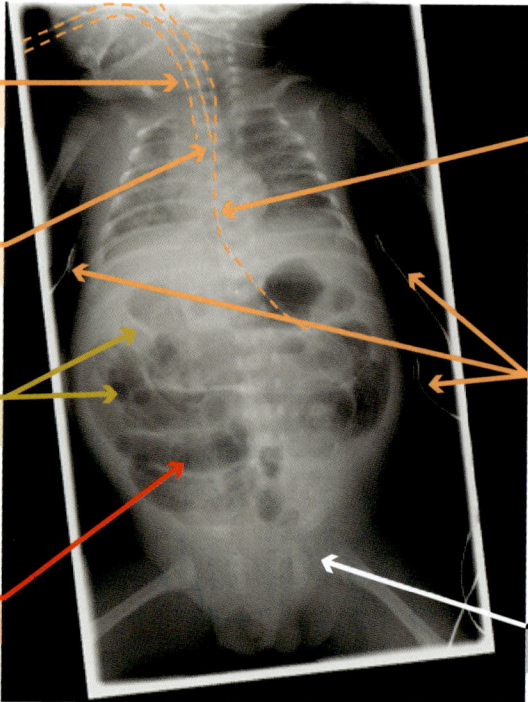

ET tube

Level of carina

Rigler's sign of pneumoperitoneum

Dilated loops of bowel

NG tube

Electrodes for cardiopulmonary monitoring

Cartilage between unfused bones

SUMMARY

This X-ray demonstrates multiple loops of dilated featureless bowel throughout the abdomen with evidence of pneumoperitoneum. Given the clinical history, findings are in keeping with bowel obstruction and secondary bowel perforation. There is likely respiratory distress syndrome in keeping with prematurity. The NG tube is in a satisfactory position, but the ET tube will need to be pulled back slightly.

INVESTIGATIONS AND MANAGEMENT

The patient should be resuscitated using an ABCDE approach.

Adequate analgesia and hydration should be provided.

The baby should be started on broad spectrum antibiotics and IV fluids and be made NBM.

Urgent bloods should be taken, including FBC, U&Es, CRP, bone profile, LFTs, coagulation, blood cultures, blood gas and group and save. A lateral shoot through X-ray would be helpful for confirmation of perforation.

The patient should be referred urgently to the neonatal surgeons for ongoing management.

SCENARIO 92

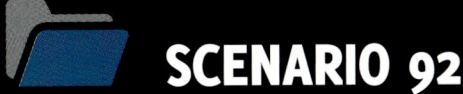

A 31 year old male is admitted on the general surgical ward following surgery for a stabbing injury. On examination, he has saturations of 98% in room air and a temperature of 37.2°C. His HR is 86 bpm, RR is 28 and blood pressure is 112/58 mmHg. The abdomen is tender and bowel sounds are present.

An abdominal X-ray is requested to assess the positions of the surgical drains.

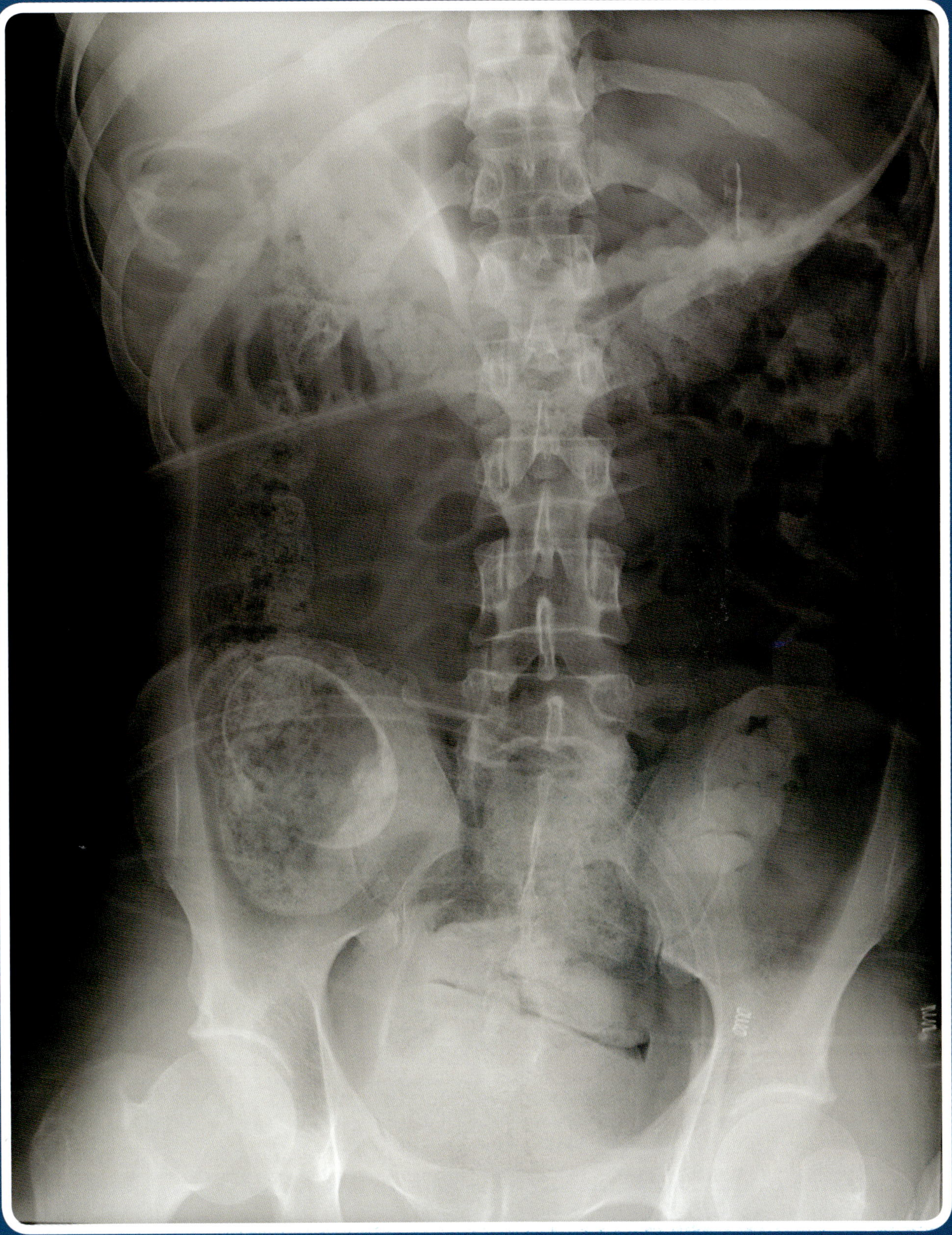

REPORT – PNEUMOPERITONEUM

REPORT
Patient ID: Anonymous.
Projection: AP supine.
Rotation: The spine is deviated to the left in keeping with mild patient rotation to the right.
Penetration: Adequate – the spinous processes are visible.
Coverage: Inadequate – the inferior pubic rami and left neck of femur have not been included.

BOWEL GAS PATTERN
The bowel gas pattern is normal.

There is a mild to moderate volume of faecal material present throughout the large bowel.

BOWEL WALL
There is no evidence of mural thickening or intramural gas within the large or small bowel.

PNEUMOPERITONEUM
There is evidence of extensive free intra-abdominal gas, in keeping with pneumoperitoneum.

Rigler's sign (double wall sign) can be seen, in keeping with air present on both the luminal and peritoneal sides of the bowel wall.

The falciform ligament sign can be seen, in keeping with air present within the abdomen outlining the falciform ligament.

SOLID ORGANS
The solid organ contours are within normal limits with no solid organ calcification.

VASCULAR
No abnormal vascular calcification.

BONES
There are no abnormalities of the imaged thoracic and lumbar spine, or within the pelvis.

SOFT TISSUES
The right psoas muscle outline is preserved. The left psoas muscle outline is not preserved, which is non-specific.

The extra-abdominal soft tissues are unremarkable.

OTHER
There is a surgical drain in situ projecting over the right upper quadrant with its tip projecting over the right L2 transverse process. There is a second surgical drain in situ projecting over the right lower quadrant with its tip projecting over the left pelvic ring.

There are further radiopaque lines projecting over the lower abdomen which likely represent external lines. There is an external artefact in the right lower quadrant as well, which may represent a dressing, although this should be correlated with clinical assessment.

There are no vascular lines or surgical clips.

REVIEW AREAS
Gallstones / Renal calculi: No radiopaque calculi.
Lung bases: Not fully included.
Spine: Normal.
Femoral heads: Normal.

Falciform ligament sign of pneumoperitoneum

Psoas muscle outline

Rigler's sign of pneumoperitoneum

Free gas

Faecal material throughout large bowel

Surgical drains

Artefact external the patient

External lines

SUMMARY
This X-ray demonstrates two surgical drains in situ as described. There is evidence of pneumoperitoneum, which is likely related to the recent surgery and penetrating trauma injury.

INVESTIGATIONS AND MANAGEMENT
The patient should undergo regular review by the general surgical team. The drain outputs should be monitored and removed at the discretion of the general surgical team.

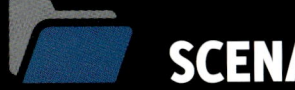

SCENARIO 93

An 18 year old female presents to ED with abdominal distension and increasing frequency of diarrhoea and passing mucus. She has a background of ulcerative colitis and is a non-smoker. On examination, she has saturations of 96% in room air and a temperature of 37.8°C. Her HR is 94 bpm, RR is 28 and blood pressure is 110/60 mmHg. The abdomen is soft and there is generalised tenderness with frequent normal bowel sounds. Urine dipstick is unremarkable and a pregnancy test is negative.

An abdominal X-ray is requested to assess for possible active colitis.

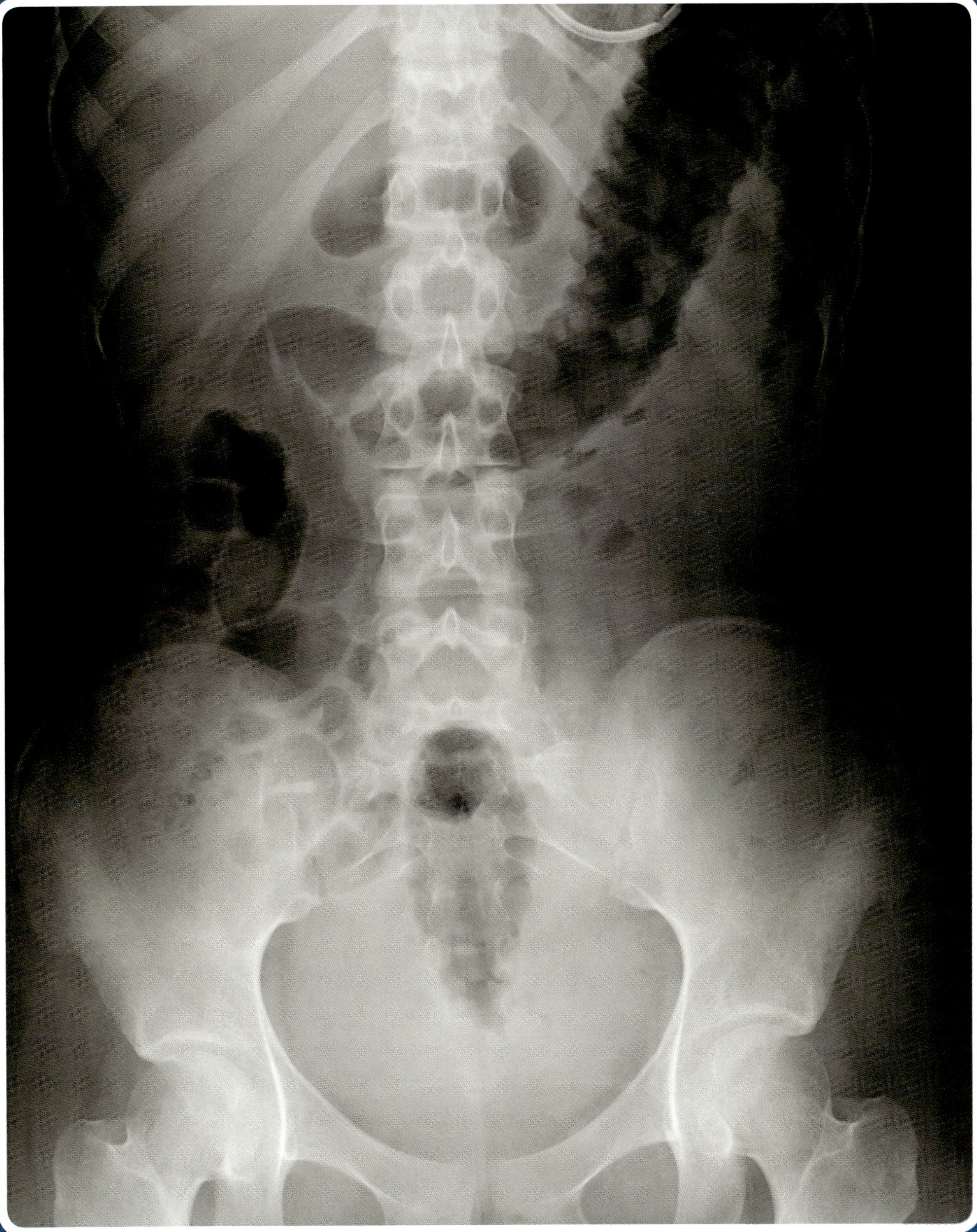

REPORT

Patient ID: Anonymous.
Projection: AP supine.
Rotation: Adequate.
Penetration: Adequate – the spinous processes are visible.
Coverage: Inadequate – the inferior pubic rami and hemidiaphragms have not been fully included.

BOWEL GAS PATTERN

There is dilatation of the transverse colon.

BOWEL WALL

There is evidence of mural thickening of the distal transverse colon in the left upper quadrant, with evidence of 'thumbprinting', in keeping with mural oedema.

There are multiple rounded areas of hyperdensity within the distal transverse colon, which may represent inflammatory pseudopolyps.

There is no evidence of intramural gas within the large or small bowel.

PNEUMOPERITONEUM

There is no evidence of free intra-abdominal gas.

SOLID ORGANS

The solid organ contours are within normal limits with no solid organ calcification.

VASCULAR

No abnormal vascular calcification.

BONES

There are no abnormalities of the imaged thoracic and lumbar spine, or within the pelvis.

SOFT TISSUES

The psoas muscle outline is visible bilaterally.

The extra-abdominal soft tissues are unremarkable.

OTHER

There is a radiopaque line seen in the upper left quadrant in keeping with an NG tube. The tip is not visualised.

There are no vascular lines, drains or surgical clips.

REVIEW AREAS

Gallstones / Renal calculi: No radiopaque calculi.
Lung bases: Not fully included.
Spine: Normal.
Femoral heads: Normal.

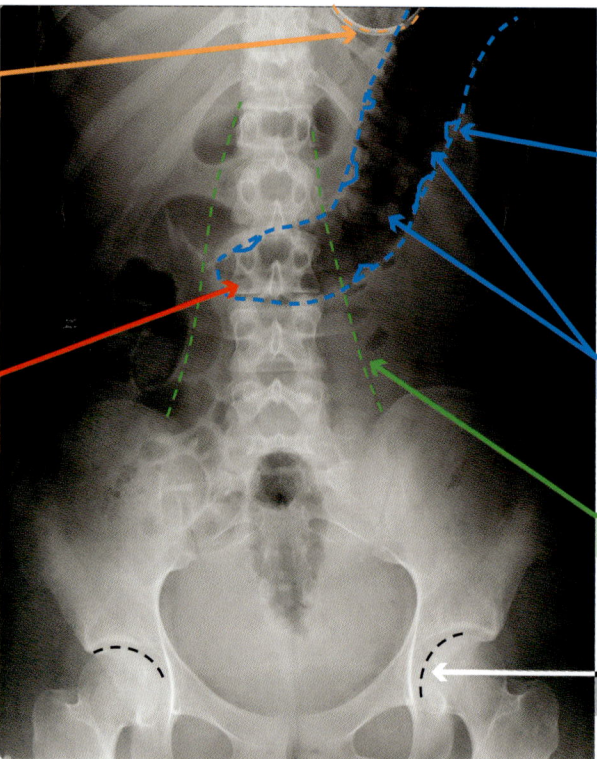

NG tube

Mural oedema of transverse and descending colon with thumbprinting

Large bowel dilatation of transverse and descending colon

Pseudopolyps

Psoas muscle outlines

Femoral heads normal

SUMMARY

This X-ray demonstrates dilatation and mural oedema of the distal transverse and proximal descending colon with evidence to suggest possible inflammatory pseudopolyposis. Given the clinical history, findings are in keeping with an acute exacerbation of ulcerative colitis.

INVESTIGATIONS AND MANAGEMENT

The patient should be resuscitated using an ABCDE approach.

Adequate analgesia and hydration should be provided.

Urgent bloods should be taken, including FBC, U&Es, LFTs, ESR, CRP, iron studies, folate, coagulation, blood gas, and group and save. A stool sample should be sent.

Urgent referral to both the general surgeons and gastroenterology team should be considered.

A CT scan of the abdomen/pelvis with IV contrast should be considered for better visualisation of the anatomy and to assess for the extent of the disease.

Treatment will depend on the results of further investigations as well as the clinical state of the patient.

SCENARIO 94

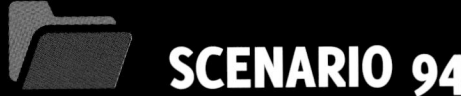

A 9 month old baby boy, born at 28 weeks gestation, develops worsening abdominal distension and vomiting. He has a PEG-J tube in situ due to severe reflux. On examination, he has saturations of 98% in room air and a temperature of 37.9°C. His HR is 180 bpm and RR is 62. The abdomen is rigid and bowel sounds are tinkling.

An urgent abdominal X-ray is requested to assess for possible bowel obstruction.

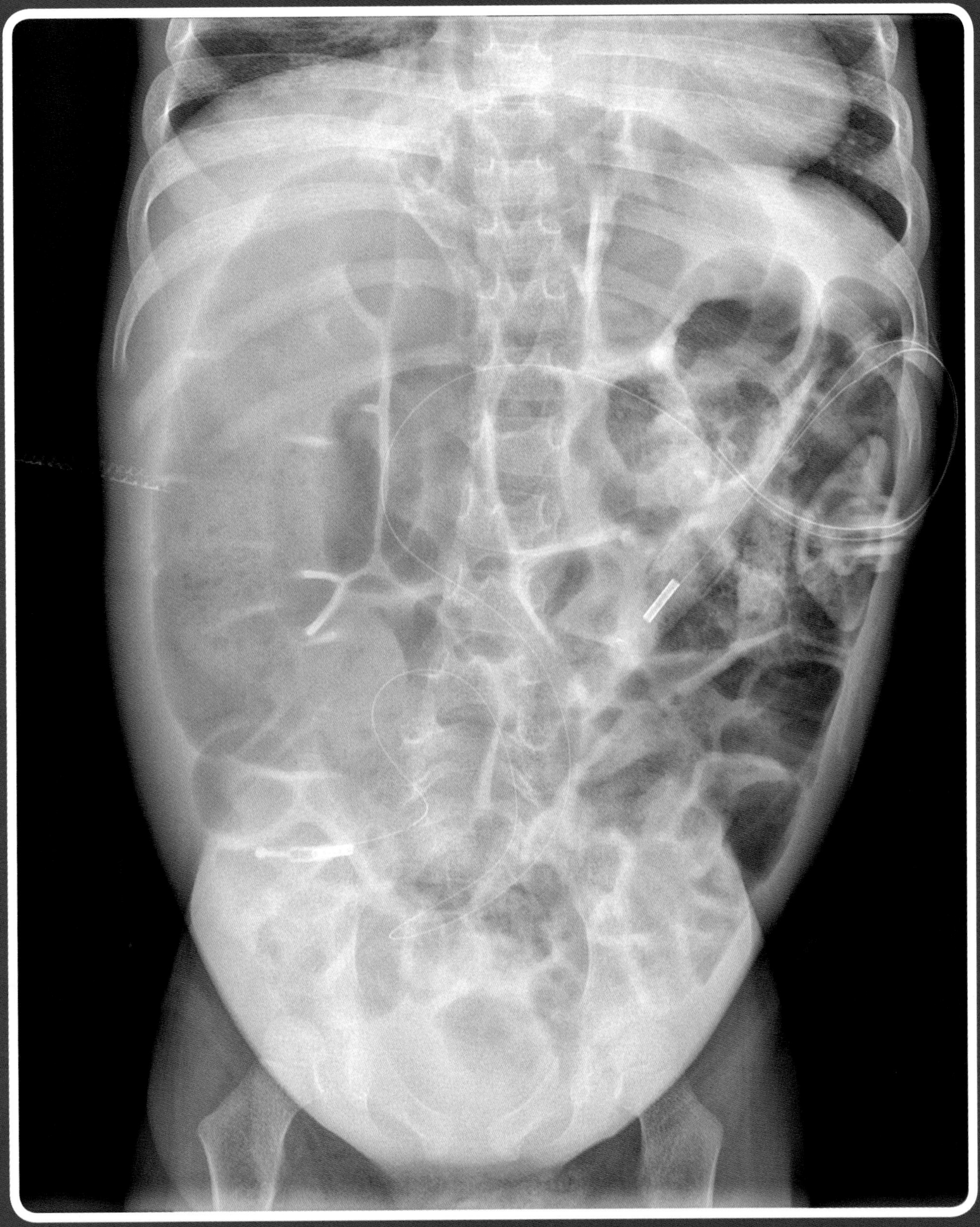

REPORT
Patient ID: Anonymous.
Projection: AP supine.
Rotation: Adequate.
Penetration: Adequate – the spine is visible.
Coverage: Adequate – the anterior ribs are visible superiorly and the inferior pubic rami are visible.

BOWEL GAS PATTERN
There are multiple loops of dilatated predominantly large bowel seen throughout the abdomen.

BOWEL WALL
There is no evidence of mural thickening or intramural gas within the large or small bowel.

PNEUMOPERITONEUM
There is no evidence of free intra-abdominal gas.

SOLID ORGANS
The solid organ contours are within normal limits with no solid organ calcification.

VASCULAR
No abnormal vascular calcification.

BONES
There are no abnormalities of the imaged thoracic and lumbar spine, or within the pelvis.

SOFT TISSUES
The psoas muscle outline is not visible bilaterally, which is non-specific, particularly in a child of this age.

The extra-abdominal soft tissues are unremarkable.

OTHER
There is a radiopaque internal-external line seen coiled across the abdomen, crossing the midline, with its tip seen in the right lower quadrant in keeping with a PEG-J tube. The PEG terminates within the stomach and the PEJ in the right lower quadrant likely within the distal jejunum. This follows an abnormal contour at the region of the duodenojejunal flexure, which is likely to represent underlying malrotation.

There are no vascular lines, drains or surgical clips.

REVIEW AREAS
Gallstones / Renal calculi: No radiopaque calculi.
Lung bases: Normal.
Spine: Normal.
Femoral heads: Normal – growth plates present.

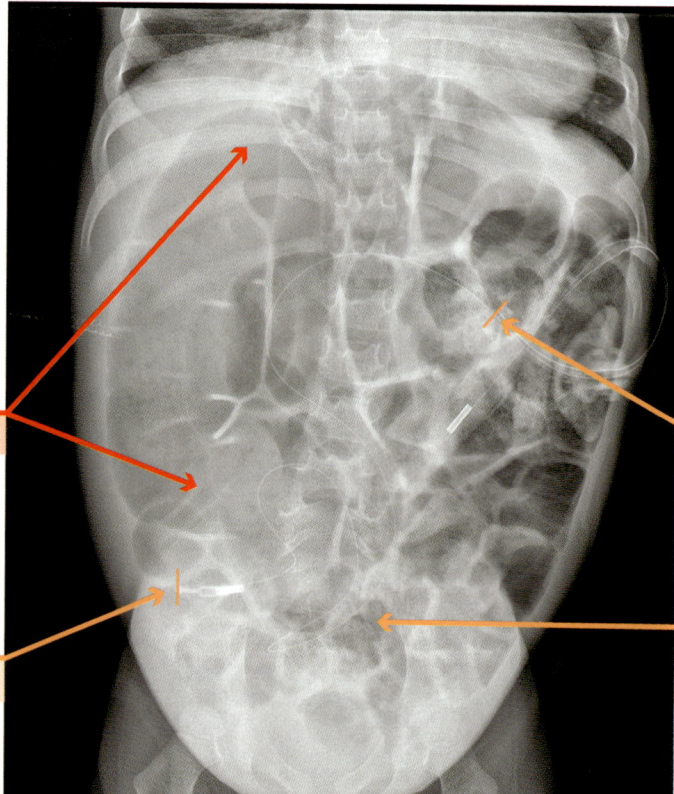

Dilated loops of bowel

PEG ends here

PEJ ends here

PEG-J (two tubes: one to the stomach one to the jejunum)

SUMMARY
This X-ray demonstrates multiple loops of dilated predominantly large bowel seen throughout the abdomen. There is a PEG-J line in situ, which follows an abnormal contour at the region of the duodenojejunal flexure, which is likely to represent underlying malrotation.

INVESTIGATIONS AND MANAGEMENT
The baby should be resuscitated using an ABCDE approach.

Adequate analgesia and hydration should be provided.

The baby should be started on broad spectrum antibiotics, be made NBM, and be started on IV fluids. The gastrostomy limb of the PEG-J should be put on free drainage.

Urgent bloods should be taken, including FBC, U&Es, CRP, bone profile, LFTs, coagulation, blood cultures, blood gas, and cross match.

The baby should be referred urgently to the surgeons for assessment and consideration of possible surgery. A contrast study would be helpful in assessing for possible malrotation.

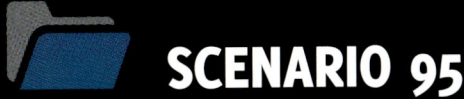
An 81 year old male presents to ED with weight loss and lethargy. He reports nausea, but has not vomited, and has significantly reduced urine output. He has no significant past medical history but complains of frequent aches and pains. He is a non-smoker. On examination, he has saturations of 95% in air, and a temperature of 36.5°C. His HR is 86 bpm, RR is 18 and blood pressure is 115/66 mmHg. The abdomen is soft and there is diffuse tenderness with normal bowel sounds. Urine dipstick is unremarkable. Early blood tests show markedly raised serum urea and creatinine, and a diagnosis of severe acute renal failure is made.

An abdominal X-ray is requested to assess for any possible bowel obstruction or abdominal lesions.

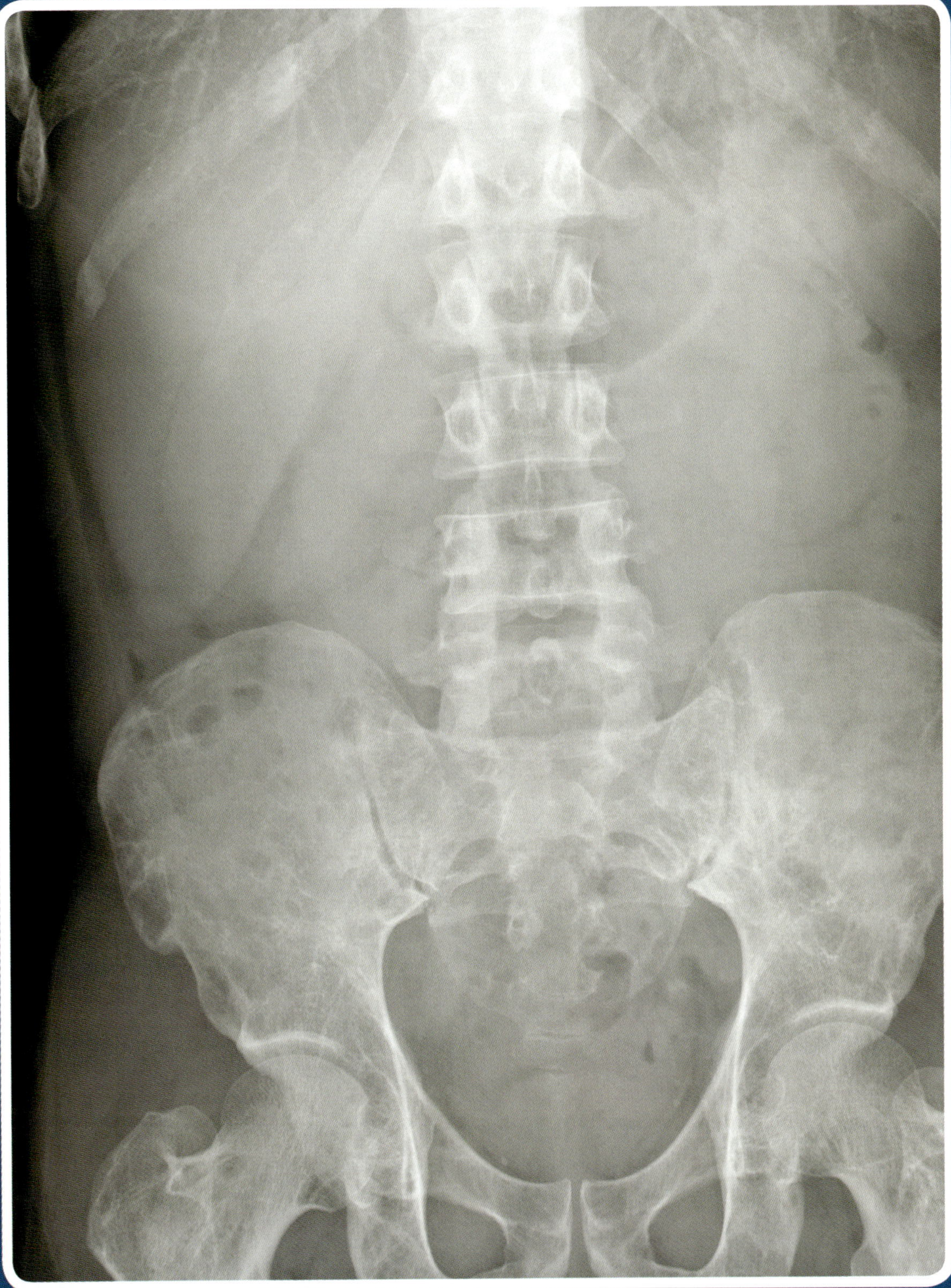

REPORT

Patient ID: Anonymous.
Projection: AP supine.
Rotation: Adequate
Penetration: Adequate – the spinous processes are visible.
Coverage: Adequate – the anterior ribs are visible superiorly and the inferior pubic rami are visible.

BOWEL GAS PATTERN

There is a paucity of bowel gas, which is non-specific.

BOWEL WALL

There is no evidence of mural thickening or intramural gas within the large or small bowel.

PNEUMOPERITONEUM

There is no evidence of free intra-abdominal gas.

SOLID ORGANS

The solid organ contours are within normal limits with no solid organ calcification.

VASCULAR

No abnormal vascular calcification.

BONES

There are no abnormalities of the imaged thoracic and lumbar spine.

There are multiple lytic lesions, some of which have sclerotic borders throughout the pelvis and both femoral heads. The zones of transition are narrow, they are not expansile, there is no obvious soft tissue component, and no periosteal reaction.

SOFT TISSUES

The psoas muscle outline is not visible bilaterally, which is non-specific.

The extra-abdominal soft tissues are unremarkable.

OTHER

There are no radiopaque foreign bodies.

There are no vascular lines, drains or surgical clips.

REVIEW AREAS

Gallstones / Renal calculi: No radiopaque calculi.
Lung bases: Not fully included.
Spine: Normal.
Femoral heads: Multiple lytic bone lesions.

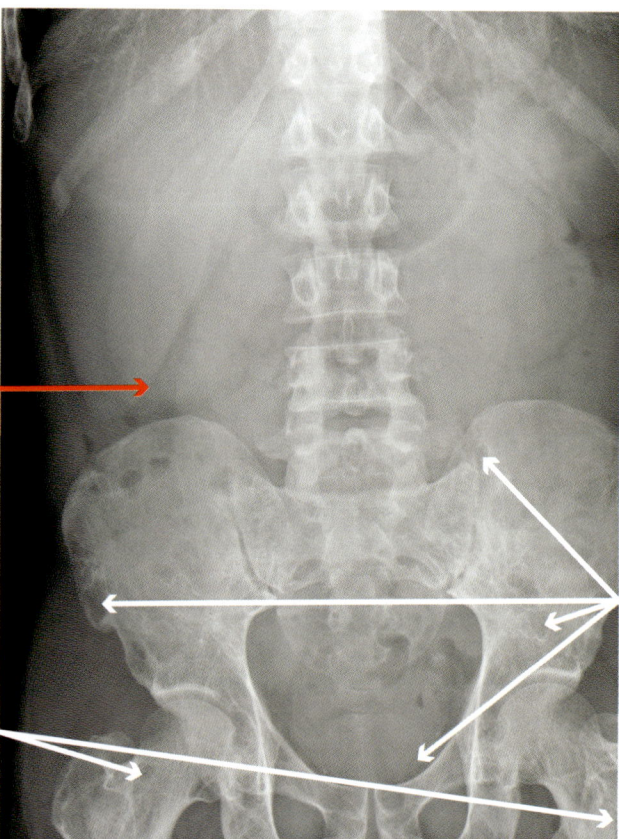

Paucity of bowel gas

Lytic bone lesions throughout pelvis

Lytic bone lesions in femoral heads

SUMMARY

This X-ray demonstrates multiple lytic bone lesions, some of which have sclerotic borders, throughout the pelvis and both femoral heads, which given the clinical history is suspicious for either metastatic deposits from an underlying primary tumour or possible multiple myeloma.

INVESTIGATIONS AND MANAGEMENT

The patient should be resuscitated using an ABCDE approach.

Adequate analgesia and hydration should be provided.

Bloods should be taken, including FBC, repeat U&Es, CRP, LFTs, bone profile, blood gas, and tumour markers.

A staging CT scan of the chest, abdomen and pelvis with IV contrast should be considered, once the acute renal failure has resolved, to identify any underlying malignancy.

Serum or urine electrophoresis should be performed to assess the presence of immunoglobulin light chains, as a diagnostic test for myeloma.

The patient should be referred to oncology services for further management, which may include biopsy and MDT discussion. Treatment, which may include surgery, radiotherapy, chemotherapy, or palliative treatment, will depend on the outcome of the MDT investigations and the patient's wishes.

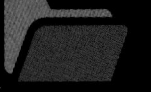

SCENARIO 96

A 60 year old female presents to ED following a collapse at home. Her past medical history is significant for advanced nasopharyngeal cancer and she is an ex-smoker. A radiologically inserted gastrostomy tube was recently inserted for long-term nutrition administration. On examination, she has saturations of 97% in room air and a temperature of 39°C. Her HR is 102 bpm, RR is 17 and blood pressure is 110/60 mmHg. The abdomen is rigid and there is widespread tenderness with normal bowel sounds. Urine dipstick is unremarkable.

An abdominal X-ray is requested to assess for possible obstruction.

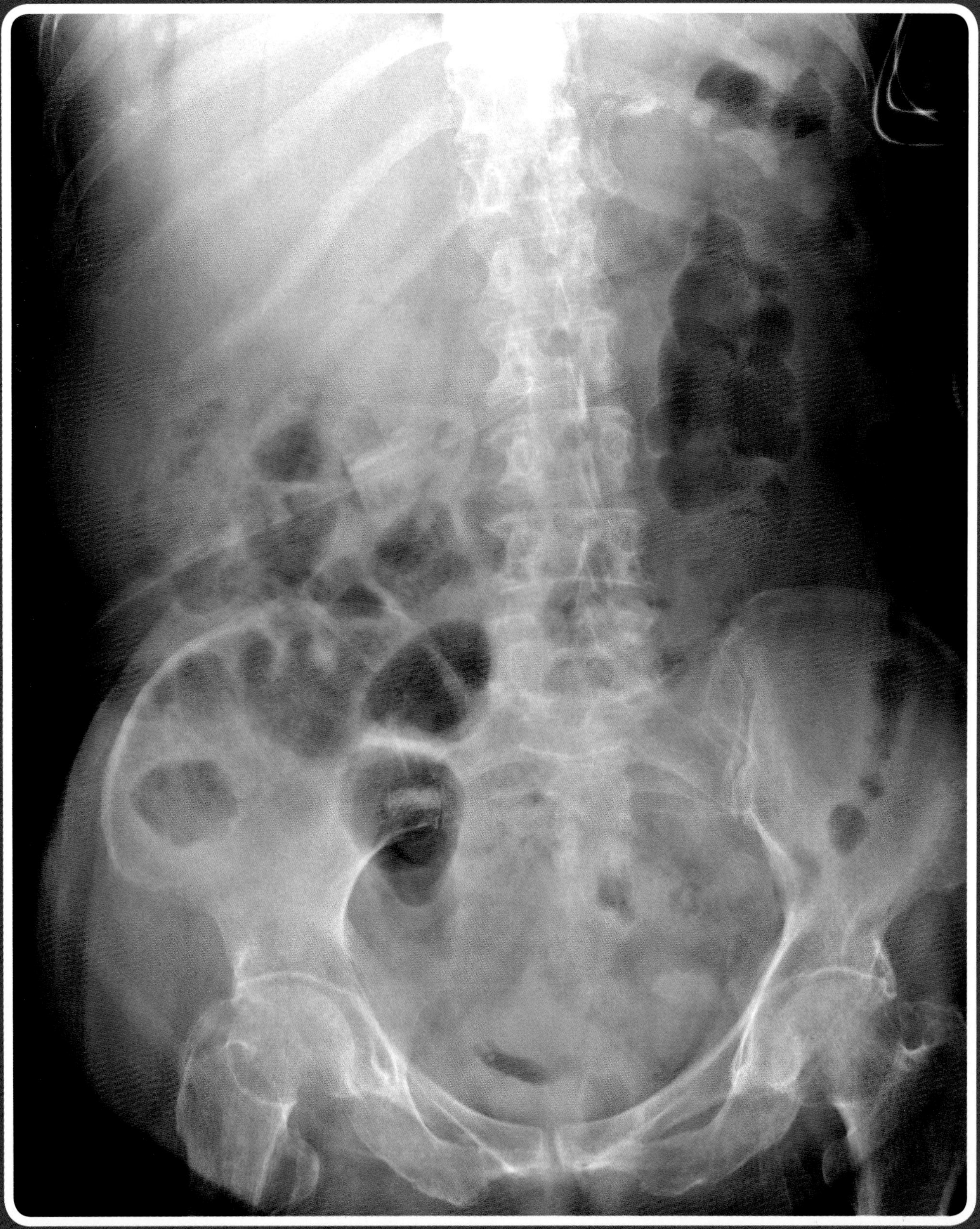

REPORT – RADIOLOGICALLY INSERTED GASTROSTOMY

REPORT
Patient ID: Anonymous.
Projection: AP supine.
Rotation: Adequate.
Penetration: Adequate – the spinous processes are visible.
Coverage: Adequate – the anterior ribs are visible superiorly and the inferior pubic rami are visible.

BOWEL GAS PATTERN
The bowel gas pattern is normal.

BOWEL WALL
There is mural thickening of the descending colon.

PNEUMOPERITONEUM
There is no evidence of free intra-abdominal gas.

SOLID ORGANS
The solid organ contours are within normal limits with no solid organ calcification.

VASCULAR
There is linear serpiginous calcification projecting over the left upper quadrant in keeping with splenic artery calcification.

BONES
There is mild lumbar scoliosis seen convex to the left, centred on the L3 vertebral body.

There is severe bilateral degenerative change in the hip joints.

SOFT TISSUES
The psoas muscle outline is visible bilaterally.

The extra-abdominal soft-tissues are unremarkable.

OTHER
There is a radiopaque tube projected over the region of the central abdomen with a triangular fixation device seen to the right of the midline. This is most likely a radiologically inserted gastrostomy tube.

There are no vascular lines, drains or surgical clips.

REVIEW AREAS
Gallstones / Renal calculi: No radiopaque calculi.
Lung bases: Normal.
Spine: Lumbar scoliosis seen convex to the left, centred on the L3 vertebral body.
Femoral heads: Both femoral heads flattened, particularly the right femoral head suggestive of previous avascular necrosis. Right femoral neck is shortened, in keeping with an old right neck of femur fracture.

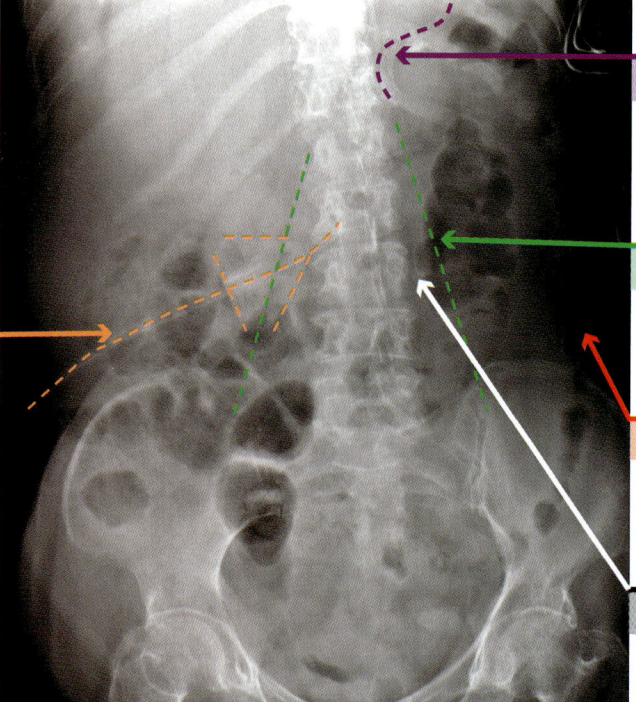

Vascular calcification

Psoas muscle outlines

Radiologically inserted gastrostomy tube (RIG)

Mural oedema

Scoliosis

SUMMARY
This X-ray demonstrates an appropriately positioned radiologically inserted gastrostomy tube (RIG). There is no evidence of pneumoperitoneum. There is some mural oedema which is non-specific, but may be related to the collapsed descending colon. It also demonstrates severe degenerative changes of the hip joints bilaterally.

INVESTIGATIONS AND MANAGEMENT
The patient should be resuscitated using an ABCDE approach.

Adequate analgesia and hydration should be provided.

Urgent bloods should be taken, including FBC, U&Es, LFTs, bone profile, CRP, coagulation, blood culture, blood gas, blood cultures, and group and save.

Broad spectrum antibiotics should be prescribed, the patient should be made NBM and started on IV fluids.

A CT scan of the abdomen/pelvis with IV contrast may be considered for further evaluation of the abdomen and surgical input should be sought.

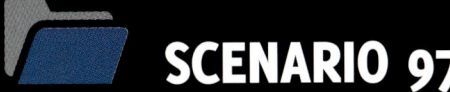

A 40 year old male presents to ED with worsening abdominal pain and 19 episodes of diarrhoea and passing mucus in the past 36 hours. He has no significant past medical history and is a non-smoker. On examination, he has saturations of 96% in room air and a temperature of 39.1°C. His HR is 103 bpm, RR is 23 and blood pressure is 140/80 mmHg. The abdomen is rigid and there is generalised tenderness with normal bowel sounds. Urine dipstick is unremarkable.

An abdominal X-ray is requested to assess for possible obstruction.

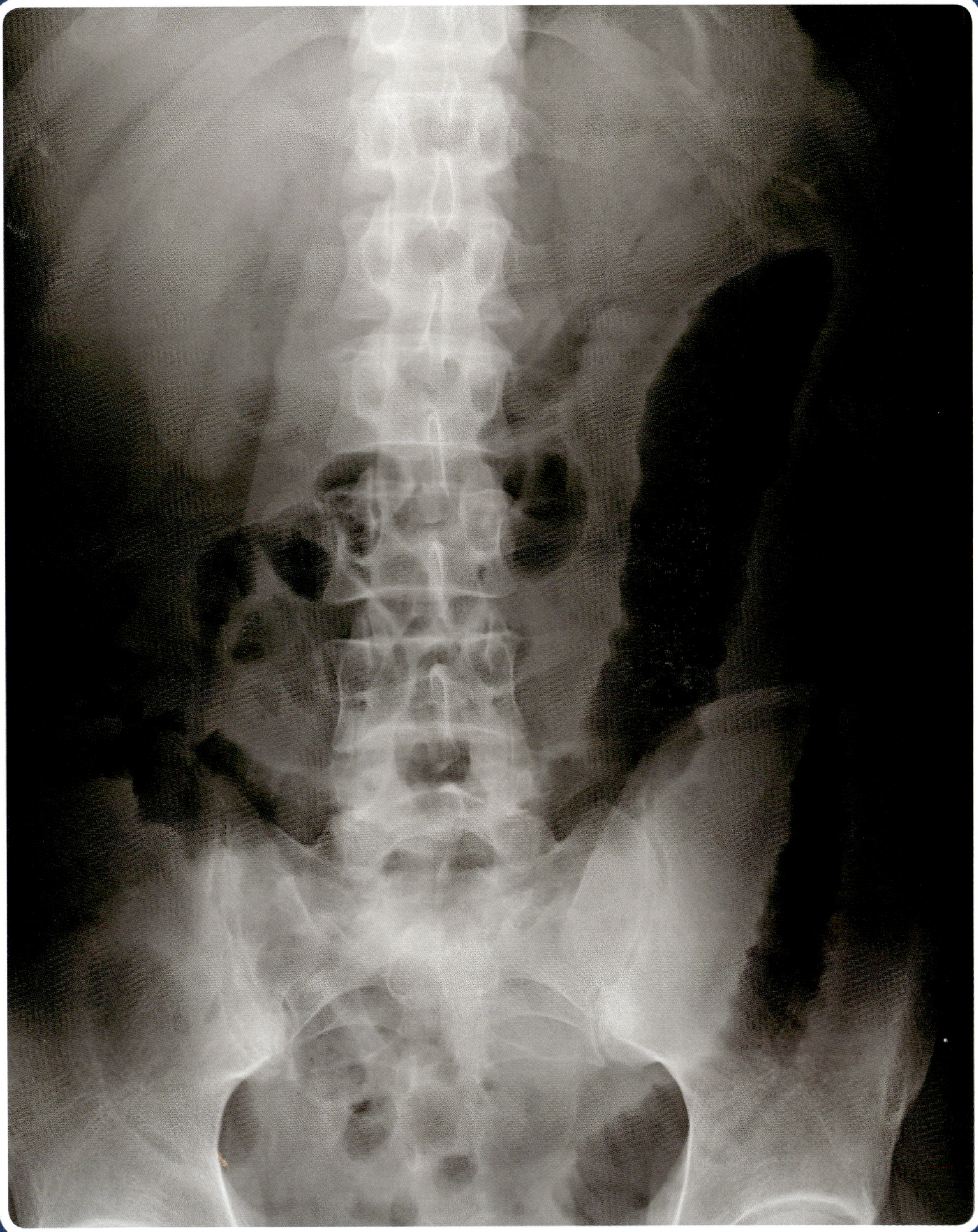

REPORT

Patient ID: Anonymous.
Projection: AP supine.
Rotation: Adequate.
Penetration: Adequate – the spinous processes are visible.
Coverage: Inadequate – the pubic symphysis, inferior pubic rami, hip joints and hemidiaphragms have not been fully included.

BOWEL GAS PATTERN

The bowel gas pattern is normal.

BOWEL WALL

There is evidence of mural thickening of the transverse and descending colon in the left upper and lower quadrants, with loss of the normal colonic haustral folds and evidence of 'thumbprinting', in keeping with mural oedema.

There is no evidence of intramural gas within the large or small bowel.

PNEUMOPERITONEUM

There is no evidence of free intra-abdominal gas.

SOLID ORGANS

The solid organ contours are within normal limits with no solid organ calcification.

VASCULAR

No abnormal vascular calcification.

BONES

There are no abnormalities of the imaged thoracic and lumbar spine, or within the pelvis.

SOFT TISSUES

The psoas muscle outline is visible bilaterally.

The extra-abdominal soft tissues are unremarkable.

OTHER

There are no radiopaque foreign bodies.

There are no vascular lines, drains or surgical clips.

REVIEW AREAS

Gallstones / Renal calculi: No radiopaque calculi.
Lung bases: Not fully included.
Spine: Normal.
Femoral heads: Not visualised.

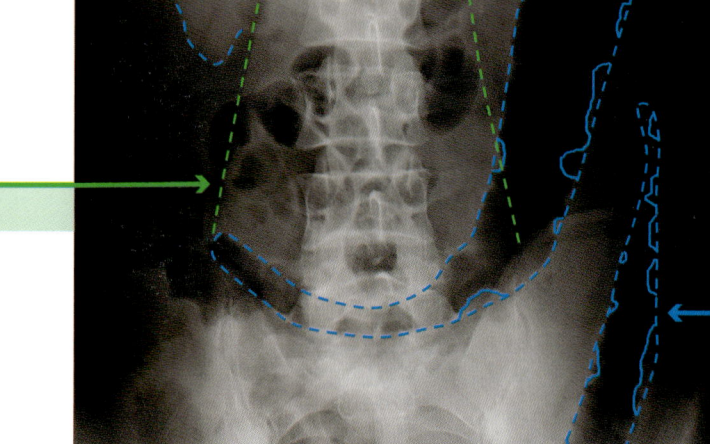

Outline of right kidney

Psoas muscle outlines

Mural oedema of transverse colon with loss of haustral folds and thumbprinting

Mural oedema of descending colon with loss of haustral folds and thumbprinting

SUMMARY

This X-ray demonstrates mural oedema of the transverse and descending colon, with loss of the normal colonic haustral folds and evidence of 'thumbprinting' in keeping with colitis. Given the clinical history, this is most likely infective or inflammatory in nature.

INVESTIGATIONS AND MANAGEMENT

This patient should be resuscitated using an ABCDE approach.

Adequate analgesia and hydration should be provided.

Urgent bloods should be taken, including FBC, U&Es, LFTs, ESR, CRP, iron studies, folate, blood gas, and group and save. A stool sample should be sent.

Urgent referral to the gastroenterology team should be considered.

A CT scan of the abdomen/pelvis with IV contrast should be considered for better visualisation of the anatomy and to assess for complications such as pneumoperitoneum and abscess formation.

Treatment will depend on the results of further investigations as well as the clinical state of the patient.

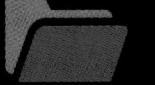

SCENARIO 98

A 10 day old baby girl, born at 28 weeks gestation, currently admitted on NICU develops severe abdominal distension and vomiting. She had bowel surgery on day 5 of life for Hirschsprung's disease. On examination, she has saturations of 98% in room air and a temperature of 36.9°C. Her HR is 170 bpm and RR is 60. The abdomen is grossly distended and bowel sounds are absent.

An urgent abdominal X-ray is requested to assess for possible perforation.

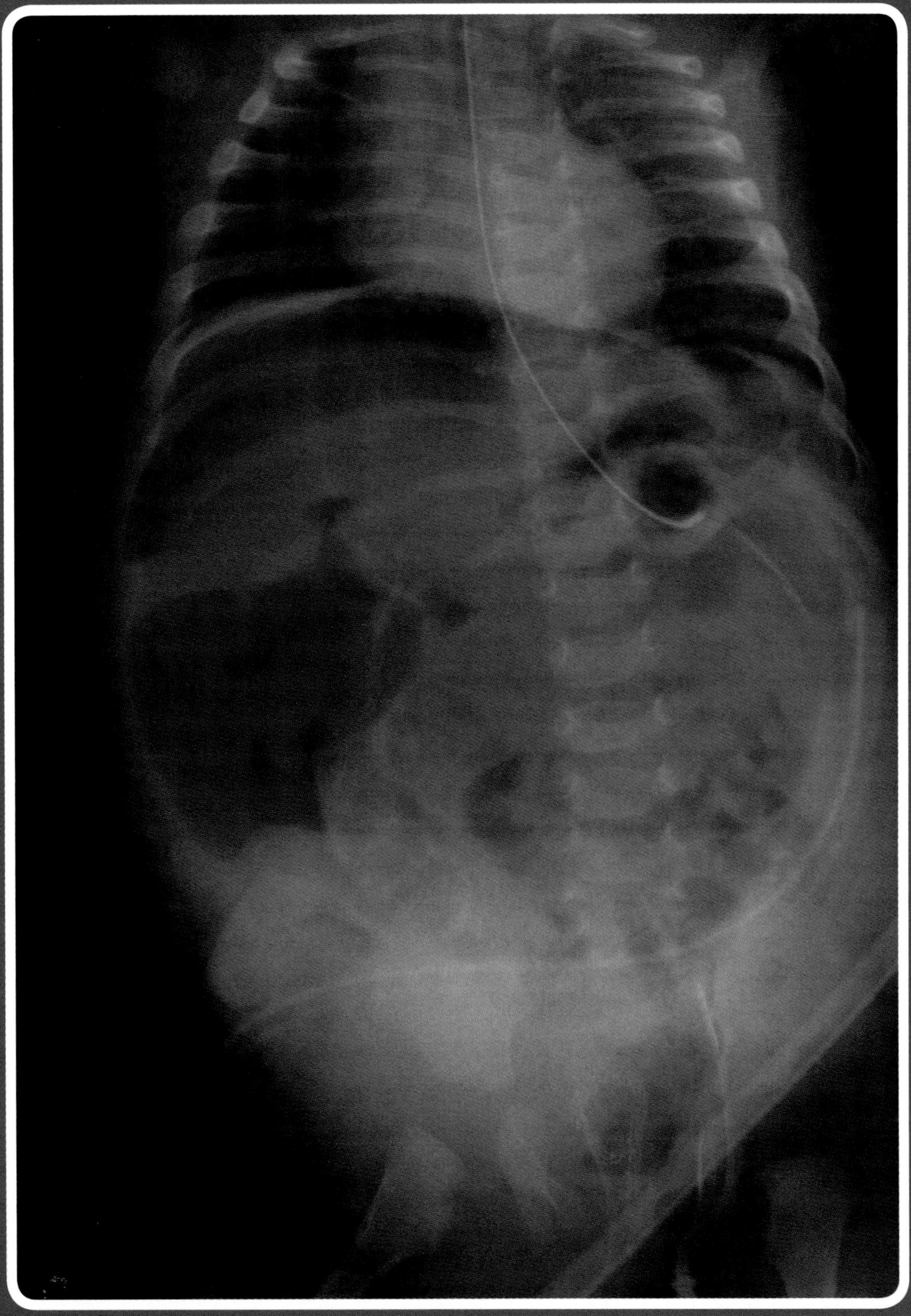

REPORT – PAEDIATRIC PNEUMOPERITONEUM

REPORT

Patient ID: Anonymous.
Projection: AP supine.
Rotation: Asymmetrical pelvis and obturator foramina due to patient rotation to the right.
Penetration: Adequate – the spine is visible.
Coverage: Adequate – the anterior ribs are visible superiorly and the inferior pubic rami are visible.

BOWEL GAS PATTERN

The bowel gas pattern is normal.

BOWEL WALL

There is no evidence of mural thickening or intramural gas within the large or small bowel.

PNEUMOPERITONEUM

There is evidence of free intra-abdominal gas, in keeping with pneumoperitoneum.

There is subdiaphragmatic free gas.

Rigler's sign (double wall sign) can be seen, in keeping with air present on both the luminal and peritoneal sides of the bowel wall.

The falciform ligament sign can be seen, in keeping with air present within the abdomen outlining the falciform ligament of the liver.

The football sign can be seen, in keeping with a large amount of air present within the abdomen outlining the entire abdominal cavity.

The lucent liver sign can be seen, in keeping with a large amount of air present anterior to the liver.

SOLID ORGANS

The liver is outlined by free gas.

VASCULAR

No abnormal vascular calcification.

BONES

The spine is deviated to the left, which is due to patient rotation towards the right.

There are growth plates at the femoral head and acetabulum (triradiate cartilage) as the ossification centres have not yet fused, which is a normal finding in a child of this age.

There is cartilage seen between vertebrae, which is a normal finding in a child of this age.

SOFT TISSUES

The psoas muscle outline is not visible bilaterally, which is non-specific, particularly in a child of this age.

Extra-abdominal soft tissues are unremarkable.

OTHER

There is an NG tube in situ, with its tip appropriately projected over the stomach in the left upper quadrant.

There is a radiopaque line projecting across the abdomen with the tip in the left upper quadrant, likely to represent an abdominal drain.

There is a radiopaque line seen projected over the region of the left hemi-pelvis in keeping with a femoral venous catheter, with the tip appropriately sited in at the level of the inferior vena cava.

There are radiopaque surgical sutures seen within the rectum, in keeping with previous bowel surgery for Hirschprung's disease.

REVIEW AREAS

Gallstones / Renal calculi: No radiopaque calculi.
Lung bases: Normal.
Spine: Deviated to the left due to patient rotation. There is cartilage between the vertebrae and the sacrum is not yet fused which is a normal finding in a child of this age.
Femoral heads: Normal – growth plates present.

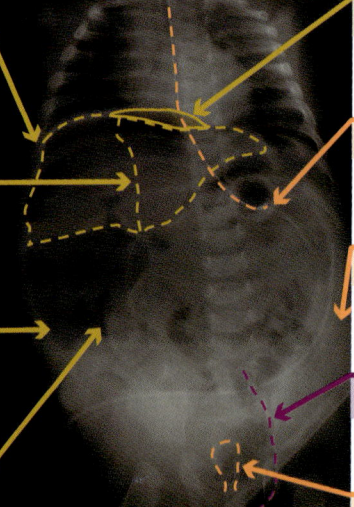

Lucent liver sign of pneumoperitoneum	Subdiaphragmatic free gas
Falciform ligament sign of pneumoperitoneum	NG tube
Football sign of pneumoperitoneum	Abdominal drain
	Left-sided femoral venous catheter
Rigler's sign of pneumoperitoneum	Surgical sutures in rectum

SUMMARY

This abdominal X-ray demonstrates extensive pneumoperitoneum. This may be out of proportion to expected post-surgical appearances suggesting possible bowel perforation. The NG tube, abdominal drain, femoral venous catheter and surgical sutures are incidental findings.

INVESTIGATIONS AND MANAGEMENT

The patient should be resuscitated using an ABCDE approach.

Adequate analgesia and hydration should be provided.

The baby should be started on broad spectrum IV antibiotics, made NBM and started on IV fluids.

Intubation should be considered in view of possible perforation and severity of illness.

Urgent bloods should be taken, including FBC, U&Es, CRP, bone profile, LFTs, coagulation, blood cultures, blood gas, and cross match.

The patient should be referred urgently to the neonatal surgeons for assessment.

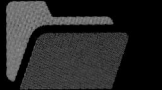

SCENARIO 99

A 16 year old female attends the gastroenterology outpatient clinic for an assessment of her bowel motility. Her past medical history is significant for chronic constipation and she is a non-smoker. On examination, she has saturations of 98% in room air and a temperature of 37.1°C. Her HR is 75 bpm, RR is 16 and blood pressure is 110/65 mmHg. The abdomen is soft and there is no tenderness with normal bowel sounds. Urine dipstick is unremarkable and a pregnancy test is negative. A patency capsule is given, but it has not as yet passed.

An abdominal X-ray is requested to assess for the position of the patency capsule.

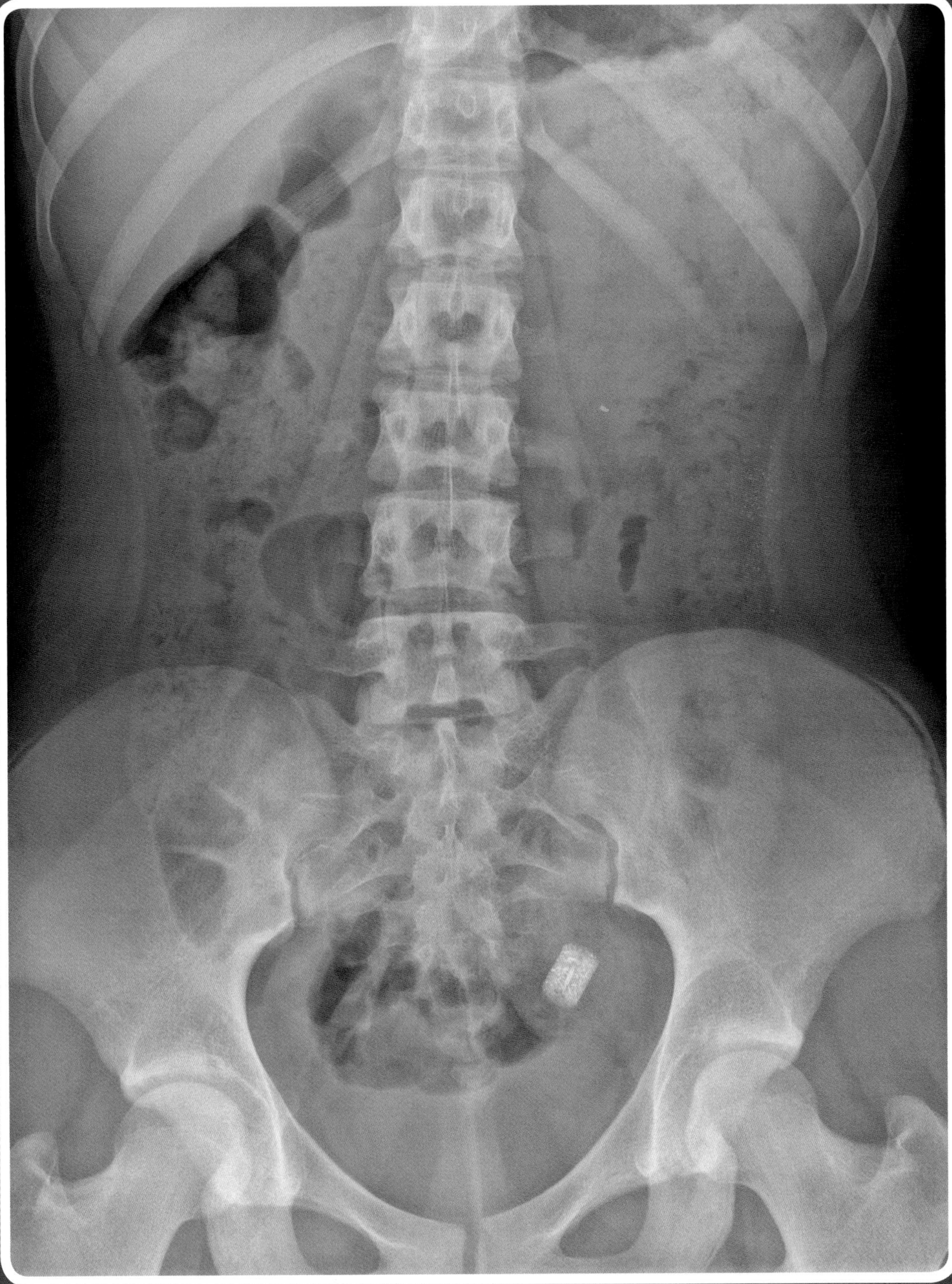

REPORT

Patient ID: Anonymous.
Projection: AP supine.
Rotation: Adequate.
Penetration: Adequate – the spinous processes are visible.
Coverage: Inadequate – the inferior pubic rami have not been included.

BOWEL GAS PATTERN

The bowel gas pattern is normal.

There is a small volume of faecal residue present throughout the large bowel.

BOWEL WALL

There is no evidence of mural thickening or intramural gas within the large or small bowel.

PNEUMOPERITONEUM

There is no evidence of free intra-abdominal gas.

SOLID ORGANS

The solid organ contours are within normal limits with no solid organ calcification.

VASCULAR

No abnormal vascular calcification.

BONES

There are no abnormalities of the imaged thoracic and lumbar spine, or within the pelvis.

An epiphyseal line can be seen at the femoral head where growth plate fusion has occured. The iliac crests apophyses are visible bilaterally. These are normal findings in an adolescent of this age.

SOFT TISSUES

The psoas muscle outline is visible bilaterally.

The extra-abdominal soft tissues are unremarkable.

OTHER

There is a cylindrical radiopaque object projected over the region of the left hemipelvis in keeping with the patency capsule, likely within pelvic small bowel or the sigmoid colon.

There are no vascular lines, drains or surgical clips.

REVIEW AREAS

Gallstones / Renal calculi: No radiopaque calculi.
Lung bases: Not fully included.
Spine: Normal.
Femoral heads: Normal.

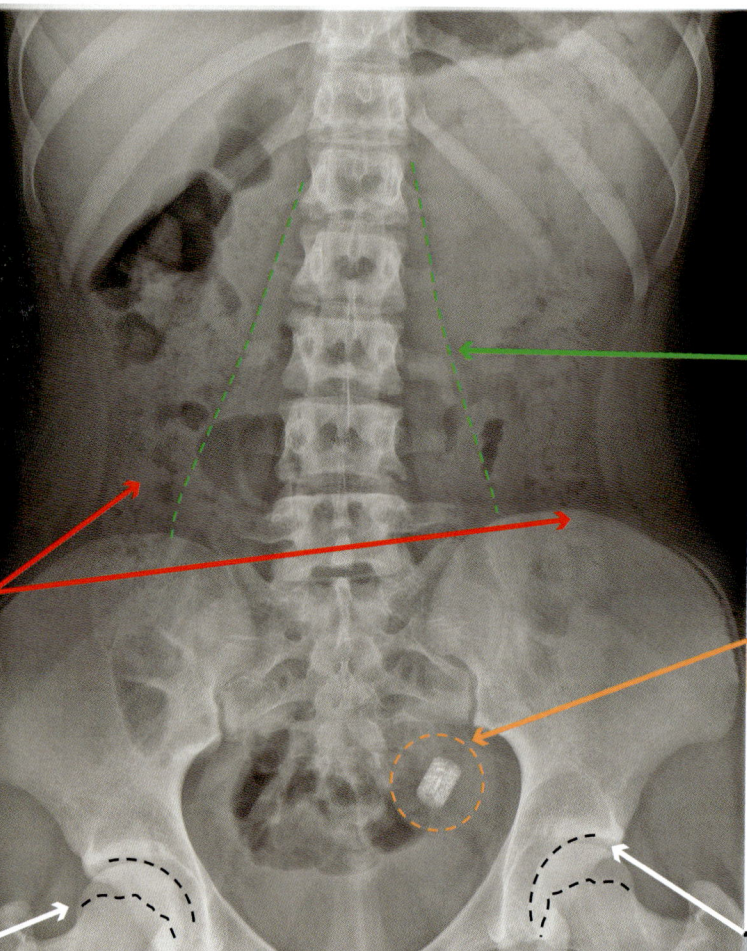

Faecal residue throughout large bowel

Psoas muscle outlines

Patency capsule

Epiphyseal lines

Femoral heads normal

SUMMARY

This X-ray demonstrates a mild volume of faecal residue throughout the large bowel. The patency capsule is projecting over the left hemipelvis likely within pelvic small bowel or the sigmoid colon.

INVESTIGATIONS AND MANAGEMENT

The patient should be advised that the patency capsule is likely to appear within the stool and should be followed up by gastroenterology.

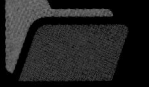

SCENARIO 100

A 68 year old male presents to ED with peritonitic abdominal pain, worsening abdominal distension, nausea and bilious vomiting. He has not passed flatus or opened his bowels for over 24 hours. He has no significant past medical history and is a non-smoker. On examination, he has saturations of 90% in room air and a temperature of 37.0°C. His HR is 110 bpm, RR is 25 and blood pressure is 125/77 mmHg. The abdomen is peritonitic and there are tinkling bowel sounds. Urine dipstick is unremarkable.

An abdominal X-ray is requested to assess for possible bowel obstruction.

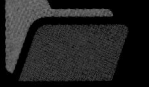

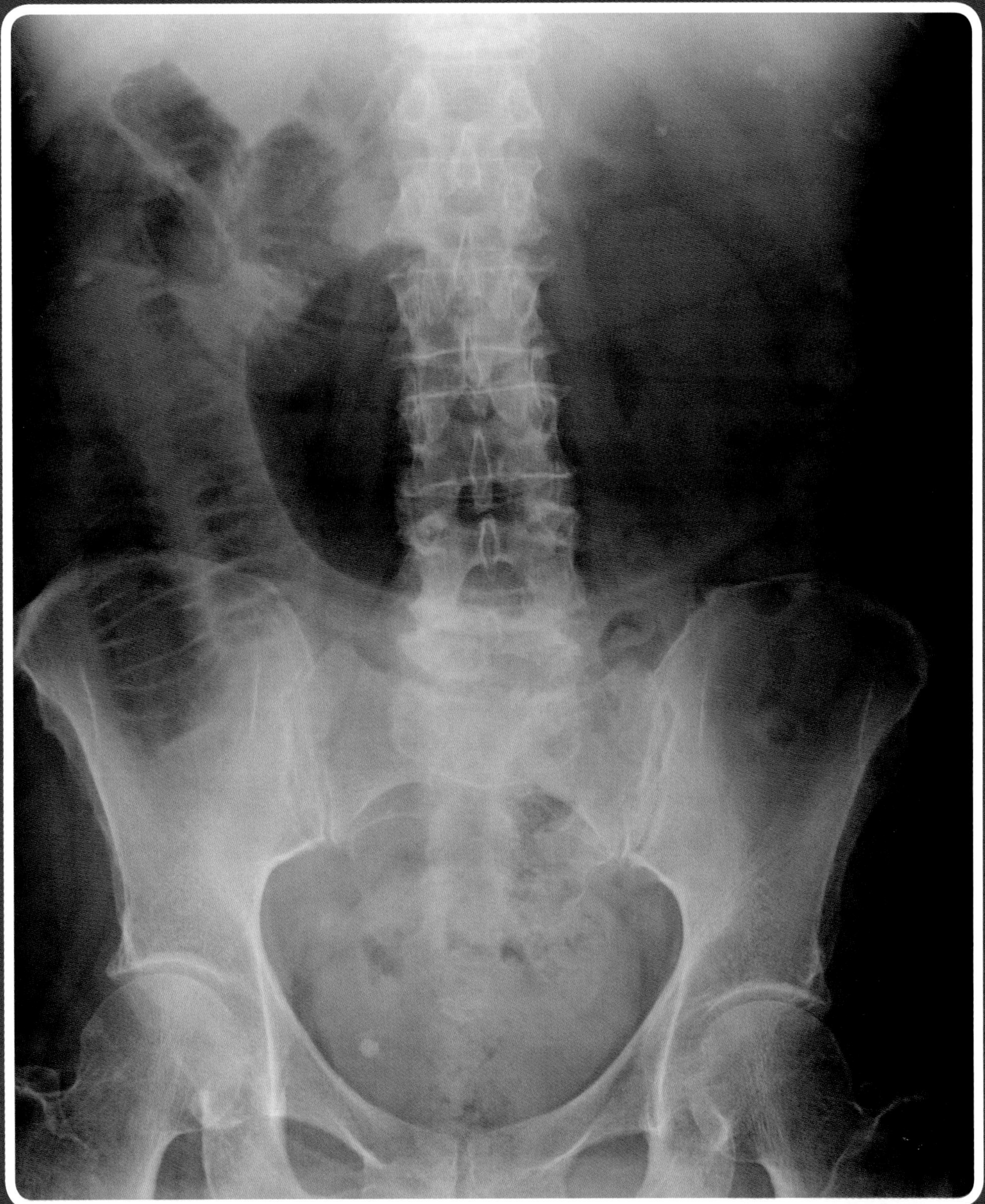

REPORT – CAECAL VOLVULUS WITH SMALL BOWEL OBSTRUCTION

REPORT

Patient ID: Anonymous.
Projection: AP supine.
Rotation: Adequate.
Penetration: Adequate – the spinous processes are visible.
Coverage: Adequate – the anterior ribs are visible superiorly and the inferior pubic rami are visible.

BOWEL GAS PATTERN

There is a large gas filled loop of bowel in the left upper quadrant and epigastrium demonstrating haustra, in keeping with caecal volvulus (a normally positioned caecum in the right lower quadrant is not visible).

There are multiple loops of dilated bowel seen within the right upper quadrant and within the right paracolic gutter demonstrating valvulae conniventes in keeping with small bowel obstruction.

The location of the caecum in the left upper quadrant and small bowel in the right paracolic gutter raise the possibility of an underlying malrotation.

There is faecal material present within the distal colon and rectum.

BOWEL WALL

There is no evidence of mural thickening or intramural gas within the large or small bowel.

PNEUMOPERITONEUM

There is no evidence of free intra-abdominal gas.

SOLID ORGANS

The solid organ contours are within normal limits with no solid organ calcification.

VASCULAR

No abnormal vascular calcification.

BONES

There are no abnormalities of the imaged thoracic and lumbar spine, or within the pelvis.

SOFT TISSUES

The psoas muscle outline is visible bilaterally.

The extra-abdominal soft tissues are unremarkable.

OTHER

There are no radiopaque foreign bodies.

There are no vascular lines, drains or surgical clips.

There is a rounded radiopaque density projected over the region of the pelvis, most likely a phlebolith.

REVIEW AREAS

Gallstones / Renal calculi: No radiopaque calculi.
Lung bases: Not fully included.
Spine: Normal.
Femoral heads: Normal.

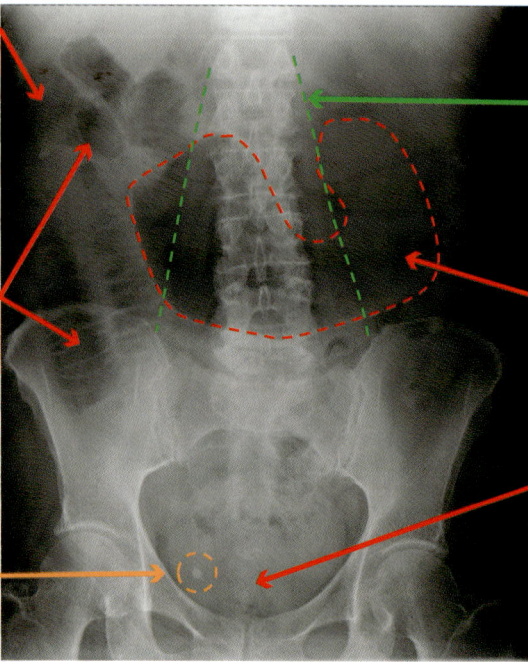

Lateral displacement of small bowel

Psoas muscle outlines

Small bowel dilatation with valvulae conniventes

Caecal volvulus

Faecal material throughout distal colon and rectum

Phlebolith

SUMMARY

This X-ray demonstrates a large gas filled loop of bowel in the left upper quadrant and epigastrium, in keeping with caecal volvulus. There are multiple dilated small bowel loops in the right upper quadrant and right paracolic gutter in keeping with secondary small bowel obstruction. The location of the caecum in the left upper quadrant and small bowel in the right paracolic gutter raise the possibility of an underlying malrotation. The pelvic phlebolith in the pelvis is an incidental finding.

INVESTIGATIONS AND MANAGEMENT

The patient should be resuscitated using an ABCDE approach.

Adequate analgesia and hydration should be provided.

The patient should be kept NBM and an NG tube inserted on free drainage to relieve the pressure in the small bowel. IV fluids should be commenced.

Urgent bloods should be taken, including FBC, U&Es, CRP, LFTs, coagulation, blood gas, and group and save.

The general surgical team should be contacted urgently and a CT scan of the abdomen/pelvis with IV contrast should be considered for better visualisation of the anatomy and further assessment. Management will be with either endoscopic decompression or surgical intervention via detorsion and caecotomy.

CASE INDEX

INDEX

*Page numbers followed by *f* indicate figures.